Modern Concepts of Communicable Disease

Modern Concepts of Communicable Disease

by MORRIS GREENBERG, M.D., M.S.P.H.

Director, Bureau of Preventable Diseases, New York City Department of Health; Assistant Professor of Epidemiology, Columbia University; Attending Pediatrician, Beth David Hospital, New York City

and ANNA V. MATZ, R.N., M.A.

Public Health Nursing Consultant in Communicable Diseases, New York City Department of Health; Lecturer in Communicable Diseases, Willard Parker Hospital, New York City Department of Hospitals

Foreword by Harry S. Mustard, M.D., LL.D.

ILLUSTRATED

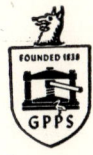

G. P. PUTNAM'S SONS   NEW YORK

Foreword

AS the authors say in their preface, there has been a very great decline in the incidence of the communicable diseases, particularly the acute ones. The old devastating epidemics, with high mortality, are pretty well things of the past in those parts of the world where, with reasonably good economic and social conditions, there is a well-trained medical profession and organized public health work. Because of this improved situation, many who have rather recently come into the field of public health are inclined to be impatient with those who continue to be interested in control of the communicable diseases.

But, in spite of progress in epidemic control, it would be a serious mistake to assume that the problem of communicable diseases is a closed chapter in man's struggle toward continuing health and longevity. Actually, only a small part of the world enjoys comparative control of the epidemic diseases and, even in the most favorable circumstances, cases of one sort or another continue to occur year after year. To some extent the great advances made in vaccines and antibiotics, applicable in prevention, cure, and control of some diseases, have tended to overshadow the still-existing gaps in knowledge in the prevention and control of the large number of diseases that still appear endemically or as mild to fairly large epidemics. The common cold is still common; and although the danger of pneumonia in influenza has been rather encouragingly offset, influenza continues to flare up. From the standpoint of prevention and specific treatment, the situation in poliomyelitis has not greatly advanced. And so it is with a number of the less dramatic communicable diseases.

These facts are likely to be forgotten in a civilization that has gained some mastery over the hazards of impure water, ineffective excreta disposal, infected food and milk, and insects. Further, where there are reasonably good housing and a community sufficiently informed to keep itself clean, the public, and even some parts of the medical profession, are inclined to forget that the present situation may be maintained only by continuing effort. In view of these circumstances it is necessary ever to remember that the balance between man and the parasites which cause communicable disease will remain in man's favor only as long as he is vigilant; that the search for new knowledge must continue in full force.

It should further be emphasized that the epidemiological approach, evidenced in this volume, offers very valuable material even to those whose interest may lie in a field other than communicable diseases, such as heart disease, cancer, or mental health. The etiology, distribution, and treatment of all these diseases must be investigated and the results assayed in terms of epidemiology; and the principles learned with difficulty in communicable diseases serve as essential and sound guides in the mass attack upon diseases due to causes other than living agents.

Those engaged in the broad field of health are greatly indebted to Dr. Greenberg and Mrs. Matz for their labors in producing this volume. In it are recorded the results of their fine scholarship and long experience. Both the student and the practitioner will now have before them an authoritative text which exhibits, in excellent proportion, basic information, objective consideration, and practical necessities. In this text one can find both philosophy and guidance.

HARRY S. MUSTARD, M.D., LL.D.

Preface

T H E tremendous reduction in mortality and the increase in the life expectancy of man that have taken place in the last half century have been due largely to the reduction in the incidence of, and mortality from, communicable diseases. This has necessitated a change in thinking about these diseases and a different orientation toward them. Some of them have ceased to have the importance they had years ago; others, which still challenge accurate diagnosis and treatment, have arisen to take their places. Knowledge about methods of prevention and of spread has increased and become more accurate. Disease is not thought of any longer as merely a clinical pathological entity caused by a definite agent. Rather, it is considered to be an imbalance between the agent on one side and the susceptible host on the other side. Frequently, this imbalance is determined by the environment. This is the epidemiological approach to disease, and it necessitates a study of the causative agent, the host, and the environment. It is the method used in this book.

It has become more and more manifest that communicable disease is not just an individual problem concerning a patient and his family; it is a community problem and can be solved adequately only if one considers all the community aspects of it. Quarantine may be an important feature of control in one community and useless in another. Patients with communicable disease are better treated in a general hospital in some communities, in special hospitals in others, and at home in still others. The problems of the communicable diseases as they relate to their communities have been stressed in the pages that follow.

A good deal of the material that follows was used in a course on epidemiology for graduate students (hospital administrators, nurses, statisticians, and some physicians) enrolled for the degree of master of science in the School of Public Health of Columbia University. Some of it was presented before the nursing staff of the New York City Department of Health as part of the staff-education program, and parts of it were used in the orientation program of newly appointed physicians in the department.

For a 2-year period one of the authors had an opportunity to explore certain problems in communicable disease while acting as chairman of a subcommittee on communicable diseases of the Curriculum Committee, New York City League of Nursing Education. The generous and stimulating discussion of the members of the subcommittee helped to clarify certain viewpoints. Special acknowledgment is made to the nursing instructors who participated in the discussions and gave valuable suggestions to the project.

It is a pleasure to acknowledge the kindness of the following people who have read and criticized different chapters of the book: Drs. Harold Abramson, Leon Buchbinder, Harold T. Fuerst, Ottavio J. Pellitteri, Arthur Robins, Nathan Sobel and Howard B. Shookhoff, and Miss Margaret A. Losty.

We wish, also, to acknowledge the aid and interest of the following, who gave assistance with the nursing aspects: Patricia I. Heely, Ruth A. Rothmayer, Corinne N. Sawyer, and Helen E. Cross of the New York City Department of Health; Helene Olandt, formerly of Queens General Hospital; Dolly M. Craven, formerly of Kingston Avenue Hospital, Brooklyn; Grace Redman of Triboro Hospital, Queens; Elsie Olson of Willard Parker Hospital; Mary M. Richardson of Lenox Hill Hospital; and La Verne Thompson of Teachers College, Columbia University. We wish to thank Miss Olga Figueroa, Mrs. Ida P. Volin, and Mrs. Sadie Koch for typing parts of the chapters, and we are particularly grateful to Mrs. Norma C. Morais for her careful typing of the entire manuscript.

Photographs of nursing technique were taken by Anne M. Goodrich, R.N. at Kingston Avenue Hospital, Brooklyn, New York, through the courtesy of Dr. I. Herbert Scheffer, General Medical Superintendent, Department of Hospitals, Dr. Louis Odessky, formerly Deputy Superintendent, Kingston Avenue Hospital and Miss Freda D. Russell, R.N., Superintendent of Nurses. The Misses Frances Chlumsky, R.N. and Margaret M. Mullen, R.N. demonstrated the techniques illustrated.

The photograph of the Unit for Collection and Distribution of Materials for Sputum Control was taken at the Triboro Hospital, Jamaica, Long Island, through the courtesy of Dr. Scheffer, Dr. H. Feinberg, Superintendent, Queens General and Triboro Hospitals, and Miss Alice Brewer, R.N., Superintendent of Nurses, Triboro Hospital.

Mr. Asa B. Elliott made our task much easier by his helpful suggestions about format and by his editorial advice.

M. G.
A. V. M.

Contents

Part I

THE BASIC PRINCIPLES OF COMMUNICABLE DISEASE

Part II

THE SPECIFIC COMMUNICABLE DISEASES

ix

Part I

THE BASIC PRINCIPLES OF COMMUNICABLE DISEASE

Chapter 1 CHANGING CONCEPTS OF
COMMUNICABLE DISEASE

THE concept of the communicability of disease has grown with the development and progress of the medical and social sciences. Various theories about disease have been advanced through periods of history, and they have been interwoven into the fabric of civilization. Tradition, cultural patterns, and religious beliefs have profoundly affected the introduction of controls for the prevention of disease. The early dogmas that sickness and epidemics were the evil work of wicked demons or the punishment by God for man's sins played a significant role in the history of man prior to the acceptance of scientific concepts.

Primitive Concepts

A review of the history of primitive man's struggle with the forces of nature discloses a belief that plagues and pestilences were the work of demons who swarmed all over the world and did their evil work out of malice. Incantations, the wearing of charms, the beating of drums, dancing, and various rituals served as barriers against such demons. Persons afflicted with disease were under the influence of evil spirits which might even have entered their bodies. Exorcism was a common practice in control of disease. This frequently involved physical hurt to the patient in an attempt to drive the devil out of his body.

Although this concept was supplanted by the belief that disease was a visitation by God to punish man for his sins, the more primitive belief in demons persisted for many years and has even continued into modern times. The trials of the witches in Salem during colonial days were an expression of this belief, and it is not uncommon, even today among simple people, to find children wearing camphor bags or pieces of garlic around their necks, so that evil spirits may be deflected by their odors.

The concept of plagues and epidemics as the expression of God's displeasure with man and as a punishment for his sins ultimately supplanted the belief in demonology as civilization progressed to faith in the Deity. Disease was still something from without imposed on man, but it was not due to the chance contact with ubiquitous spirits of evil. There was plan and reason for illness in the individual

3

and in the mass. It was the result of God's anger for man's sinfulness. It was for the purpose of giving man a chance to purify himself, to leave the paths of evil, to become just and upright. When man strayed from righteousness, punishment was his due, and this was meted out by the Lord in the form of sickness in the individual or a plague on an entire group. To get well, to limit the spread of an epidemic, to control disease, one had to pray to God, to admit one's sins, and to make amends by leading a just life.

This concept of disease has also come down to modern times. The belief that human beings who are ill with communicable disease and communities which are suffering from epidemics of disease have displeased the Deity and are being punished for their sins still finds expression today. Throughout the rise of civilization, the rational concept of disease as a result of physical, chemical, and biologic influences has had to struggle against the twin beliefs of primitive men that disease is due to the whim of demons or that it is a punishment of man by an all-wise God.

Ancient Concepts

Religion was an integral part of the lives of ancient people. Illness was related to the supernatural, and so was the healing of disease. The physician was a man of God who could lead lesser men into righteous paths and thus cure them of their diseases. It was inevitable that the priests should also be the physicians. It was also inevitable that observation and experience would soon bring about the introduction of rational therapy combined with, and confused by, the more primitive beliefs. In Egypt the physicians knew something of inspection and palpation as part of diagnosis, and they used plants of various kinds in treatment.

The ancient Hebrews lived under a theocratic regime, and it is no wonder, therefore, that the priests were also the healers as they were the lawgivers. It is also not surprising to find the concept that outbreaks of disease were a punishment of men by an angry God for the sins that they committed. Disease was related to dirt and impurity. He who was impure in mind before God was also impure in body. To purify him was a religious function and was the province of the priests. Purification of the body is closely related to sanitation, and it is probably because of the stress laid on purification that a system of sanitary hygiene grew up among these people. No one could enter the temple unless he was clean, and bathing was essential to keeping clean. The ritual bath became an important feature of the daily life, and it has persisted among orthodox Jews to the present time. Baths must be taken on the day before the Sabbath; baths must be taken by a woman at the termination of the uncleanliness of her menstrual period. Similarly, since soldiers depositing their excrement in the field might soil themselves and become unclean, they were required to cover such excrement with earth, or to bury it.

Although the sanitary regulations of the Hebrews were based on religious rather than rational concepts, they nevertheless were of a high order. They embraced concepts of isolation and quarantine, disposal of excreta, sex hygiene, nutrition, and rest. In essence, the regulations were disciplinary and prophylactic. There was practiced the social principle that, since man is part of a community, he must not do things which will endanger the rest of the community, even if the restrictions are unpleasant or irksome to him.

An example of the detailed procedures imposed on persons with skin diseases, particularly leprosy, is found in Leviticus, chapter 13, verses 2 to 13. A person with a skin eruption reported to the priest, who examined him. Detailed descriptions of the rash are given and information to the priest as to when the rash should be considered leprosy and when not; also, when to isolate the patient and when to permit him to go free. If the patient was isolated, he had to be re-examined by the priest at fixed intervals until such time as isolation and quarantine could be terminated. When this happened, terminal disinfection was practiced, and the precise methods used, such as shaving of the head and beard, bathing, and changing into clean clothes, are given in detail.

Greek Medicine

Among the early Greeks ideas about medicine followed the pattern of other ancient peoples. They were a blend of belief in demons and belief in Gods. Aesculapius, son of Apollo, was the God of Medicine. He is pictured with a serpent, which was his symbol, and which has remained to the present day as a symbol of physicians. As among the Hebrews, the priests were the healers in ancient Greece. Treatment consisted largely of baths, massage, and diet, interspersed with incantations and magic.

It was during the fifth century B.C. that the idea of disease as a natural phenomenon asserted itself among the Greeks. It found its greatest exponent in Hippocrates (460–355? B.C.), known as the father of medicine. According to his doctrine, the universe is formed of four elements—air, earth, water, and fire—and they possess four elementary properties—hot, cold, moist, and dry. The body has four humors—blood, phlegm, yellow bile, and black bile—and when these are perfectly mingled man is healthy, but when one of the humors is defective or in excess or improperly proportioned to the others, disease results.

Hippocrates was greatly concerned with climate and weather and their influence on epidemic disease. He realized that respiratory diseases occur more often in the winter, and intestinal and malarial diseases in the summer. He laid stress on the importance of physical diagnosis and described certain symptoms with great accuracy.

Roman Influence

Another great figure in classical medicine is Galen (A.D. 130–200). He was born in Asia Minor, but he migrated to Rome and exerted much of his influence while there. Like Hippocrates, he discarded completely the supernatural concept of disease; he dissected animals and performed physiological experiments. His fame rests chiefly, however, on his voluminous philosophical discussions of disease. The ideas which he propounded with great authority, many of which were wrong, carried considerable weight for many centuries.

The great contribution of the Romans to medicine was in the field of environmental sanitation. They carried out extensive hygienic measures such as the drainage of swamps, the improvement of soil, the building of houses, the transmission of good drinking and bathing water by aqueducts, and the construction of public baths.

Medieval Concepts

Following the collapse of the Roman Empire, Europe experienced a period lasting many centuries, frequently referred to as the Dark Ages, when civilization seemed to retrogress. Hygiene and sanitation were neglected, water supplies became polluted, dirt and filth were rampant, public bathing was discouraged. No great men arose to carry on the work begun by the Greeks and Romans. It was an age of intellectual darkness, with superstition taking the place of reason.

Disease was common and swept Europe in waves of catastrophic epidemics. Leprosy assumed alarming proportions, and only feeble attempts at isolation were made here and there. It became particularly widespread with the return of the soldiers from the Crusades. Various regulations, some of great cruelty, were invoked to keep lepers segregated and excluded from normal society. The force of some of these measures has continued to the present day, when the term "leper" still strikes fear in the hearts of many people.

It was plague, the Black Death, however, that wiped out a large part of the population of Europe. It was introduced from Asia in the fourteenth century, spread from Turkey and Greece to Italy,

France, and Spain, and then to England, Germany, and the Netherlands. It marched on to engulf Scandinavia and Russia, and when it had finished its work, half to three quarters of the population had succumbed. The dislocation in the economy of Europe was very great. There were no workers to till the fields or to provide food, no merchants to carry on industry. That superstition, greed, and intolerance prevailed is not surprising.

The plague was so obviously a contagious disease that all writers of the time were impressed by this, although the exact method of spread was a mystery. The idea of an animate cause did not occur to anyone. The notion that the air was polluted and noxious and spread its poisonous effects was the predominating view of those who thought about the matter. It was a view which prevailed to the time of Budd and Snow in the nineteenth century. Nevertheless, the idea of isolation of the sick and of quarantine of homes and ships was thought about. Venice forbade infected ships to enter its harbor in 1374 and established a quarantine station in 1403.

As might be expected, leprosy and plague were not the only epidemic diseases that occurred during the Dark Ages. The soil was ready for many others. They are the two, however, which caused the greatest havoc. The Black Death, especially, is probably the greatest scourge that ever attacked man.

The Renaissance

By the middle of the fifteenth century the dark haze that had covered Europe began to lift, and a new, liberal spirit began to spread. This had its effect on medical thought as well as on the arts. The two great physicians of this period were Fracastoro (1483–1553) and Paracelsus (1493–1541). Paracelsus was the first physician to lecture in the popular vernacular rather than in Latin. He was greatly impressed by the medicinal value of metallic salts. Paracelsus was a mystic, and he unfortunately drew on magic, astrology, and alchemy to support his theses. Fracastoro is usually associated with the disease syphilis which he studied intently and to which he gave its name. He made notable contributions to the study of contagion. He distinguished three methods of spread—direct, from a distance, and by means of fomites. He recognized that disease was transmissible and that the transmitted agent propagated itself and was specific for each disease. To treat a disease it was necessary to destroy the agent, neutralize it, or extrude it from the body. Many of Fracastoro's views on contagion are accepted today.

Progress was also made during the Renaissance in freeing medical thought from the dicta of Galen. Leonardo da Vinci and Vesalius made dissections of the human body and showed that the anatomy of man differed from that of the lower animals, and a number of workers began the study of physiology which was brought to a high point by the work of Harvey in the seventeenth century.

Anton von Leeuwenhoek (1632–1723) is one of the outstanding figures of the seventeenth century. He was not a physician but was greatly interested in lenses. He built better and better microscopes and used them to examine all objects that came to his hand. He wrote down his findings and reported them to the Royal Society of London. He described blood cells, spermatozoa, protozoa, and bacteria. Sydenham (1624–1689) was essentially a clinician. He gave very good descriptions of a number of diseases but followed Hippocrates in his conception of the causes of epidemic disease.

Epidemics continued to take their toll in the seventeenth century. Plague still spread from country to country, malaria was epidemic in Italy, and typhus was prevalent in many countries. Smallpox occurred not only in Europe but on the American continent, and scarlet fever and diphtheria were recognized. Although sanitary legislation was begun, there was no active or concerted movement for its advancement. Streets were still dirty, no provisions were made for a clean water supply, and the disposal of sewage was quite primitive.

Eighteenth Century

It was not until late in the eighteenth century that progress began to be made in environmental sanitation and preventive medicine. John Howard, Sheriff of Bedfordshire, devoted a large part of his life to the cleaning up of English jails and the introduction of sanitary procedures. Edward Jenner (1749–1823) made his famous observation that cowpox prevented the occurrence of smallpox and vaccinated his first patient in 1796. The method rapidly spread over Europe and was first used in America by Benjamin Waterhouse in 1800. Thus began the first example of the eradication of a dangerous disease by a simple prophylactic measure.

Modern Concepts

The concepts of the method of spread of communicable disease had made little progress in the eighteenth and even into the nineteenth century. In England, Sydenham's philosophy held sway. In America, Benjamin Rush (1745–1813), one of the greatest doctors of his day, argued vehemently that yellow fever was caused by morbid exhalations and noxious effluvia from putrid vegetables and from ponds. This concept of disease as being due to emanations from filthy and decayed and putrid matter was strongly supported by Noah Webster, the lexicographer, who, although not a physician, was greatly interested in epidemiology. It was, indeed, the prevailing philosophy of the times.

Although the theory was undoubtedly wrong, it did focus attention on environmental sanitation. The work of John Howard has been mentioned. The outstanding figure in this field in the nineteenth century was Edwin Chadwick (1800–1890), the first great sanitarian. Chadwick was secretary of the Poor Law Board in England and made an extensive study of social conditions. As a result of this, a great campaign for sanitary measures was inaugurated, with stress on clean water, proper disposal of excreta, and proper ventilation. What Chadwick did in England, Lemuel Shattuck (1793–1859) did in America. His Report of the Sanitary Commission of Massachusetts still serves as a model for sanitarians.

The break in the long-held concept that epidemic disease was caused by a miasma from decayed matter was made by John Snow (1813–1858). His epidemiological investigation of the outbreak of cholera in London was carried out in the modern manner. He proved conclusively that cholera was spread from the infected ill person to the susceptible well person, that the agent of disease must multiply in the body of the person attacked, and that it was present in the discharges from the intestinal tract. He went on to argue that transmission occurred by the contamination of the water supply, and he proved his point by statistical evidence. He indicated furthermore, that communicability, in the modern sense, was true not only of cholera but also of such diseases as syphilis, measles, scarlet fever, smallpox, typhoid, yellow fever, plague, and dysentery.

William Budd (1811–1880) supported Snow's thesis. His own investigations were made on typhoid fever. He worked in a country district and was able to trace the infection from patient to patient. He noted that the disease could be spread by hands, water, and milk contaminated with fecal discharges, and he advised the disinfection of linens and stools and the boiling of water.

Snow and Budd had the genius to entertain the modern concept of communicable disease. It is to their credit that this occurred before anything was known of the method of growth and reproduction of microorganisms and before there was any demonstration that each infectious disease is caused by a specific living agent. Such proof was not long in coming. Although a number of workers prepared the field, the name that stands out above all is that of Louis Pasteur.

Pasteur (1822–1895) began as a chemist but soon became interested in what is now known as "microbiology." He proved that infections were caused by microorganisms, that these were specific, and that spontaneous generation of life was a myth. He performed experiments in immunization, and the Pasteur treatment of rabies is still used, in a modified form, to this day.

Pasteur's teachings in bacteriology were ably carried on by a host of workers, the most famous of whom was Robert Koch (1843–1910), the discoverer of the tubercle bacillus, who developed methods for isolating and cultivating bacteria. The application of Pasteur's discovery in bacteriology to the control of infections in humans was first made by Joseph Lister (1827–1912) who conceived the notion of applying carbolic acid to infected tissue in order to disinfect it.

No history of the achievement of medicine in the nineteenth century is complete without mention of Florence Nightingale's (1823–1910) pioneering efforts in the field of nursing. The famous Lady of the Lamp was a woman of great force and determination. It was due to her persistence that a female nursing service was established in the military hospitals of Scutari and Balaklava during the Crimean War. Her stressing of cleanliness and gentleness in the care of the injured helped to minimize the deleterious results of infection in war wounds.

Contemporary Concepts

Although a large number of bacteriologists, using Koch's postulates, increased the current knowledge of disease by discovering specific agents for the different communicable diseases, the filth theory of disease was not quickly annihilated. It was still necessary to explain how an individual who had never been in contact with a case of communicable disease nevertheless fell a victim to it. The concept of the carrier of disease had to be established. This was not the work of a single individual but of many workers in the field of bacteriology. One of the most important workers in the field was William H. Park (1863–1939), the first director of laboratories of the New York City Department of Health. He proved, by the actual swabbing of throats, that diphtheria bacilli could persist long after the recovery of the patient. From this, the next step was logical. The throats of healthy children who had had no contact with diphtheria were cultured, and diphtheria bacilli were found in a small proportion.

The carrier state in other communicable diseases was soon demonstrated by other workers. The proof that typhoid fever may be transmitted by a carrier handling food that others eat was dramatically shown by Soper, a sanitary engineer, in the case of Typhoid Mary, the first chronic typhoid carrier in the files of the New York

City Department of Health. Carriers have been demonstrated in a host of diseases—cholera, typhoid and paratyphoid fevers, amebic and bacillary dysentery, pneumonia, diphtheria, streptococcal sore throat and scarlet fever, meningococcus meningitis, poliomyelitis, yellow fever, malaria, and infectious hepatitis.

The discovery of the carrier state indicated how it was possible to become ill with a communicable disease without being in contact with a person suffering from the disease. The converse of this had to be explained. How was it possible to be in close, continuous, intimate contact with a case of communicable disease like malaria and still not get it? A new idea was introduced—the idea of a vector, capable of transmitting disease from an infected to a noninfected individual or from an infected animal, the reservoir, to a human being. One of the earliest workers to explain this method of infection was the American, Theobald Smith (1859–1934), who demonstrated the transmission of Texas fever in cattle by a tick. A little later Ronald Ross (1857–1932) demonstrated the transmission of avian malaria by mosquitoes, and Grassi proved the same in humans; still later, Walter Reed showed that a different mosquito transmitted yellow fever.

Vector transmission has been shown to occur in a number of diseases, some of virus etiology, some bacterial, and others protozoan. Examples of the first are yellow fever and typhus; of the second, plague and tularemia; and of the third, malaria and kalaazar. Although the commonest vector is the mosquito, there are others such as fleas, lice, ticks, and flies.

The discovery of the part played by human carriers and by animal vectors in the spread of infection has rounded out the modern concept of communicable disease. It is always caused by a living agent, and the agent is specific for the disease. It is transmitted from individual to individual by contact of the healthy susceptible person with the sick person, or through the medium of a healthy carrier, or by an animal vector. In some diseases, like measles and chickenpox, direct contact is the only method of spread; in others, such as diphtheria and meningitis, spread may occur by contact either with a case or with a healthy carrier; in still others, for example malaria and yellow fever, spread occurs only through the intervention of an intermediate animal, usually an arthropod vector.

Communicable diseases may, of course, be transmitted by water, milk, or food, but that is only because such water, milk, or food has been contaminated with the agent of disease by a case or a carrier. Except in rare instances, microorganisms of disease do not live a saprophytic existence outside the animal body. While it is conceivable that inanimate objects, when recently seeded, may transfer infection from one person to another, as in the case of the same handkerchief used by two individuals one of whom has a cold, this is an unusual occurrence. Most microorganisms die when in the dried state, and they dry out rapidly when exposed to air. For many years it was a regulation of the Department of Health of New York City to seal all coffins of persons dead of a communicable disease and to forbid funerals in such deaths. This was undoubtedly a throwback to the miasmatic concept of infection. It is true that some bacteria are spore bearers, and that spores may exist outside of the animal body for long periods of time. Anthrax, for instance, has been transmitted by shaving brushes. Sporeforming bacilli are few in number, however, and play a comparatively small part in the total body of communicable disease.

That infected air may play a part in the transmission of communicable disease has been demonstrated in comparatively recent years by Wells and others with the use of the air centrifuge. It appears possible, theoretically, to infect a person who has not been exposed to another individual suffering from the same disease. It has been shown, for instance, that in a room inhabited by individuals with a respiratory infection, droplet nuclei of bacteria from the individuals' throats and noses may be disseminated in the air and may float about for various periods of time. Furthermore, heavier droplets which sink to the floor or rest on furniture may evaporate and become lighter nuclei which are swept up in a current of air and float about, infecting others in the room. Cross infection on a ward has been explained on this basis. Attempts to control such air-borne infection have been made with the use of ultraviolet irradiation and various chemical vapors. Careless judgment may confuse such air-borne infection with the medieval notion that disease was spread by noxious emanations from decaying matter. The concept of air-borne infection is that the air surrounding an individual may serve temporarily as a medium for the transfer of living agents of disease from one person to another in the same way that milk, contaminated by a typhoid carrier's fingers, may serve as a medium for the transfer of organisms inhabiting his body to the body of a healthy person.

Increase in the Life Span

In 1919, the death rate in New York City was 13.4 per 1,000 individuals; in 1949, the rate had been reduced to 9.2, a saving of 4.2 lives out of every 1,000 persons. With a population of 8 million people, this represents a saving of 33,600 lives a year. Since the saving was chiefly in the lives of young people, the population is longer lived. In 1911, the expectancy of life at the time of birth was 46 years; in 1949, an infant could expect to live 67 years. How did this saving in lives come about? Chiefly as a result of the conquest of communicable disease. Deaths in the first month of life were more than three times as high in 1919 as in 1949. The saving in these lives was chiefly in the reduction of mortality from respiratory infections and diarrhea. The deaths from some of the commoner communicable diseases 30 years ago and recently in New York City are given in the accompanying table.

| | DEATHS | |
DISEASE	1919	1949
Diphtheria	1,239	2
Measles	218	7
Whooping cough	161	13
Scarlet fever	136	1
Typhoid fever	121	1
Meningococcus meningitis	171	30
Pulmonary tuberculosis	7,395	2,364
Pneumonia	10,977	2,408
Total	20,418	4,826

In this group of diseases alone, if the rates of 1919 had applied in 1949, there would have been 15,592 more deaths. The saving in lives has been tremendous.

The Rise of Bacteriology

An analysis of the influences that brought about this condition indicates that the prime factor was the change in concept of infectious disease from the mystical to the rational. Disease ceased to be vague, mysterious, supernatural. It was the result of the action of tiny living agents that attacked the body, multiplied in it, and as a result destroyed its economy, brought about pathological processes, and so destroyed its normal physiological processes as to cause death. There was a great rush to the laboratory. Following the epoch-making discoveries of Pasteur and Koch, a host of brilliant minds began the study of microbial agents, learned of ways to grow them in the test tube, classified them, and identified them with specific diseases. They learned their ways of behavior in and out of the body; they subjected them to various methods of attack; they studied the injuries caused when the agents were injected into laboratory animals. Methods of staining were developed so that differentiation became a simple technique, the need or lack of need of oxygen for multiplication was evaluated for the different germs, and the thermal death points were clearly established. Better and better microscopes were built to study the anatomy of the microorganisms and their architectural arrangements. It became a simple matter to differentiate not only bacilli, cocci, and spirochetes, but to separate the lance-shaped coccus of pneumonia from the round streptococcus, and to distinguish the latter which grew in chains from the equally round staphylococci that grew in clumps.

The Development of Immunology

Gradually, there grew up the ancillary science of immunology. The research workers discovered that when an active agent of disease attacked the body, defense mechanisms were developed within the body, and these were frequently strong enough to overcome the attack and destroy the invaders. Furthermore, in many instances the defense mechanisms that were built up outlasted the disease and were strong enough to withstand a later attack by the same agent. The defense mechanisms were as specific as the infecting agents. An attack by the diphtheria bacillus brought out defense agents against that bacterium but not against the typhoid bacillus, and, conversely, an attack of typhoid fever protected the individual against further attacks by the typhoid bacillus but not against the diphtheria bacillus or the pneumococcus. The defense mechanism began to be studied more and more intently, with better and more precise methods. It was found that the body protected itself in a variety of ways—by developing antibodies which could dissolve the bacteria, or clump them, or neutralize them, or destroy them in other ways. Thought was given to the possibility of developing a defense mechanism within the body before it was attacked by an agent of disease.

A beginning in this direction had already been made in 1796. Edward Jenner had observed that people who had had cowpox did not take smallpox, and he developed the simple method of preventing smallpox by inoculating healthy people with the virus of cowpox. Now cowpox was either a modified form of smallpox or a related disease. The idea took root that it might be possible to use organisms which were so attenuated that they were harmless to cause disease but yet active enough to stimulate bodily defenses against their more virulent brothers. It was soon discovered that even organisms which had been completely killed by heat or a chemical could, when injected into an animal body, stimulate the development of antibodies against the homologous living organisms. Certain organisms such as the diphtheria bacillus did not do their greatest damage by multiplication in the body but by the elaboration of a toxin which was more destructive than the organism itself. If this toxin was injected into animals in increasing doses, the animals developed an antitoxin. This antitoxin could be combined with the toxin, and the resulting mixture was harmless when injected into the human body but quite potent in causing the development of antitoxin. William H. Park was one of the pioneers in the use of the toxin-antitoxin mixture in mass immunization of children in New York City. Later, Ramon showed that it was not necessary to inactivate the toxin with antitoxin. If the toxin was treated with Formalin its toxicity was destroyed, but its immunizing property remained and was greater than in the toxin-antitoxin mixture. As a result, such a product, known as toxoid, was introduced and is now used universally in immunization against diphtheria.

Sanitation

Hand in hand with the development of the sciences of bacteriology and of immunology came the development of the science of sanitary engineering. In its early beginnings it was largely a housekeeping job, cleaning up filth and dirt and garbage, teaching simple rules of personal hygiene, encouraging the use of water within and without, and the proper disposal of excrement. It soon developed into more precise and complicated methods which enveloped large-scale measures. The purity of water supplies had to be ensured, and this was accomplished by protecting the sources of supply and by the development of the process of water purification. The proper disposal of sewage, either by means of sewage treatment plants or by diverting it into channels which would not contaminate drinking or bathing waters, was another major accomplishment. Swamps were effectively drained. Methods of garbage disposal in large communities, such as by incineration, were introduced. The pasteurization of milk, the introduction of proper methods of preparing and processing foods and preserving them by refrigeration, the proper ventilation of buildings, the construction of sewers, and the introduction of sanitary plumbing were all measures which changed the environment and aided man in his struggle against agents of disease.

The Discovery of Antibiotics

From earliest times man sought for drugs to combat illness. Discoveries were often purely accidental. The use of mercury in the treatment of syphilis antedated the knowledge of the cause and nature of the disease. Peruvian bark, or quinine, was used to treat quotidian fever or malaria when that disease was thought to be due, as its name implies, to bad air. With the development of bacteriology came the ordered search in pharmacological laboratories for specific drugs to destroy specific agents of disease. One of the most famous researches in the field of specific therapy was that of Ehrlich, who, after 606 attempts, discovered a drug which could be injected into man and destroy the spirochetes of syphilis in his body without harming him. No discovery of similar importance in the therapy of infectious disease occurred until Domagk reported his results with sulfanilamide in the treatment of mice infected with the pneumococcus. The next great discovery was that of Fleming who, in 1929, called attention to the fact that a culture plate of gram-positive organisms which had been accidentally contaminated by the mold *Penicillium notatum* failed to show the usual growth of colonies. The development of penicillin by Chain and Florey in 1938, some 13 years after Fleming's observations, the introduction of streptomycin by Waksman in 1944, and the rapid development of a number of new antibiotics have added to the physician's armamentarium a number of agents which can be injected into or fed to man without causing him harm, but which have the miraculous quality of destroying the disease agents which attack him.

Only within the past 10 years a chemical has been introduced in the field of sanitation which has the power of destroying insects and other arthropods, but which is comparatively harmless to man. This drug, DDT, can be sprayed in homes, dusted on the human body, and widely disseminated in animal houses, barns, stables, and on large bodies of water and thus can aid in the destruction of those arthropods which serve as vectors of certain communicable diseases. Man has learned to recognize the agent of disease which attacks him, to use effective measures for its destruction, to develop powers of resistance within himself, and to alter the environment so as to aid him in the struggle.

The Epidemiological Approach

In the modern concept, communicable disease is a result of the interaction of three factors—the agent, the host, and the environment. As long as an equilibrium exists among the factors, health is realized. When the equilibrium is disturbed, disease results. Neither the agent alone nor the host alone nor the environment alone causes disease; it results only from a disturbance in the relationship of all three. The agent of disease may be present without causing disturbance, as when diphtheria is introduced into a well-immunized community. Or it is possible to have a susceptible host and not have disease because the agent is lacking, as was the case in the Faroe Islands where measles had not occurred for 60 years because the community was isolated and no one had introduced it. When a case of measles was introduced, almost everyone on the island came down with the disease. Even when agent and host are both present, the proper environment is necessary for disease to assert itself. A community may have a number of typhoid carriers living in it and a large number of susceptible persons, but if the water supply, the sewage disposal, and the food supply are properly supervised, if the carriers are educated to practice strict personal hygiene and are not permitted to handle food for others, no typhoid fever will break out in that community.

The great reduction in mortality from communicable disease in the past 50 years has been due largely to notable improvements in methods of attacking the agent of disease, of bolstering up the defenses of the host, and of so improving the environment as to make it difficult for the agent to survive. Chronologically, improvement began in the last category first. Its beginnings were discussed in the historical review. Its progress has been continuous, and today civilized communities have regulations governing water supply, garbage disposal, sewerage, pasteurization of milk, preparation and distribution of food, sanitary plumbing, and other environmental matters which affect health and life. The proper control of these factors has probably been more effective than anything else in reducing incidence and mortality from diseases, such as typhoid fever, that are commonly spread by fecal contamination.

In point of time, the next advance was in strengthening the defenses of the host. The science of immunology is still very young, but already a tremendous amount of information has been gathered, and practical methods have been developed to immunize susceptible individuals to a number of communicable diseases such as smallpox, diphtheria, whooping cough, tetanus, cholera, plague, and typhus and to confer limited immunity to other diseases such as measles. There is every reason to believe that progress will continue in this field and that the time is not far off when active immunity to diseases like poliomyelitis and mumps will be developed.

The last of the triad against which a frontal attack has been made is the agent. Attempts to destroy the agent after it has lodged in man's body have been made since early historical times. These efforts have been chiefly on an empirical basis. The use of Peruvian bark in the treatment of malaria was an accidental discovery. So was the use of mercury in the therapy of syphilis. The first systematic attempt at chemotherapy was the series of experiments carried out by Ehrlich which culminated in his discovery of salvarsan. However,

this drug was effective against spirochetes only. Many other bactericidal drugs have been tried since then, but in each instance it has
been found that the drug injured the host as much as the agent did
and had to be discarded. The introduction of the sulfonamides
added a drug which inactivated the agent and was harmless to the
host. The recent addition of the antibiotics has given the physician a
powerful weapon with which to attack agents of different kinds even
after they have established a firm foothold in the body, without
affecting the host's other powers of defense. The feverish activity in
numerous research laboratories and the frequent addition of newer,
improved antibiotics lead one to believe that further refinements
may be expected and a more extensive number of microscopic agents
may come under attack.

It must be realized that the antibiotics so far isolated have had
no effect on diseases caused by viruses. No antibiotic has as yet been
found to have any effect on viral diseases like the common cold,
measles, mumps, or chickenpox, or on any of the viral diseases affecting the central nervous system, such as poliomyelitis or encephalitis.
However, some of the newer antibiotics like Aureomycin, chloramphenicol (Chloromycetin), and Terramycin show definite activity
against rickettsiae, which are midway between the viruses and the
bacteria, and there is even some evidence that the large viruses, like
that causing psittacosis, may be adversely affected by the antibiotics,
so that there appears reason to believe that viruses also may soon be
destroyed, or prevented from multiplying, by an antibiotic.

The outlook for the control of communicable diseases appears
very bright. With the methods at hand and in prospect of destroying
the agent, with the host adequately immunized against attack, and
with the environment made more and more hazardous for survival
of infectious agents, the prospect that communicable disease may
some day be completely eliminated becomes more than a silly, idle
dream.

Changes in Control Measures

It is obvious that, as a result of the newer knowledge, the mechanics of control should have undergone many changes. In former
years great stress was laid on isolation of the patient and quarantine
of the contacts and the patient's home, since it was felt that by confining the disease to a single group and excluding members of the
group from commerce with others there would be no spread. When
more exact knowledge of carriers was obtained, there came about
the realization that it was not very sensible to shut up a few household carriers and allow many other carriers in the community at
large. During an epidemic of scarlet fever, for instance, as many as

10 to 15 per cent of the population may carry in their throats the streptococcus responsible for the disease. It is estimated that from 10 to 100 times as many normal individuals carry the virus of poliomyelitis as there are people sick with the disease. There is no practical or feasible way of picking out the carriers, and the numbers of them would be too great to confine. Hence, quarantine of contacts has been largely discarded as a method of control. In New York City quarantine of contacts is imposed only in the case of smallpox and diphtheria, and it is doubtful whether in the latter disease it is necessary. Furthermore, there are no carriers in some of the communicable diseases. There appears to be no reason for keeping a contact to measles or chickenpox, for instance, away from his fellows, unless he develops the disease, since these diseases are not carried by a symptomless person. It is much better control to let him play with his fellows and watch for symptoms at the end of the incubation period. If he develops any, he is isolated at that time. In 1941, contacts to cases of measles were still being excluded from school in New York City, yet the largest epidemic of measles in the history of the city occurred in that year, and 80,000 cases were reported. The exclusion of contacts from school was abolished that year, but the cyclic occurrence of the disease has continued as in the past, and in no year since 1941 have even half as many cases been reported. On the other hand, isolation of the patient is still a worth-while control measure, since the number of organisms thrown out by the patient is vastly greater than those sent out by the carrier, and, in some diseases, they are more virulent.

Another change that has resulted from increased knowledge is a modification of the period of isolation. In general, this has been in the direction of a shortening of the time. It has resulted from a better knowledge of the nature of some diseases, a more correct understanding of transmission, and a realization that certain infectious diseases have become milder and that treatment with antibiotics has shortened the period of communicability of others.

Placarding of the premises of cases of communicable disease has been discarded as a method of control. It is ineffective, costly, and psychologically unsound. There is no reason for placarding an apartment, since it is the patient and not the apartment that spreads the disease. To avoid the possibility of contracting a communicable disease spread by the respiratory tract, the family should be taught not to permit susceptible individuals to come in contact with the patient. Careless people are not deterred by a placard. Public-minded people will keep susceptible people away from the patient, whether a placard is on the door or not. Placarding premises takes up considerable time which can be used to better advantage in other ways. A placard on a door is psychologically a poor educational procedure. It frightens neighbors and makes the mother and siblings of the patient pariahs. We have not observed the placard to do more than scare away delivery boys. The discarding of placards by the New York City Department of Health has not arrested the downward trend of communicable disease in the city.

There is still less to be said in favor of the barbarous method of tagging cases and contacts of certain communicable diseases. For a period there existed the quaint custom in certain communities of putting an arm band on children with whooping cough and on their siblings. The theory back of this was that the children could be out in the fresh air and yet other children could be kept away from them. It is hardly necessary to point out how wrong such a method is, educationally and psychologically. It is doubtful if it has any police value, either.

The newer knowledge of communicable disease indicates that the routine taking of cultures from the throats of all children, and of vaginal smears of all girls admitted to hospitals, institutions, day-care agencies, shelters, or camps should be discouraged. As a public health procedure it is not of much value. It wastes considerable time by holding up admissions, and it has exerted little influence in the reduction of diphtheria and gonorrhea. In the case of diphtheria, many routine positive cultures are found to be avirulent. The emphasis should be shifted to the proper immunization of all children. In a community of immunized children, the fear of spread of diphtheria is negligible. Vaginitis is easily controlled by sulfonamides and antibiotics. A child who, on admission, shows clinical symptoms of diphtheria or gonorrhea should be isolated, properly diagnosed, and adequately treated, but routine cultures should be abolished.

The reduction in incidence of communicable diseases, the response of many of them to treatment with sulfonamides, and the more exact knowledge of the methods of spread have tended to simplify nursing procedures. Terminal disinfection has lost its former appeal. Since organisms generally dry out rapidly and die when shed by the human body, there seems little reason to worry about the disinfection of clothes, furniture, floors, and walls after patients have recovered. Stress should rather be laid on concurrent disinfection, since the discharges from the patient are infectious and should be properly disposed of. Furthermore, the elaborate nursing procedures adopted in former years, the mystic rite of the basin of smelly disinfectant into which the nurse carefully dipped her fingers before leaving the room, the sprinkling of disinfectant solutions on walls and floors, the hanging up of sheets which had been soaked in dilute carbolic solution have all been shown to be elaborate mumbo jumbo. Nursing in communicable diseases is essentially the same as nursing in other diseases. Stress should be laid on proper hygienic measures to prevent spread and on proper medical measures to prevent complication. The nurse should be aware of modern trends so that she can instruct the patient and the family not only about hygienic measures but also about questions of immunity and other protective measures.

The rational approach to communicable diseases has brought about a psychologic change in the attitude of the public. When epidemics were considered the work of demons and when later they were thought to be the punishment of God, individuals ill with communicable disease were thought of as cursed. Decent people kept away from them. With the increase in knowledge and the development of bacteriology, it became clear that the difference between one communicable disease and another was the difference in bacterial agent. Various factors in the host and the environment determined the manner and rate of spread. The control of epidemics depended not at all on rituals but on the effective control of spread and of proper strengthening of the host's defensive mechanism. It would be idle to say that senseless fear has been completely abolished. People still want to run when they hear the word polio, although they have no clear notion what good running will do. However, a more rational attitude, based on information rather than on mysticism, is gradually spreading among people. Words like tuberculosis and syphilis can be pronounced out loud and even discussed in newspapers.

The continued reduction in the number of cases of communicable disease has brought about an administrative change in their care. When huge numbers were listed and many deaths occurred, when knowledge of the spread was uncertain, when methods of defense were only tentatively being worked out, and when there were no specific drugs to combat the diseases, the facilities needed to house cases of contagion were great. General hospitals refused to take such cases because they shared in the popular taboos and they were not sure that they could confine the diseases and prevent their spread to other patients. Pesthouses were consequently built on the edge of town, and all cases of communicable disease were confined in them. In time, these hospitals became quite respectable and efficient. The Willard Parker Hospital in New York and the Herman Kiefer Hospital in Detroit, for instance, have built up enviable reputations. Their need, however, has lessened with the times. Cases are fewer and their care is less arduous. Since communicable diseases are seasonal in occurrence and since outbreaks occur at times which cannot be predetermined, the special communicable-disease hospitals find themselves with a tremendous load at certain times and with practically no patients at other times. Furthermore, the increase of old people in the population has brought about greater need for care of diseases of old age. The old people with degenerative diseases are knocking at the doors of these hospitals which are practically vacant in certain seasons. In addition, there is another important factor to consider. With the decrease in incidence of communicable diseases, physicians and nurses rarely get an opportunity to see cases unless they are attached to the special hospitals. Interns and student nurses may go through their entire training without ever seeing a case of measles or diphtheria. For educational, administrative and economic reasons there has therefore begun a trend to disband special hospitals for communicable diseases and to open up general hospitals for their care under certain safeguards. It is reasonable to believe that this movement will continue with greater force in the years ahead.

REFERENCES

1. Castiglione, A.: *A History of Medicine*, Alfred A. Knopf, Inc., New York, 1947.
2. Dubos, R.: *Louis Pasteur*, Little, Brown & Company, Boston, 1950.
3. Galston, Iago: *Progress in Medicine*, Alfred A. Knopf, Inc., New York, Chaps. II and III, 1940.
4. Garrison, F. H.: *An Introduction to the History of Medicine*, 4th ed., W. B. Saunders Company, Philadelphia, 1929.
5. *Holy Bible*, Book of Leviticus, Chaps. 13 and 15.
6. Shattuck, L.: *Report of the Sanitary Commission of Massachusetts, 1850*, Harvard University Press, Cambridge, Mass., 1948.
7. Smith, G.: *Plague on Us*, Commonwealth Fund, Harvard University Press, Cambridge, Mass., 1943.
8. Snow, J.: *On Cholera*, Commonwealth Fund, Harvard University Press, Cambridge, Mass., 1936.
9. Winslow, C-E. A.: *The Conquest of Epidemic Disease*, Princeton University Press, Princeton, N.J., 1943.
10. Zinsser, H.: *Rats, Lice and History*, Little, Brown & Company, Boston, 1944.

Chapter 2 COMMUNITY CONTROL

THE control of communicable disease is a governmental function similar to the maintenance of peace or the protection of private property. It is obvious that such a function cannot be left to individual physicians or groups of doctors, nor can it be entrusted to voluntary agencies interested in public health. It is only the citizenry as a whole, as represented in the government, that can take efficient and necessary action to protect the public health, since such protection may involve certain restrictions in the conduct of particular individuals. Laws governing the conduct of members of a community should not be entrusted to anyone but the responsible legislators elected by the community.

The United States is a Federal government. Under the Constitution, the individual states are independent and make their own laws. The Federal government has only such powers as have been delegated to it by the states in the Constitution. Laws governing the health of citizens are reserved to the states. The Federal government is, however, given explicit power in the Constitution to regulate commerce with foreign nations and between the states and to provide for the general welfare of the United States. These powers have been interpreted rather liberally, so that a considerable public health service has been built up by the Federal government.

National Health Services

A marine hospital service was organized in 1798 to give medical care to American seamen, and the latter were required to contribute part of their wages for the service. As far as public health was concerned, the Federal service limited itself to the control of communicable diseases by imposing maritime quarantine whenever necessary. This was carried out in co-operation with the health department of the port of entry. The marine hospital service was the beginning of the United States Public Health Service, which has gradually expanded until it has become one of the largest health services in the world.

Public Health Service

The United States Public Health Service was organized in 1902 as the United States Health and Marine Hospital Service. At the same time a laboratory was established in connection with it and was given the name of National Hygienic Laboratory. The services were placed in the Treasury Department and remained there until 1939 when they were moved to the Federal Security Agency.

The functions of the United States Public Health Service have been expanded from time to time by acts of Congress. Thus, in 1912, the Service was given authority to make investigations and administer research projects, to control interstate sanitation, to carry on investigations in methods of public health administration, and to distribute Federal aid to state and local health departments. The last of these functions was increased tremendously under the Social Security Act of 1935. Large sums have been allotted annually to the Service to be used as grants-in-aid to the states in order to improve and strengthen local health services.

Further expansion of the Public Health Service has resulted from specific acts of Congress. At present the functions include, in addition to those already mentioned, the examination of aliens entering the country, the medical care of Federal prisoners and narcotic addicts, the care of lepers at the national leprosarium in Carville, La., and the treatment of tuberculous and neuropsychiatric patients. Other functions that have been added are research in and control of a number of specific diseases.

The Service is manned by commissioned officers, who are technical men and women. They are physicians, dentists, nurses, sanitary engineers, pharmacologists, zoologists, chemists, veterinarians, etc. They are appointed by the President, with the consent and advice of the Senate. There are various grades and ranks, and promotions are made from rank to rank on the basis of good work, time in the Service, and the results of promotion examinations. The pay is patterned after that in the Army. In addition to the regular corps, there is a reserve corps from which men and women are drawn in times of special need. The total number of commissioned and other employees in the Service is about 15,000 persons.

ORGANIZATION

The head of the United States Public Health Service is the Surgeon General, who is appointed by the President, with the consent of the Senate, for a term of 4 years. He directs the affairs of the Service and advises the United States government on matters of health both in this country and abroad. He receives advice from several boards, such as the National Advisory Health Council, National Advisory Cancer Council, National Advisory Heart Council, National Advisory Mental Health Council, Federal Hospital Council, National Advisory Dental Research Council, and the Water Pollution Control Advisory Board. These councils and boards are made up of men prominent in their field, who are appointed by the Surgeon General and who serve without fee.

The administrative work of the Service is divided into four bureaus, each headed by a chief, responsible to the Surgeon General. These are:

1. Office of the Surgeon General
2. Bureau of Medical Services
3. Bureau of State Services
4. National Institutes of Health

Office of the Surgeon General

This bureau is directed by the Deputy Surgeon General and is the administrative part of the Service. It is concerned with management, personnel, finance, supplies, etc. It is divided into eight divisions, each headed by a chief. These are the Divisions of (1) Commissioned Officers, (2) Finance, (3) Management Services, (4) Personnel, (5) Supply, (6) Public Health Methods, (7) International Health, and (8) Civilian Health Requirements. The Division of Public Health Methods, in addition to its other duties, publishes the monthly scientific journal *Public Health Reports,* in which appear the results of the findings of most of the technical investigations carried on by various members of the Service. The Division of International Health co-ordinates and directs the activities of the Service in the international health field. One of its functions is to act as liaison officer between this government and other governments, as well as the World Health Organization, in matters of health.

Bureau of Medical Services

The manifold activities of this bureau are performed through seven divisions. They are Divisions of (1) Hospitals, (2) Hospital Facilities, (3) Medical and Hospital Resources, (4) Nursing Resources, (5) Dental Resources, (6) Foreign Quarantine, and (7) Administrative Management. The Division of Hospitals administers nineteen marine hospitals and clinics, two hospitals for the care of psychotic patients and narcotic addicts, two tuberculosis hospitals, and one leprosarium, as well as the health activities of the Coast Guard. The Division of Hospital Facilities plans and administers the program for aid to states in the hospital construction program. The Divisions of Nursing, Dental, and Medical and Hospital Resources are concerned with the broad questions of national policy relating to nursing education and service, dental health, and hospital and medical care. The Division of Foreign Quarantine carries the burden of the inspection of persons, imports, and conveyances arriving in United States from foreign countries; it promulgates rules to prevent the introduction of certain diseases and vectors into the country, prescribes certain health precautions to be observed by carriers arriving at any port from foreign countries, examines aliens entering the country and applicants for visas at foreign ports, and carries out international agreements relating to matters of quarantine. To prevent the entry of cases of communicable disease, it was the custom to order ships to anchor in the harbor of the port of entry until a proper examination of persons and cargo had been made by an officer of the Service. Since this caused great delay and was not necessary for control, the practice of radio pratique has developed. According to this plan, the ship's surgeon radios to the quarantine office concerning health conditions on his ship. If they are satisfactory, the ship is permitted to dock, and examinations are then made on board boat. International agreements require the quarantining of only five major diseases—smallpox, cholera, typhus, plague, and yellow fever. A boat arriving with a case of one of these diseases is usually required to anchor off shore or at the quarantine station until it has been boarded by the quarantine officials and arrangements have been made for the disposition of the case and the other passengers and crew. Cases of other acute communicable diseases, such as measles, diphtheria, etc., which are not detainable, are turned over to the health authorities of the port of entry. The rules of quarantine apply to incoming persons from foreign countries, irrespective of whether they arrive by boat, train, or plane.

The Bureau of Medical Services, in addition to the functions administered through its divisions, is also responsible for supervising Service personnel which it assigns to various bureaus in other Federal departments. These include the Bureau of Indian Affairs in the Department of the Interior, the Bureau of Prisons in the Department of Justice, the Division of Foreign Affairs in the Department of State, the U.S. Coast Guard in the Treasury Department, the Bureau of Employees' Compensation, the Office of Vocational Rehabilitation, the Social Security Administration in the Federal Security Agency, and the U.S. Maritime Commission.

Bureau of State Services

This bureau operates through the medium of fourteen divisions. These are (1) the National Office for Vital Statistics, the Divisions of

(2) Public Health Nursing, (3) Public Health Education, (4) State Grants, (5) Chronic Disease and Tuberculosis, (6) Dental Public Health, (7) Venereal Disease, (8) Sanitation, (9) Industrial Hygiene, (10) Engineering Resources, and (11) Administrative Management; and the (12) Communicable Disease Center, (13) Environmental Health Center, and (14) Arctic Health Research Center. The Bureau of State Services also controls the regional organization of the Public Health Service. The manifold activities of the bureau can be surmised from the mere listing of the divisions. The National Office of Vital Statistics collects, tabulates, analyzes, and publishes vital statistics on the incidence of communicable disease in the different states, and information on mortality from these diseases. Special studies on certain aspects of morbidity and mortality are also made. The Division of State Grants co-ordinates the administration of all grants to state and local agencies. The other divisions are concerned with the study, planning, control, and consultative aid to states of the specific activities assigned to them. The three centers consist of offices and laboratories for the investigation of communicable disease, environmental health, and health in arctic regions, respectively. The Communicable Disease Center is located in Atlanta, Ga., and the laboratories are in nearby Chamblee, Ga., and in Montgomery, Ala. This center is staffed with individuals able and prepared to cope with all aspects of communicable disease, including epidemiologists, statisticians, entomologists, veterinarians, nursing consultants, etc. It is ready to undertake the investigation of unusual occurrence of disease in any part of the country or to assist any state in the study and control of any aspect of communicable disease within its boundaries. Its laboratories in Chamblee and Montgomery will receive specimens for diagnosis from state health departments. Many states do not have facilities for special types of laboratory procedures or for the laboratory diagnosis of certain rare diseases. The Communicable Disease Center encourages the state laboratories to send specimens which they are unable to process.

The Regional Organization is an administrative setup in the Service. The country is divided into a number of regions, and a Regional Medical Director is placed in charge of each. He and his staff represent the Service in its relationship with the states or with local agencies in connection with grants-in-aid programs or other co-operative projects. In other words, he acts as a liaison officer between the Service and the states.

National Institutes of Health

The expansion in the laboratory bureau has kept pace with the expansion of the other activities of the Public Health Service.

Originally, the National Hygienic Laboratory was a modest organization for the performance of essential laboratory work in public health. It grew and became the National Institute of Health, which functioned as a research and diagnostic laboratory for the Service. Further expansion has converted it into a large bureau known as the National Institutes of Health, occupying a great many acres of land and buildings in Bethesda, Md. The director has charge of seven different institutes, one division, and a clinical center. These are the Institutes of (1) Microbiology, (2) Cancer, (3) Heart, (4) Arthritis and Metabolic Diseases, (5) Dental Research, (6) Mental Health, and (7) Neurological Diseases and Blindness; the Division of Research Grants; and the Clinical Center. The various institutes comprising the National Institutes of Health carry on fundamental research in their particular fields in order to improve diagnosis, treatment, and prevention of disease. In six of the institutes research is directed to a particular disease or disease group—cancer, heart disease, dental disease, mental disease, neurological disease, including blindness and arthritic diseases. In the last, research is also directed toward fundamental problems such as metabolism, nutrition, biochemistry, chemotherapy, pathology, toxicology, and pharmacology. The National Microbiological Institute conducts investigations in all aspects of growth and survival of microorganisms, as related to public health, with the purpose of obtaining information on the transmission, control, and prevention of infectious disease. This institute is also charged with the responsibility of setting up standards and administering the Congressional act which regulates the manufacture and interstate transmission of biologicals. The Division of Research Grants administers the program of grants for research to institutions and individuals, in support of basic study in medical fields. The Clinical Center is a large hospital with facilities for several hundred patients and for necessary laboratory facilities and operating and treatment rooms. Patients suffering from any of the diseases under investigation are admitted to the clinical center and receive the benefit of the known diagnostic tests and the latest discoveries in therapy.

The expansion of the activities of the Public Health Service has required increasing funds for its operations. For the year ending June 30, 1952, the approved budget of the Service amounted to $228,362,408. This was divided into funds to be paid as grants to the states amounting to $148,290,300, and funds for direct operations amounting to $80,072,108. The grants to the states were made for hospital construction ($82,500,000) and for other activities such as general health, venereal disease, tuberculosis, water-pollution control, cancer, mental health, heart disease, and a special grant to Alaska. The amount allotted for direct operations was separated into moneys to be used for construction ($7,035,540) and funds to be used for research and investigations ($14,545,688), technical assistance to states, medical care, and other direct operations.

It will be noted that all aspects but one of a well-rounded public health program are carried on by the United States Public Health Service. The one exception is in the field of maternal and child health. The omission of this function is not an act of carelessness. It is a deliberate one. The promotion of child and maternal health is a function of the Children's Bureau, an agency completely separate from the Public Health Service. From the point of view of administration, it appears illogical to maintain an independent bureau for one of the many functions of a public health service. However, historically, there is logic in the arrangement. The Children's Bureau was originally established as a result of the activities of many women who were concerned with the problem of child labor. It has grown rapidly. The individuals guiding the bureau have been such able persons and the caliber of service that the bureau has given is of so high a standard that there has been reluctance to merge it with the Public Health Service.

Children's Bureau

The Children's Bureau was established by an act of Congress on April 9, 1912, for the purpose of investigating and reporting on all matters pertaining to the welfare of children and child life, and especially infant mortality, birth rate, orphanages, juvenile courts, desertion, dangerous occupations, accidents, diseases of children, and employment and legislation affecting children in the several states and territories. It was placed in the Department of Commerce and Labor. The next year, when separate departments were created, the bureau was placed in the Department of Labor and remained there until 1946, when it was transferred to the Federal Security Agency, the same agency of which the Public Health Service is now a part.

The functions of the bureau are (1) to investigate and report on matters relating to the welfare of children, (2) to administer grants-in-aid to the states under provision of the Social Security Act, and (3) to co-operate with other American republics in the program of the Interdepartmental Committee on Scientific and Cultural Cooperation.

ORGANIZATION

The actual work of the bureau is administered by a chief, with the help of assistants, through several divisions. The Office of the Chief directs all activities, develops programs, formulates policies, and co-operates in national and international programs concerned with children. The seven divisions of the bureau are the Divisions of (1) Research, (2) Health Services, (3) Social Services, (4) Reports, (5) International Cooperation, (6) Administrative Services, and (7) Grants Fiscal Services. The Division of Research conducts investigations in all aspects of a child's life and develops standards. The Division of Health Services develops policies and recommendations for health services to mothers and children and services to crippled children and administers the grants to states for such services. The Division of Social Services performs the same functions with reference to social services to children, such as foster care, adoption, guardianship, day-care centers, treatment of neglected or delinquent children, etc. The Division of Reports is the public health education branch of the bureau. In addition to the writing and distribution of pamphlets, leaflets, and other material concerned with child life and acting as an information center for the bureau's activities, it publishes a monthly periodical, *The Child*. The Division of International Cooperation co-operates with other countries in programs for child care, gives consultation services to other countries, and exchanges technical information with other countries on questions of child life. The Divisions of Administrative Services and of Grants Fiscal Services are the auditing branches of the bureau. The first concerns itself with budgets, supplies, accounting, maintenance of records, etc., and the second is concerned especially with the budgets, reports, and records of monies granted to states under the Social Security Act.

When it was first organized the Children's Bureau received an appropriation of $25,640 and had a staff of 15. It has expanded rapidly. For the fiscal year 1950–1951, Congress appropriated $1,500,000 for salaries and expenses of the bureau, which employed a staff of 260 at that time. In addition, a large fund was granted to the bureau for grants-in-aid to states. Such grants were first made available in 1921, when Congress passed the Sheppard-Towner Act. This provided $1,240,000 for the states to assist in reducing maternal and infant mortality and protecting the health of mothers and infants. The control of the program was given to a board consisting of the Chief of the Children's Bureau, the Surgeon General of the Public Health Service, and the Commissioner of Education. In 1935 the Social Security Act was passed. It provided federal funds as grants to the states for maternal and child health services, crippled children, and child welfare. These programs are administered by the Children's Bureau. For the fiscal year 1950–1951, Congress appropriated $30,250,000 for such grants. It was broken down to provide $13,2000,000 for maternal and child health services, $9,975,000 for services to crippled children, and $7,075,000 for child welfare services.

The amount of money that goes to each state is determined by the Children's Bureau according to certain formulas. For maternal and child health these are based on the state's need, the number of live births in rural areas, and the ratio of live births in the state to total live births in the country. For crippled children the formula is based on the state's need, the number of children in the state, and the number of children in rural areas. To obtain grants for both these programs the states must match half the grants. For child welfare services there is no definite amount for the state's share. This is determined by the ratio of youths under 18 years old in rural areas to the total rural child population. To qualify for any grant the state agency must submit its program to the bureau for approval. If approval is denied, the agency may appeal to the Federal Security Administrator.

Department of Agriculture

There are a number of other federal agencies that are concerned with the control of communicable disease. Among these is the Department of Agriculture. It carries on scientific studies of diseases and parasites peculiar to domestic animals, and thus attempts to prevent and control those diseases which are transmissible to man. Meat that is sold in interstate commerce for human consumption is inspected for freedom from disease. Also, rules and regulations for the production and handling of milk in interstate commerce have been established by this department. This department is also concerned with the study of insects and methods for their eradication and control. Much of the knowledge of the effectiveness of DDT as a measure of control in vector-borne disease of man has come from studies carried out by members of this department.

Department of Interior

Two agencies of this department carry on activities which stress the control of disease. One is the Fish and Wildlife Service, which is concerned primarily with programs to protect wildlife and fish.

Such programs involve the destruction of rodents and the elimination of hazards to fish in streams and lakes. The other is the Bureau of Indian Affairs, which makes available medical, nursing, and public health services to Indians living on reservations. In addition to the operation of hospitals, where Indians can obtain medical care, there are programs for the control of disease, particularly tuberculosis, among Indians. As already indicated, medical personnel is assigned by the Public Health Service to this bureau.

Department of Defense

The health of the officers and enlisted and conscripted men and women of the department of defense is an important responsibility of the department. There are three general divisions of the military service, those of the Army, Navy and Air Force. The medical care of the personnel in each of the services is entrusted to the Surgeon General of that branch of the Service. Hospitals for the care of men and women in service who are injured or ill have been established at a number of posts. In addition, the services carry on investigations in various aspects of the control of communicable disease.

Veterans Administration

This is an extremely large service which is concerned with the health and welfare of veterans. As part of its function many large hospitals have been built in various parts of the country where veterans can obtain medical care. In these hospitals, as in other well-run hospitals, research in various aspects of medicine, including communicable disease, is constantly going on.

State Function in Community Health

Since the state, in our Federal form of government, is the sovereign unit, the authority to prevent disease and to further active health among its citizens and the responsibility for doing so rest upon it. All states in the Union have a constitution, which is a statement of basic principles guiding the state in its many functions. The power to pass laws which will guard the health of its citizens is granted to the legislatures of the states by their constitutions. The types of laws passed by the legislatures and the manner in which the public health functions of the state have been organized vary from state to state. This is bound to be so, since climate, geography, size and type of population, density, industrialization, wealth, and other factors differ in the different states. A health law which is workable in a tightly packed urban community may be altogether unwieldly in a sprawling rural community. It is, therefore, not at all surprising that methods for the control of communicable disease vary from state to state. On the contrary, it is surprising that there is so much unanimity. It indicates a high degree of good will and co-operative effort on the part of health officers the country over.

Organization of a State Department of Health

A state department of health covers so many fields of activity that, unless properly organized, it would not function efficiently. After many years of experiment a similar plan of organization has been adopted by most states. This is to divide the department of health into a number of units, usually called bureaus, each headed by a director, and to assign a specific type of activity to each bureau. The six fundamental services that are considered essential for all departments of health, local as well as state, are (1) vital statistics, (2) control of communicable diseases, (3) environmental sanitation, (4) laboratory service, (5) maternal and child hygiene, and (6) public health education. Depending on their size and variety of activity, state health departments have added other bureaus. Most of them have a bureau of general administration. In many, all nursing activities have been grouped in a bureau of public health nursing. Some have bureaus of dentistry and of nutrition. Some departments have expanded to include services which do not strictly refer to communicable disease, and have established bureaus of medical care or of cancer. Each state department must determine what particular health problems are of concern to its communities. An important health problem in one state may be of no significance in another state. Hence, there cannot be a uniform number of bureaus in all state health departments. The six mentioned above are, however, basic and should be found on the organizational chart of every health department.

State Health Officer

All states have health departments. These are, as a rule, under the administrative supervision of a state health officer. He is known under different titles in different states, but the one most commonly used is commissioner of health. He has general supervision over the department of health and is usually responsible to the governor for its activities.

STATE BOARD OF HEALTH

In most of the states a board of health has been created by specific act of the legislature. This body usually consists of five to seven men interested in the public health, several of whom are physicians, and all of whom serve without pay. The state health officer is a member of the board, in some states acting in an ex officio capacity. The board of health is vested with the power, by the legislature, of formulating a sanitary code, whose rules and regulations have the force of law and are the guiding basis of the health department's work. Boards meet once a month, as a rule, listen to reports, pass on suggested amendments to the code, initiate new regulations, and perform such other functions as are assigned to them by act of legislature. In some states the board of health is known as the public health council.

FUNCTIONS OF A STATE DEPARTMENT OF HEALTH

Assistance to local health units

By and large, the main function of a state health department is to supervise, advise, and strengthen local health services. This is done, to a considerable extent, by state subsidies. Local health services do not, as a rule, have sufficient funds to support a good health program. Subsidies from the state frequently help them to get needed personnel, necessary construction, or the addition of services which they could not afford without the subsidies. In recent years the funds have been increased by grants made to the states by the Federal government for specific purposes, such as building hospitals and establishing programs for venereal diseases, cancer, tuberculosis, and other diseases and for carrying on necessary research.

In addition to funds, the state department of health offers skilled advice on technical health matters to the local units. Obviously, it is neither economical nor practical for most local health units to employ a skilled epidemiologist or a statistician or a fully equipped laboratory or many other costly services. These can be maintained by the state, and the local health units can call upon them for advice or assistance. Of course, if the state finds that a particular health unit is uninterested in the local health, is unwilling to face problems and try to solve them, or is neglecting necessary health services, it may step in and supervise the services or even supersede the local health officers. Such drastic action is rarely necessary.

Maintenance of intercommunity services

There are some health services which, of necessity, affect more than one local health unit. It might be a large water reservoir serving two or more adjacent local units, or a river draining the areas of a number of communities, or a state park open to all the citizens of the state, or a public bathing beach which draws people from a number of near-by communities. Occasionally, the adjacent local units will combine forces and pool their resources to keep the service going efficiently. Sometimes they are unable to afford it, and sometimes local jealousies interfere. Occasionally, serious disputes arise, as when a community complains that its bathing facilities are being polluted by the dumping of wastes into the stream by the community upstream. In such cases the state department of health steps in to adjust amicably the differences that have arisen, or, if the cost is too great for the local communities or their rivalries are too acute, to take complete charge of the service.

Maintenance of standards

The state department of health is the leader of public health in the state. It can afford the services of experts in the various fields of public health, it has prestige, and it has the opportunity to recommend to the board of health legislation which has the power of law. It is thus able to set standards in all aspects of public health and compel local communities to adopt these standards as a minimum. Regulations governing isolation and quarantine of cases of communicable disease, the treatment of water supplies, the pasteurization of milk, the hospitalization of certain cases of communicable illness, and similar matters are promulgated by the state health authorities and are usually embodied in the sanitary code. They become the law of the state, and all local health units must abide by them. Frequently, the state department of health issues advice to the local units in the form of a memorandum of departmental policy. The local units may or may not follow such advice. As a rule, if the state department of health merits respect, the local units adopt the advice because they know it is a result of superior experience or knowledge and because they are afraid to take the consequences, in the form of loss of prestige, if the state's advice is not followed.

Direct services

There are certain health services which must be uniform, which cannot be run on a small scale, which require the expenditure of large funds, and which require expensive equipment and skilled personnel. Such services must be run directly by the state and offered to all citizens within its boundaries. Among these services the one that stands out is that of gathering information on births, deaths, and other vital statistics. To be of value, uniform certificates must be used. They must be stored in a proper place for preservation, there must be facilities for reproducing them when needed, and skilled statisticians and expensive machines are needed to tabulate and to interpret them. Another essential service is a laboratory. Here, too, there is need for proper space, expensive equipment, and skilled personnel to perform the multitudinous tests that are frequently necessary to make a correct diagnosis. A community may need the services of skilled sanitary engineers who can figure out the amount of water that it will need, the best way of obtaining it, and methods of impounding, filtering, and chlorinating it; who can determine the best way to prevent the pollution of streams, to dispose of sewage, to keep bathing beaches clean and healthy, and to tackle similar hygienic problems. There are the epidemiologists, or medical detectives, who ferret out the source of epidemics, prevent their spread, and offer measures for their control. There may be a need for a hospital to care for tuberculous individuals, and yet no local community may have sufficient funds to build and maintain it or enough patients to fill it. All such services must be maintained by the state and must be offered alike to all citizens through their local health departments. These may freely call on the state for technical assistance or request needed services when necessary.

Cooperation with other state and Federal agencies

There are many health matters which concern several neighboring states or that concern all the states and the Federal government. An example of the former is the control of rabies in counties bordering on two adjacent states. An example of the latter is a uniform method of reporting communicable disease to the Federal government. Matters like these are discussed by the respective health departments of the states, with each other, and with the Federal government.

Local Health Services

It is in the field of local health services that most confusion exists and where great differences of organization are found, not only in different states but in each state. A study of local health services was undertaken by a committee of the American Public

Health Association, and its report was filed in 1945. Its investigation showed that about 40 million people in the United States were living in communities with no local health services or with part-time health services. Tradition has had a great deal to do with the way in which public health activities are managed. In New England, for instance, the tradition in government has been for each city, town, or village to have its own unit of government. In the South and West the county is commonly the unit. Since cities, towns, and counties vary in size and population, it is obvious that some units will be too small to afford a good service. The committee decided to survey each state, determine its public health practices and needs, and, after consultation with state health commissioners and other interested persons, offer suggestions for the organization of the local health services. It took as its guide three basic principles: that each local health unit be completely covered with a basic minimum, full-time service; that the units have a large enough population to support such a service—approximately 50,000 persons to a unit; that the cost approximate $1 per capita. Using these criteria, it recommended the establishment of 1,197 local health units in the United States. Some were single-county units, some multicounty, some county-district, and others city units.

A local health department, the committee advised, should have a board of health appointed by the local executives, consisting of five to seven members, two or three of whom should be physicians. The board should advise the health officer, establish policies, legislate local ordinances not inconsistent with the state public health law, and hold hearings when citizens complain of certain actions of the health officer. As an example, the health department in a community of 50,000 inhabitants may have, as a minimum, the following full-time personnel: one medical health officer; one sanitary engineer; one sanitary inspector; ten public health nurses, of whom one should act as supervisor; and three clerical employees. Clinical services could be run by part-time personnel. Consultations in the field of public health, such as statistics, engineering, and epidemiology, could be obtained from the state department of health. The minimal services that a local department of health should offer are the six basic ones mentioned on page 33. In communities with populations larger than 50,000, additional staff may be added. The functions of some of the basic services might be given to full-time medical men or women, who would act as chiefs of bureaus. There would, of course, have to be added additional public health nurses, sanitarians, and clerks. The larger the community, the more extensive would be the demands for public health services and the greater the number of full-time employees. Some very large local communities have health departments which are larger than many of the state health departments. In New York City, for instance, the staff of the department consists of about 4,000 full-time and 1,000 part-time employees.

The functions of the bureau of communicable diseases in the local health unit consist of:

1. The receipt of reports of communicable disease as listed in the sanitary code
2. The tabulation of these reports according to sex, age, and other epidemiological characteristics for the purpose of having bases of comparison and knowledge about the areas where greater efforts at control are necessary
3. The establishment of rules and regulations for the isolation and quarantine of cases of communicable disease and for concurrent and terminal disinfection
4. The epidemiological investigation of outbreaks of disease and of single cases of certain diseases to determine the source, prevent the spread, and establish control
5. The investigation of animal diseases which are transmissible to man, and the establishment of rules and regulations for their prevention and control
6. The carrying on, within the limits of its budget and personnel, of studies in the field of communicable disease which will shed light on causation, spread, relationships, and control.

Voluntary Health Agencies

There are many private, nongovernmental health agencies in the United States. Some are organized on a national basis, with local chapters. Others function on a state basis, and still others on a local basis only. Many limit their activities to a single disease, such as the National Tuberculosis Association or the National Foundation for Infantile Paralysis. Some have a wider scope and cover a number of conditions, such as the Association for the Aid of Crippled Children. Still others are interested in the broad aspect of general health, like the American Red Cross, or in some particular aspect of public health, such as the visiting nurses' services. In the early history of the country they served a very useful function. State and local public health services were very weak. These agencies fought for greater public support of health activities, established clinics, arranged for home nursing, carried on programs of health education, and performed many other services which most health departments are now expected to perform. At present they still serve a useful function, but this is chiefly in the field of education, demonstration of new activities, relief, and subvention of research. No voluntary agency should attempt, and no community should allow, the usurpation of functions which the local or state health department has been organized to perform. Often, there is close and harmonious co-operation between a health department and a private agency. For instance, in most communities there is a visiting nurses' service, which provides nursing care to patients who cannot afford full-time nursing service. In the same communities the health department may send public health nurses to make home visits in cases of communicable disease, and to instruct the family in techniques of isolation, quarantine, etc. With increasing shortage of nurses, many communities have found it profitable to make a co-operative arrangement, so that public health nurses from the visiting service caring for a case of communicable disease will also undertake to teach the family the public health aspects of the disease and the principles of isolation, quarantine, etc., thus eliminating the visit of a public health nurse from the health department. In return, the latter, visiting a case of communicable disease will, in addition to her educational work, give nursing care to the patient or instruct someone in the family about necessary procedures.

There are, in addition to the voluntary agencies, a number of foundations interested primarily, or to some extent, in public health. Such foundations have usually been established by wealthy, socially minded persons. They are incorporated, nonprofit organizations. Most of them do not take a direct part in the public health field but supply funds as grants-in-aid to individuals, hospitals, schools, or health departments for special studies in some particular aspect of public health.

REFERENCES

1. Emerson, Haven: *Local Health Units for the Nation,* Commonwealth Fund, Harvard University Press, Cambridge, Mass., 1945.
2. Federal Security Agency: *Organizational Chart, Public Health Service,* Washington, D.C., 1951.
3. Lenroot, K. F.; Bain, K.; Glasser, M. A.; and Larson, N.: *Current Program of Children's Bureau,* Federal Security Agency, Washington, D.C., 1950.
4. Shepard, W. P.: *Essentials of Public Health,* J. B. Lippincott Company, Philadelphia, 1948.
5. Smillie, W. G.: *Preventive Medicine and Public Health,* The Macmillan Company, New York, 1947.

Chapter 3 EPIDEMIOLOGY

IN the narrowest sense, epidemiology may be defined as the science of epidemics. Originally, the function of the epidemiologist was to investigate epidemics, trace their source, limit their spread, and introduce control measures to prevent their recurrence. This is still an important function of the epidemiologist. However, the concept of the term "epidemiology" has become broadened to include disease as it applies to masses of people, irrespective of whether it occurs as an epidemic or endemic phenomenon. Even with the broadening of the definition, epidemiology was still thought of almost exclusively in relationship to communicable disease. Only in comparatively recent years has it been realized that the tools the epidemiologist has learned to forge in order to conquer communicable disease can also be used in the study of noninfectious disease. The modern concept of epidemiology is that of a science concerned with the relationships of disease in the aggregate—what has been called "crowd diseases." Such a science must concern itself with the agent and the host and with the influence that is exerted on them by the environment in which they operate.

It becomes clear that the science and art of epidemiology need not be limited to communicable disease. There are other diseases which attack large masses of individuals. Cancer is an example. Surely there is an agent of this disease even if it is not definitely recognized, and there are human, susceptible hosts. The interaction of one on the other, and the influence of the environment on both can be studied in the same way that they have been studied in communicable disease. It is, therefore, as reasonable to speak of the epidemiology of cancer as of that of diphtheria or tuberculosis.

The epidemiologist treats disease in the mass much as the physician treats a single individual. When a patient presents himself, the physician tries to find out what his complaint is. He then attempts to establish a diagnosis by getting a good history, examining the patient, learning about his background, and obtaining assistance from the laboratory. If the diagnosis is established and the cause of illness determined, he treats the patient with specific or symptomatic medication and attempts to remove the source of illness. The epidemiologist, studying the occurrence of disease in a community, attempts to establish the nature of the disease. He obtains a careful history of the community, learns about its previous experience with this and related diseases, and observes characteristics of the disease as they affect individuals. He obtains data from the laboratory, the sanitarians, and others, which help him to determine the cause and spread of the illness. He observes the geographic distribution, the number and kinds of people under attack, and the time relationships of the occurrence of the disease in groups of individuals. He is now ready to make an attempt at control either by attacking the agent, by increasing the host's resistance, or by modifying the environment. Often he is successful. Occasionally, as in the case of the clinician with a single patient, he is only partly successful. Like the clinician, he cannot work alone. He needs the assistance of the bacteriologist, the chemist, the sanitarian, the geographer, the biologist, the statistician, and others.

There are three factors that must be considered in any epidemiological investigation. These are the agent, the susceptible host, and the environment. All three may be present and yet live with each other in peace and contentment, and no disease occur. Let there, however, be a disturbance in any one of them to disrupt the balance, and mass disease will appear and spread. One can think of this graphically as a balanced scale in which one of the pans represents the agent, the other pan the host, and the weights the environment. If the agent and host balance each other, the scale remains at rest. If either pan gets heavier, or if weights are added to one side without an equal counterbalance, one side or the other will tilt. An example of such imbalance is offered by the epidemic of diphtheria in Europe in the 1940's. Between World Wars I and II, Europe had learned to balance agent against host, and diphtheria had all but disappeared. In central and western Europe this was brought about largely by strengthening the host through immunization programs. In the Scandinavian countries, where migrations were at a minimum, it was brought about largely by elimination of the agent and keeping the environment the same. The disruption brought about by invasion, mass migrations, and interruption of immunization programs caused an imbalance. In central and western Europe this was due largely to weakening the host; in the Scandinavian countries it was largely due to change in environment. Both caused a disturbance of the equilibrium, with the result that diphtheria became widespread. It is essential.

therefore, in a study of epidemiology, to consider each of the three factors and their interplay.

The Causative Agent

The causative agent is usually thought of positively as a factor, such as a microorganism, whose presence causes disease. However, one must think of it negatively, too, as a factor whose absence may cause disease. Thus, scurvy will occur in a community if there is an insufficient intake of vitamin C. Agents of disease may be classified as physical, chemical, and biological.

Physical agents may be mechanical, thermal, or radiant. One of the commonest examples of mechanical agents causing illness is the motor vehicle, which is responsible for numerous deaths each year. Thermal agents may cause extreme heat or cold, either of which is deleterious to the human organism. Radiant agents were represented largely by the X ray; in recent years, other rays which are produced as a result of atomic fission have begun to play an increasingly larger role. Any of these agents may cause widespread disease.

Chemical agents may cause illness in a variety of ways—by inhalation, by ingestion, or by contact. Death from carbon monoxide poisoning is a good example of an accident due to inhalation. Outbreaks of food poisoning in which a food was contaminated with a chemical such as arsenic or fluorine are examples of illness caused by ingestion of chemicals. So are overdosages of certain drugs. Nutritional disturbances such as obesity, malnutrition, hypervitaminosis, scurvy, and rickets are caused by the overabundance or lack of one or more necessary elements in the diet, and they make up a type of disease that may be classified under chemical agents.

The biologic agents have played a major role in the causation of disease and are still an important factor. They include multicellular organisms like worms and insects; single-celled organisms such as the ameba or the *Plasmodium* of malaria; fungi, for example, ringworm; microscopic forms of life like bacteria; and viruses, which are too small to be seen under the ordinary microscope. All have played an important part as agents of disease, and some still do.

A thorough knowledge of all agents is not possible for a single individual, but the epidemiologist should have a working knowledge of their composition or structure, their manner of spread, the portals of entry and exit in the human, and the possibility of their avoidance or destruction by man.

The Host

The factors which influence the susceptibility of a host to injury by an agent are many and varied. Habits and customs play a part. Certain religious groups are forbidden to eat pork. They cannot, obviously, suffer from trichinosis. In countries where little milk is drunk, brucellosis presents no problem. People who are clean in their habits and surroundings will not fall prey to epidemic typhus.

The defense mechanism of the host is a varied and complicated thing. It is built up, like an army, in several layers. One might think of the first line of defense as anatomic, consisting of external structures such as the skin, hair, nails, and secretions, which offer a bar to entry of toxic agents. A second line of defense is largely physiologic. The cough reflex, the feeling of nausea, the ability of the liver to detoxify, of bones to store certain metals, and of body fluids to alter acid-base relationships, the heat regulating mechanism, the local tissue reaction—these are some of the manifold abilities of the host to prevent noxious agents from overwhelming the body. Finally, one can think of the last line of defense as that of immunity, a complicated line whose greatest activity is seen under attack by biological agents. This is discussed at length in Chapter 4.

Other, more general, factors of the host enter into the defense mechanism. There are those of age, sex, and color. It is hardly necessary to point out that certain diseases affect certain age groups more than others and one sex or color group more than another. There are reasons why this is so, and these must be analyzed separately for each condition. There are other factors, such as the host's constitution, his heredity, and his previous experience with the specific agent, that enter in the determination of the host's ability to withstand attack from a specific agent.

The Environment

The causative agent and the susceptible host do not carry on their struggle *in vacuo*. The environment under which they live may be favorable to one or the other. Changes in the environment, natural or man-made, may shift the balance from one to the other and may help to determine whether the host will survive or succumb. A knowledge of the environment is essential in all epidemiological investigation.

The physical environment is largely a matter of geography. The location of a community on land that is fertile or unproductive, near or far from a water supply, will determine the type of flora and fauna that can grow and multiply, and the ability of these to maintain a population. Closely allied to geography are season and climate. They are particularly important in determining whether certain vectors of disease can or cannot survive. Obviously, malaria cannot be a problem in the arctic, since the temperature is too cold for the survival of mosquitoes. Season and climate may play a part indirectly in the causation of illness or death. Drownings are obviously more common in summer than in winter, while automobile accidents are more common in icy or rainy weather.

The social and economic environment of a society frequently determines not only its level of education but its desire and ability to undertake community health measures and to provide facilities for medical care. The level of sanitation, provision for a good water and milk supply, proper waste disposal, and proper housing facilities are among the measures that are essential for healthy community life. Flood control, prevention of soil erosion, and reforestation programs are of great importance in certain localities, and their effectiveness depends on the extent to which the community has developed socially and economically.

The biologic environment is of particular importance in the epidemiologic investigation of disease caused by living organisms. It is important to know the types of fauna present. Yellow fever will not make much headway in a community if the *Aedes* mosquitoes are not found there. A community that has a good rat-eradication program will not suffer much from murine typhus.

Epidemiologic Method

The more information the epidemiologist has regarding the agent, host, and environment as they relate to the particular problem in hand, the easier will be the solution of the problem. But information alone is not enough. The data acquired must be marshaled in a meaningful way in order to shed light on the particular problem studied. There must be a definite reason for the investigation, and this should be stated clearly and succinctly. Data must be collected. The type of data, their manner of collection, their source, and the method of recording must be clearly considered in advance. Great care must be exercised in the choice of the personnel who will be used in collecting information, in the determination of ways in which the necessary data will be obtained, and in the precautions taken to exclude unconscious bias. The data must then be classified and arranged in certain categories, such as age, sex, occupation, exposures, etc. They are then tabulated either manually or by machine. An analysis of the tables is now made. The skill and experience of the epidemiologist will often determine whether the tables are so arranged as to bring out common factors or clues for the solution of the problem. The analysis, if adequately done, will lead to hypotheses which can be tested either in the field or in the laboratory. The solution of the problem may be complete or partial. Further data, or further analysis of the data already gathered, may be required. The fundamental data and methods of epidemiology are the same for all who use them. The success attained in their use depends, as in other disciplines, on the individual who uses them.

Chapter 4 INFECTION, RESISTANCE, AND ALLERGY

Infection

BY infection is meant the invasion of body tissues by pathogenic organisms, resulting in injury to the body. One of the ways in which the body attempts to protect itself against such injury is by producing antibodies to engage the infectious agent and to destroy it or make it harmless.

The commonest types of infectious agent that we are familiar with are the bacteria and viruses. One should remember, however, that infectious agents may be much larger. In order of increasing size, they may be classified as viruses, rickettsiae, bacteria, fungi, protozoa, and metazoa. Examples of diseases in which the types of infectious agents mentioned are the cause of illness are measles, typhus fever, pneumonia, ringworm, malaria, and tapeworm infestation.

For an infectious agent to cause damage to tissues, it is necessary that it gain entrance to the organs of the body. It may do this through the respiratory tract, digestive tract, skin, or mucous membranes of the mouth, eyes, urethra, vagina, or rectum. Each of these portals of entry has certain mechanisms which offer a first line of defense. These must be broken through. What these defense mechanisms are will be explained later.

Resistance

By resistance is meant the ability of an animal body to protect itself against the entry of, and the injury caused by, agents of disease.

General Defense Mechanisms

A body threatened by an infectious agent attempts to defend itself in a variety of ways. First one may mention the *natural barriers*. The skin is a firmly knit tissue which, unless it is injured, resists strongly the passage of agents of disease. The hairs in the nose and the cilia in the upper respiratory passages tend to entangle material carrying infectious agents. Some of the secretions of the mucous membranes are bactericidal for many organisms, and other secretions, like tears, act mechanically to wash out foreign material settling on the conjunctiva. The exposed mucous membranes tend to have a flat epithelial layer, offering greater resistance to the passage of foreign bodies than do the lower layers. These barriers are extremely effective. How effective they are can be judged by the readiness with which infection occurs after an injury to the outer part of the body.

Another line of defense against invading organisms is the *filtering mechanism* of the body. Scattered widely over the body are small lymph glands which drain specific parts of the body. An agent of disease that has gained entrance by breaching the first barrier is frequently caught in the meshes of the lymph structure and annihilated there. It is common knowledge that when an infection of the hand occurs, a red streak may be seen extending up the arm to the armpit. The gland in the armpit enlarges and is tender. This is due to the inflammation resulting from the struggle between the infectious agent and the defense mechanism in the gland. As a rule, the defense mechanism is the victor. Other glandular structures serve similar purposes. The tonsils help to keep infection from descending to the lungs. The liver filters out ingested toxic material which may cause severe damage to the body, and the spleen plays a similar role. All of these are part of the secondary defense mechanisms of the body.

If the infective agent has managed to breach the two walls discussed above, the body will offer another defense which is known as *inflammation*. Most people think of inflammation as injurious. Actually, it is another method of defense used by the body. There are dilatation of blood vessels, an outpouring of blood and tissue fluid and of blood cells to surround the infectious agent, and an attempt by the body to create a wall around the struggling mass to keep the infection from penetrating farther. As a result of all this activity, the inflamed area becomes hot and swollen and tender. If the body defenders are victorious, the infection is overcome. Some of the cells that have wandered into the battle area from the blood vessels and tissue spaces engulf and digest the destroyed microorganisms. This is known as "phagocytosis." The mass of debris resulting from killed organisms, broken-down blood cells, and body fluids is thick and creamy-looking and known as "pus." It is absorbed by the body, or it is extruded either by breaking through to the surface or as a result of an incision made by a surgeon. The struggle is ended. The body has won.

There are other defense mechanisms which protect the body against invasion by microorganisms. The mechanism of some of these is not well understood, although the effect is known. One group of these mechanisms may be discussed under the heading of *constitutional factors*. Race is one of the factors. It has been shown, for instance, in many outbreaks of poliomyelitis, that Negroes are not affected in the same ratio as are white people; on the other hand, the reverse is true of tuberculosis. Why this is so is not quite clear. There have been various theories to explain it, and numerous discussions have been held to determine whether the influence of race on resistance is due to heredity or environment. There is no need to review all of this here. Suffice it to say that the fact remains that race may exert an influence on resistance to infection. Heredity is another factor which exerts an influence for which there is no adequate explanation. It is possible, for instance, to breed a strain of mouse that becomes highly resistant to a particular microorganism. Clinical observation seems to indicate that this also holds true in man. The familial occurrence of rheumatic fever has been noted by many investigators.

Then there are the factors of age and sex which play a part in the defense mechanism. It is well known that measles rarely occurs in a child under 6 months of age; it is also well known that poliomyelitis is uncommon in people above the age of 40. There is considerable discussion in the literature to explain this age susceptibility and resistance, but we need not discuss it here further than to note that it does occur. Differences in resistance by the sexes to certain infectious diseases has also been noted. It is well known that a proportionately larger percentage of males than of females is susceptible to poliomyelitis, while the reverse is true of whooping cough.

Endocrine factors play a part in the determination of resistance. Diabetics are notoriously susceptible to skin infections. Changes in metabolism likewise play a part. The state of nutrition of an individual often determines his susceptibility or resistance to certain infections. The tremendous increase in tuberculosis in the central European countries following World Wars I and II, when the nutritional state of the population was low, is an example of the importance of this factor.

Fatigue and chilling are other constitutional factors which appear to lower resistance to infection. Experimentally, both these factors have been shown to lower the resistance of monkeys to poliomyelitis. Recent controlled observations in humans indicate that those who engage in active exercise at the onset of poliomyelitis tend to get a more serious form of the disease than those who take to bed at the beginning of illness.

The defense mechanism of the body is also influenced by species resistance. Although all animals are susceptible to infections, they vary in their susceptibility to different organisms. Thus, the lower animals are resistant to typhoid fever but are susceptible to the salmonella organisms, closely related to the typhoid bacillus. On the other hand, man is resistant to the virus of Newcastle disease, while fowl are quite susceptible to it. Some diseases may attack both animals and man, but in different degrees. Glanders, for instance, is common in horses but comparatively rare in man. Finally, there are certain diseases that affect man and animals regularly, but different strains affect different species. Tuberculosis affects humans, cows, and birds. Man is susceptible to the human and the bovine types but not to the avian type. It should also be pointed out that some infectious agents may attack two or more species but do not cause illness in all. The plasmodium of malaria attacks both man and mosquito, but it causes illness in man only. The plague bacillus may infect humans, rats, and fleas, but only the humans and the rats become ill with the disease.

Immunity

Immunity refers to the specific resistance brought about in an animal body by the interaction of a foreign agent and the host's cells, body fluids, and blood.

The study of immunity is comparatively recent, but already a wealth of material explaining the process has been published. Much remains to be done. Immunity results essentially from an antigen-antibody reaction. It is, therefore, necessary to clarify the meanings of these terms.

An *antigen* is a substance which, when introduced into animal tissues, stimulates the formation of an antibody, and which reacts specifically when mixed with the antibody. Thus, when diphtheria toxin is introduced into the tissues, diphtheria antitoxin is produced by the body, and the antitoxin combines with the toxin, fixing it, and preventing it from damaging the body. Antigens are specific; this means that each antigen calls forth a specific antibody which will combine only with that antigen. They are large molecules, usually coming from heterologous species, and are usually protein in character. Antigens may be extremely small, like toxins, small viruses, or simple proteins, or they may be larger, like blood cells, bacteria, or large viruses.

Antibody is the substance appearing in the blood or body fluids as a result of stimulation by an antigen, which reacts specifically with antigen. Antibodies resulting from the stimulation of toxins are spoken of as *antitoxins*. Almost all antibodies are found in that fraction of the blood serum known as gamma globulin. The antibodies are apparently elaborated by the cells of the body as a result of stimulation, are produced in large numbers, and are poured out into the tissue fluids and blood stream.

There are different kinds of antibodies. Whether these represent different ways of manifesting the same antibody or not is not quite clear. The most commonly demonstrated antibodies, which are used practically in tests in the laboratory, are agglutinins, precipitins, lysins, neutralizing antibodies, and complement-fixing antibodies. Experience has indicated which one of the antibodies is more easily demonstrated in the various infective diseases. In some of them no antibody can be demonstrated, because antigen appears to be lacking. This may be due, as in measles, to the fact that the virus has not been successfully grown in culture or obtained in animals, or it may be due to technical difficulties. In those diseases in which antibody can be demonstrated, it is usual for the antibody to be absent at the beginning of illness and to increase in titer until the height is reached in convalescence. By getting a specimen of blood early and late in the disease, a significant rise in antibody titer for a specific antigen can be demonstrated. This is usually considered good evidence that the disease was caused by the agent from which the antigen has been obtained. Bacteriologists usually consider a fourfold increase in titer as significant.

One of the ways of demonstrating antibodies in an individual's blood is to mix in a test tube a small amount of his serum with the antigen. If a precipitin is present in the blood, the antigen-antibody reaction will manifest itself as a cloudy precipate at the bottom of the tube, or as a cloudy ring at the junction of antigen and antibody. The Kahn and Mazzini tests for syphilis are examples of precipitin reactions. In the agglutinin reaction a clumping of bacteria occurs when they are mixed with the patient's immune serum. A good example is the Widal test for typhoid. Living typhoid bacilli are mixed on a glass slide with serum from the suspected patient. If the patient has typhoid fever and immune bodies are present in his blood, the typhoid bacilli will gradually lose their motility and become clumped. The clumped bacilli can be observed under the microscope.

Lysins are antibodies which dissolve the antigen. Such antibodies are present in the convalescent blood of cholera patients. They dissolve bacteria and are, therefore, known as "bacteriolysins." Some lysins dissolve red blood cells; these are known as "hemolysins." Hemolysins are used indirectly in the performance of the complement-fixation test, which is a test for the presence of complement-fixing antibodies. Complement is a substance normally present in the blood serum of most animals, which takes part in the antigen-antibody reaction. When antigen and antibody combine, complement becomes fixed in the reaction. Complement is destroyed if the serum is heated to 56° C. for 30 minutes. The complement-fixation test is used for diagnostic purposes in many diseases and was first popularized in the diagnosis of syphilis where it is commonly spoken of as the "Wassermann test."

In performing the complement-fixation reaction an indicator system is used. This consists of sheep red cells and serum from a rabbit that has received injections of sheep red cells and has consequently produced anti-sheep-cell hemolysins. If the sheep cells and the rabbit antiserum are mixed in a test tube, the cells will be hemolyzed if complement is present:

(1) Sheep red cells + anti-sheep-red-cell rabbit serum + complement = hemolysis

If any of the three factors is absent, hemolysis will not result. When the indicator system is used in the complement-fixation test, the rabbit immune serum is heated to destroy complement. When sheep red cells are added, no hemolysis occurs:

(2) Sheep red cells + anti-sheep-red-cell rabbit serum = no hemolysis

Suppose a complement-fixation test for syphilis is to be performed. Serum from the suspected person is obtained. A small amount of this is heated in a test tube to destroy complement. Syphilitic antigen and a measured amount of complement are added. If the suspected individual has syphilis, his serum will contain syphilitic antibodies. They will react with the antigen, and the complement will become fixed in the reaction. The indicator system (2) is now added. No hemolysis results, since the complement is fixed and therefore unavailable—the Wassermann test is positive. If the suspect does not have syphilis there are no antisyphilitic antibodies in his blood. When syphilis antigen and complement are added to the serum, the complement remains available. When the indicator system is added, hemolysis results as in (1)—the Wassermann test is negative.

The neutralization test depends on the principle that when antigen and its specific antibody combine, the antigen is neutralized and cannot do any more damage. Suppose a patient has recovered from an illness suspected to be poliomyelitis. A sample of his blood serum is obtained and mixed with poliomyelitis virus. The mixture is injected into a monkey. If antibodies against poliomyelitis were present in the serum, they will have neutralized the antigen, and the monkey will remain well. If such antibodies were not present, the antigen was not neutralized, and the monkey will come down with poliomyelitis. The neutralization test can also be demonstrated in the test tube. Influenza virus has the property of agglutinating the red blood corpuscles of fowl and some other animals. If an individual is suspected of having had influenza, he must have antibodies against influenza in his blood serum. If some of the serum is taken and mixed with influenza virus, it will neutralize the virus and thus inhibit it from agglutinating red blood corpuscles. This test is often spoken of as the "Hirst test" or the "agglutination-inhibition phenomenon." It is a fairly rapid test and is used practically in a number of laboratories in the epidemiological investigation of outbreaks of suspected influenza and in the differentiation of types of influenza.

One other term requires definition. This is opsonin. It is a substance present in normal serum which has the property of acting on bacteria and increasing their susceptibility to phagocytosis. Bernard Shaw, in the preface to his play *The Doctor's Dilemma,* refers to the opsonins as having the property of "buttering" the bacteria. In testing for opsonins, serum, white blood cells, and bacteria are mixed in capillary tubes and incubated at 37° C. for 30 minutes. The contents are then expelled on slides. Films are made and stained, and the bacteria in 50 to 100 random leukocytes are counted. The relative opsonic effect of two serums can then be expressed as a ratio of the numbers of bacteria engulfed by the same number of white blood cells in the two serums. The test has a high degree of error, and it is not used widely. Some investigators have used it in the diagnosis of brucellar infections.

An antigen-antibody reaction which was widely used for typing pneumococci before the introduction of antibiotics is the capsular swelling reaction or quellung phenomenon. If antipneumococcus-type specific rabbit serum is mixed with pneumococci of that type, the capsule of the pneumococcus swells and, particularly if stained, can be distinctly seen under the microscope. The test is simple and rapid and was widely used when type-specific rabbit antiserums were employed in the treatment of pneumonia. The beneficial therapeutic effect of the antibiotics on all types of pneumonia has done away with the need of the test. The principle, however, remains and may be used in other bacteria that have a capsule surrounding them, such as *Hemophilus influenzae.*

APPLICATIONS OF PRINCIPLES OF IMMUNITY

Now that the underlying principles of immunity have been explained, their practical application to disease can be discussed. Immunity to a disease may be active or passive.
Active immunity
  1. Naturally acquired
    a. By recovery from active infection
    b. By contact with infection

2. Artificially induced
Passive immunity
  1. Naturally acquired
  2. Artificially induced

Active Immunity

Active immunity results when an antigen is introduced into a body. The body responds by producing antibodies to destroy the antigen. Active immunity may be acquired naturally. This happens when an individual recovers from an infectious disease. An individual who gets measles develops antibodies against measles; a person recovering from typhoid fever has antibodies against typhoid. Active immunity may also occur as a result of close contact with a case of infection. This may be due to an infection of the contact that is so mild that it causes few symptoms—what is known as a "subclinical" infection—or it may be due to the fact that the contact receives small doses of infection over a considerable period of time and thus becomes immunized as he would if he were injected with minute doses of the causative bacteria. We see this phenomenon frequently in contacts to a case of typhoid fever. If their stools are cultured frequently, positive specimens will be obtained now and then, yet no illness results. Apparently, they receive very mild doses which are not sufficient to make them sick but are sufficient to immunize them.

Active immunity can be induced artificially. Such immunity is induced by injecting the antigen against which immunity is desired. The types of antigen used to induce artificial immunity are either vaccines, mixtures of toxin and antitoxin, or toxoids. Vaccines are the living or killed bodies of bacteria and viruses. When living vaccines are used, they are so manipulated in the laboratory that their ability to cause disease is destroyed, but their antigenic powers are retained. Examples of such vaccines are smallpox, yellow fever, and BCG vaccines. Most vaccines consist of bacilli or viruses that have been killed by heat or chemicals. Examples are pertussis, typhoid, and typhus vaccines. Some bacteria cause disease chiefly by elaborating a poison or *toxin* which is absorbed. Tetanus germs, for instance, are in themselves harmless; but they elaborate a toxin which is deadly. If tetanus organisms are introduced into a deep wound, they do their damage not by invading the tissues but by producing a toxin which is absorbed and which causes severe damage to nervous tissue. To protect a person against tetanus it is necessary to protect him against the toxin of tetanus. Similarly, in diphtheria most of the damage caused by the infection is due to the toxin which is absorbed from the membrane in the throat where the diphtheria organisms lodge and multiply. The toxins can be obtained by grow-

ing the germs in a liquid medium in a bottle. After a certain length
of time the medium is filtered. The germs are held back, and the
toxin is obtained in the filtrate. When antitoxin is added to toxin
in sufficient quantity to neutralize the poisonous action of the toxin
but not completely to destroy its antigenic activity, the mixture can
be used to immunize human beings. It is known as *toxin-antitoxin*.
In diphtheria, this was the first type of immunizing mixture used
for large-scale programs of active immunization. The main disadvantage of its use lies in the fact that it is not completely stable,
so that separation of the toxin may result and cause injury to the
injected individual. A second objection is that failure to immunize
with this mixture occurs in a fair percentage of individuals injected.

The next development in the active immunization against toxins
was to treat the toxin with a chemical, Formalin. This destroyed the
toxic property of the toxin but retained its antigenicity. A toxin so
treated is known as *toxoid* or fluid toxoid. In Europe it is frequently
referred to as *anatoxin*. It is perfectly safe, and it has the further
advantage of greater antigenicity, so that a larger percentage of
individuals becomes immune when injected with toxoid than when
injected with toxin-antitoxin.

A further development in methods of active immunization was to
add alum to the toxoid mixture. This causes a precipitation of the
toxoid; it is known as *alum-precipitated toxoid*. The British refer to
it as A. P. T. It is a more potent immunizing agent than fluid toxoid.
This is probably due to the delayed absorption of the toxoid from
the site of inoculation where it is held by the alum, thus prolonging
the immunizing stimulus.

Tests for the titer of antitoxin in a person's blood are usually done
by the neutralization method, as previously described. A simple
method of determining immunity in diphtheria without using the
complicated neutralization method is to do a *Shick test*. This consists
of injecting a minute amount of diphtheria toxin intradermally in
the flexor surface of one arm. A reading is made after 4 to 7 days.
If the person tested is immune, the injected toxin will have been
neutralized by the person's antitoxin, and no reaction will occur at
the site of injection. If the individual is not immune, a raised, reddened area will result. This gradually fades after a few days, leaving
an area of brown pigmentation with desquamation. It is customary
to do a control test with heated toxin in the opposite arm.

A similar test has been devised to determine the susceptibility of
individuals to the scarlet fever toxin which causes the rash. It is
known as the *Dick test*. This test, however, determines only the susceptibility to the scarlet fever rash and not susceptibility to infection
with the hemolytic streptococcus, which causes scarlet fever. It is,

therefore, not so valuable a tool as the Shick test for immunity to diphtheria and is not employed very widely.

The discussion of toxins has been limited so far to those easily separated by simple filtration from the bacteria which produce them. Such toxins are spoken of as *exotoxins*. They are extremely poisonous, even in small quantities, and cause definite, recognizable symptoms in the host. There are other toxins produced by bacteria which remain attached to the bacteria and can be separated from them only by such vigorous methods as grinding, alternate freezing and thawing, and dissolving with various chemicals. They are known as *endotoxins*. They are not so highly poisonous as the exotoxins, and the exact way in which they damage tissues is not clear. They do not readily stimulate the production of antitoxins as the exotoxins do. Examples of exotoxins are those of diphtheria and tetanus, and the botulinus bacilli. Examples of endotoxins are those of cholera, and the typhoid bacilli, meningococci, and streptococci. Some bacteria produce both exotoxins and endotoxins. The staphylococci, for instance, in addition to an endotoxin, produce an exotoxin which is a common cause of food poisoning.

The development of antibodies as a result of active immunization takes considerable time. Experience and experiment have taught how concentrated a vaccine should be used, how large a dose should be given, how many doses are necessary, and at what intervals the injections should be made. Field and laboratory investigations have also established the period of time after immunization that must elapse before the antibody titer is high enough in the serum to combine with specific antigen that may be introduced and thus prevent disease with that antigen. They have also determined the period of time in which the titer of antibody remains high enough to be effective. If the antibody in the serum has decreased to a titer so low as to be ineffective, it can be revivified and brought back to its original high titer, or even a higher one, by an additional injection of a small quantity of the specific antigen. This is called a "booster" or "recall" injection. The advantages of active immunization are, therefore, that it can be planned in advance, when the person to be immunized is well, that it is reasonably long-lasting, and that when the antibody titer declines it can be brought back by a booster dose.

Passive Immunity

Occasions arise when a susceptible person, especially a child, is exposed to a disease against which he has not been actively immunized, although substances for such immunization are available. In such cases it is necessary to use for injection serums from individuals or animals that contain antibodies to the disease which threatens.

This is passive immunity. The antibodies which are introduced have no power to stimulate antibody production by the host, as happens when antigens are injected, and they usually disappear from the circulation in a comparatively short time. While they are present in the circulation, however, they are as effective in combining with antigen as are actively formed antibodies.

Like active immunity, passive immunity may be naturally or artificially acquired. Since the blood circulation of a pregnant woman is intimately related to the circulation of the fetus she carries, allowing for the passage of gases and fluids from the one to the other, antibodies possessed by the mother also pass to the fetus. At birth, therefore, the infant possesses all the circulating antibodies of the mother. They persist in the infant's blood for a period of approximately 6 months. Thus, children born to mothers who have previously had measles are immune to this disease for the first half year of their lives. Similarly, newborn infants are usually immune to diphtheria and remain so for about 6 months, since their mothers usually have immunity to this disease. Passive immunity which is so acquired by an infant is spoken of as "natural passive immunity" or "congenital passive immunity."

Acquired passive immunity is the immunity which results when immune serums are injected into a susceptible person. Such immune substances are obtained from humans who have had the disease before or from humans and animals that have previously been actively immunized. Blood taken from large groups of humans, most of whom have had measles, contains antibodies against the disease. This blood is fractionated, and one of the fractions, *gamma globulin,* contains the antibodies in a highly concentrated form. If a child is exposed to measles, he is given an injection of gamma globulin and can thus be prevented from getting the disease, or, if a smaller dose is given, he will get a modified form of measles which will hardly make him ill. To obtain antibodies against whooping cough, individuals giving a previous history of the disease are immunized with whooping cough vaccine. After a certain length of time their blood is tested for antibodies against whooping cough. If these are in high titer the blood is drawn and fractionated and the gamma globulin is obtained. This is then used for children not previously immunized against whooping cough who are intimately exposed to a case. It is known as *pertussis hyperimmune gamma globulin* or by the trade name Hypertussis.

It is obviously not practical and is too expensive to use human beings for the purpose of obtaining antibodies. In the case of diphtheria, tetanus, and some other diseases, animals are used for the production of specific antibodies. In diphtheria, horses are injected with increasing doses of antigen. When their blood shows high titers of antitoxin it is drawn, and the serum is separated, refined, and standardized. If the serum is kept in the refrigerator, the antitoxin titer will remain high for a long time. Such antitoxin can be used prophylactically to protect a child who has been exposed to diphtheria and has not previously received active immunization. Antitoxins are also effective in the treatment of disease if they are used early and in sufficient amounts.

The advantages of passive immunity are that the serum is prepared in advance, that it is readily available, and that it confers immediate immunity. The disadvantages are that the immunity is temporary, lasting only about 3 weeks, and that it has to be used repeatedly with subsequent exposures. Another disadvantage of animal serums is that they are foreign substances and can cause severe serum reactions.

Immunizing Agents

There are a number of immunizing agents in common use for active and passive immunization. A short description of their properties and method of production is given below. The table on page 62 gives the dosages and intervals of administration.

For Active Immunization

Smallpox

A vaccine is used which is prepared from material collected from vaccinal lesions on the skin of calves. There is active, living virus in this vaccine.

Diphtheria

Diphtheria toxoid is a filtrate of diphtheria bacilli grown in a flask to which has been added 0.3 to 0.5 per cent Formalin. If alum is added, the toxoid is precipitated by the alum. Either the fluid or the alum-precipitated toxoid may be used for active immunization.

Pertussis

A vaccine is used which is prepared from virulent, Phase I pertussis bacilli which have been killed. In the fluid form there are 20 billion killed bacilli per cubic centimeter. If alum is added, the bacilli are precipitated by the alum. Either fluid or alum-precipitated vaccine may be used.

Tetanus

Tetanus bacilli are grown in a fluid medium. The filtrate contains tetanus toxin. Formalin is added to convert the toxin into toxoid. If alum is added, the toxoid is precipitated. Either fluid toxoid or alum-precipitated toxoid may be used for active immunization.

Combined pertussis vaccine and diphtheria and tetanus toxoids

A combination of pertussis vaccine and the toxoids of diphtheria and tetanus, alum-precipitated, is put out by a number of firms and can be used to immunize against all three diseases.

Typhoid fever

A saline suspension of typhoid bacilli killed by heat is used. It is standardized to contain 1 billion organisms per cubic centimeter.

Typhoid-paratyphoid vaccine

A mixed vaccine containing typhoid, paratyphoid A, and paratyphoid B organisms is used for combined immunization against all three diseases. It contains 1 billion typhoid bacilli and 750 million paratyphoid A and paratyphoid B bacilli per cubic centimeter.

Rabies

The spinal cord of rabbits infected with rabies virus is used in active immunization. In the original Pasteur treatment the spinal cords of infected rabbits were dried for varying periods of time. The virus thus became inactivated but was still alive. Several types of vaccine have been used. The most frequently used vaccine in this country is the Semple vaccine in which the infected cord is treated with phenol and the virus is thus killed.

Epidemic typhus

The rickettsiae of typhus fever are grown in the yolk sac of developing chick embryos, and are killed before being standardized for use.

Rocky Mountain spotted fever

Either of two types of vaccine may be used. One of them is made from the tissues of infected ticks and the other is made from rickettsiae grown in the yolk sac of developing chick embryos. In both, the rickettsiae are killed prior to use.

Yellow fever

An attenuated but living yellow fever virus, grown in developing chick embryos, is used. In this country the vaccine is not produced commercially but will be administered by the Public Health Service to anyone who requires it.

Cholera

A vaccine of killed, culture-grown cholera organisms is employed.

Plague

A vaccine of killed, culture-grown *Pasteurella pestis* is employed.

Tuberculosis

A vaccine, known as BCG (Bacillus Calmette Guérin), is employed. This is a vaccine of whole, living bovine tubercle bacilli which have been grown in culture and have become attenuated.

Influenza

Influenza virus is grown in chick embryos. The allantoic fluid of the embryos is obtained, purified, and inactivated. The vaccine now sold contains a few strains of influenza A and influenza B virus.

Pneumonia

Immunization is performed with a vaccine made from the polysaccharides of the pneumococcus capsule. Several types of pneumococci are used.

FOR PASSIVE IMMUNIZATION

Diphtheria

Over a period of time, horses are injected with diphtheria toxoid. When the titer of antitoxin in the blood is high, the horses are bled and the serum is separated, purified, and standardized for use.

Tetanus

Antitoxin is prepared as in diphtheria, except that the immunizing agent is tetanus toxoid.

Botulism

Botulinus antitoxin is prepared in a similar manner to diphtheria and tetanus antitoxin. Since the toxins produced by different strains of *Clostridium botulinum* are specific, a different antitoxin can be produced for each of the strains. In this country the strains A and B are the most common. A combined antitoxin against these two strains is available.

Measles

Gamma globulin is the fraction of blood containing the antibodies. Blood is obtained from human donors and is pooled. The gamma globulin fraction is separated, purified, and bottled. Since most adults have had measles, their blood contains antibodies against this disease, and these are present in the gamma globulin fraction.

Hyperimmune pertussis serum and gamma globulin

Individuals giving a history of pertussis are further injected with pertussis vaccine. When their serums show a high titer of antibodies they are bled and the serum is separated from the blood cells and purified. The serum may then be used for passive immunization against whooping cough, or the serum may be fractionated and the gamma globulin obtained and used. Obviously, when whole serum is used, a much larger dose is needed than when gamma globulin is used.

Of the procedures used for active immunization, those against smallpox, diphtheria, and whooping cough are generally employed routinely for infants and young children. Tetanus is included with these immunizations in many communities. Vaccination against typhoid fever should be advised for contacts to cases or carriers of typhoid, for all people who plan to travel outside the country, and for individuals in a community where an epidemic of typhoid fever exists or where typhoid fever is endemic. Antirabic vaccine should be recommended for individuals who have been bitten by a rabid animal or an animal suspected of being rabid. It is also recommended for individuals bitten by a stray dog in a community where rabies in dogs is endemic. Vaccination against epidemic typhus, yellow fever, cholera, and plague is advisable for persons traveling to countries where these diseases are endemic. People living in comunities where Rocky Mountain spotted fever is endemic, whose occupations or habits may bring them in contact with infected ticks, should be vaccinated against this disease. Vaccination against influenza and pneumonia may wait until vaccines are prepared which contain sufficient strains to assure their effectiveness. BCG vaccination should be limited to those who have a negative tuberculin test and are exposed to active cases of tuberculosis, for instance, nurses on a tuberculosis ward.

Passive immunization should be used against measles in young susceptible children who are intimately exposed to the disease and in older children or adults who have not had measles and whose physical condition is such that measles will present an extra hazard. Hyperimmune pertussis serum or gamma globulin should be used in young children intimately exposed to whooping cough who have not had the disease and who have not been actively immunized. If they previously received active immunization, on exposure they should be given a booster dose of pertussis vaccine. Children exposed to diphtheria who have not been previously immunized with diphtheria toxoid should be given diphtheria antitoxin; if they have previously been immunized with toxoid, they should receive a booster dose of diphtheria toxoid. Individuals who suffer a trauma causing a deep, lacerating wound should be given a prophylactic dose of tetanus antitoxin unless they have previously been immunized actively with tetanus toxoid, in which case they should be given a booster dose of tetanus toxoid. Individuals who have eaten food known or suspected to be contaminated with botulinus toxin should receive a prophylactic injection of botulinus antitoxin A and B. The antitoxins for diphtheria, tetanus, and botulism may be used in the treatment of the respective diseases as well as for prophylaxis.

Allergy

Under immunity there were discussed the reactions which a body develops to protect itself against a living agent or its products when such an agent invades the body. There is another phenomenon that occurs in which the body becomes hypersensitive as a result of the introduction of an antigen. This may result in injury to rather than in protection of the body. It manifests itself in one of several forms.

Anaphylaxis

Anaphylaxis is a term used to indicate an acute systemic hypersensitiveness that occurs in animals as a result of properly spaced multiple injections of a foreign substance. If a small amount of egg white is injected into a guinea pig, the animal becomes sensitized to this substance. Nothing happens to the animal at this time. If, however, a second injection of egg white is given to the pig intravenously or intraperitoneally about 10 days later, symptoms of hypersensitiveness result; the animal gets restless, sneezes, has difficulty in respiration, and may get convulsions and die. This is known as "anaphylactic shock." Other experimental animals also develop anaphylaxis under similar circumstances, but the symptoms of anaphylactic shock differ greatly in different species of animals. In each animal the symptoms are the same, whatever sensi-

IMMUNIZING PROCEDURES

Active Immunization

Diseases	Agent Used	Number of Doses	Each Dose	Interval between Doses	Booster Dose
Smallpox	Smallpox virus	1	1 capillary tube	......	1 capillary tube
Pertussis	Pertussis vaccine, alum	3	0.5 cc. (1 cc. = 20 billion organisms)	1 month	1 cc. fluid vaccine or 0.5 cc. alum vaccine
	Pertussis vaccine, fluid	3	1 cc., 1.5 cc., and 1.5 cc. (20 billion organisms per cc.)	1 month	1 cc. fluid vaccine
Diphtheria	Toxoid, alum	2	1 cc.	1 month	0.1 cc. fluid vaccine
	Toxoid, fluid	3	1 cc.	1 month	0.1 cc. fluid vaccine
Tetanus	Toxoid, alum	2	1 cc.	4–6 weeks	1 cc. fluid toxoid
	Toxoid, fluid	3	1 cc.	4–6 weeks	1 cc. fluid toxoid
Typhoid	Typhoid vaccine	3	0.5 cc.	1 week	0.1 cc. intradermal
Rabies	Semple vaccine	14	2 cc.	1 day	1 cc.
Epidemic typhus	Typhus vaccine	2	1 cc.	1 week	1 cc.
Rocky Mountain spotted fever	RMSF vaccine	3	1 cc.	1 week	0.5 cc.
Yellow fever	Yellow fever vaccine	1	0.5 cc.	Once	1 cc.
Cholera	Cholera vaccine	2	0.5 cc. and 1 cc.	1 week	1 cc.
Plague	Plague vaccine	2	0.5 cc. and 1 cc.	1 week	1 cc.
Influenza	Influenza vaccine	1	1 cc.	Once	1 cc.
Tuberculosis	BCG vaccine	1	0.1 cc.	Once	?

Passive Immunization

Diseases	Agent Used	Number of Doses	Each Dose	Interval between Doses	Booster Dose
Diphtheria	Antitoxin	1	500–1,000 units	Once	None
Tetanus	Antitoxin	1	1,500 units	Once	None
Measles	Gamma globulin	1	2 cc.	Once	None
Pertussis	Hyperimmune gamma globulin	1	2½ cc.	Once	None
Botulism	Antitoxin	1	2,500–5,000 units	Once	None

tizing agent is used. Animals that have been sensitized to an antigen can be desensitized if small amounts of the antigen are injected repeatedly over a short period of time. Anaphylactic shock may occur in humans also, but it is comparatively uncommon.

There are several theories to explain anaphylactic shock. The most commonly accepted one is that in anaphylaxis, as in immunity, the injection of an antigen stimulates the production of antibody. If there is a sufficient concentration of antibody in the circulation, it will combine with the later introduction of antigen and neutralize it in the blood stream; an immune state results. If there is insufficient antibody in the circulation, some of the antigen which is introduced later gets to the cells, reacts with antibody there, and injures the cells. As a result of the cellular injury, a substance known as "histamine" is liberated by the cells. This causes the shock symptoms.

Allergy in Man

Allergy is a hypersensitiveness which manifests itself by heightened reactivity to a specific antigen. The most common clinical symptoms of allergy in man are asthma, hay fever, and urticaria. The antigen need not be a toxic substance. Thus, egg is a food which has good nutritional value and which most people eat and enjoy. There are certain individuals, however, who are sensitive to egg protein. When they eat egg they develop urticarial lesions. Similarly, certain persons are sensitive to pollens. During the season when the grass or weed to which they are sensitive pollinates, the pollens are widely disseminated in the air, are absorbed through the nasal mucosa, and cause hay fever.

The terms "allergy" and "allergic" have been used very loosely by many people. One hears people say that they are allergic to all drugs or that they are allergic to rich foods. These uses are incorrect. In allergy, as in anaphylaxis and in immunity, the antigen, or allergen, as it is commonly called, which brings out the hypersensitive state is a specific substance. An individual may be sensitive to a number of specific substances but not to a vague group of unrelated substances. A person may be sensitive to certain protein foods, like egg and chicken, for instance. That does not mean, however, that he is sensitive to all protein foods.

The mechanism which is responsible for allergy in man appears to be closely related to, if not identical with, the mechanism that operates in anaphylaxis in experimental animals. Certain investigators have pointed out differences in the two phenomena. They note that allergy often is exhibited on first contact with an allergen, whereas this is not so in anaphylaxis. Also, allergy appears to be an inherited state and runs in families, but this is not true of anaphylaxis. Although differences do exist between the two conditions, the points of similarity are greater than the discrepancies. It appears probable that both represent a similar type of reaction which is essentially an antigen-antibody reaction. The presence of antibody in the circulation of allergic individuals can be shown in the *Prausnitz-Küstner reaction.* This is performed by bleeding a person who is allergic to a certain substance, say egg white, and injecting a small amount of the blood serum intradermally into the arm of a nonallergic individual. If egg white is injected into the same spot 24 hours later, a marked local reaction occurs. No such reaction is seen if the egg white is injected into an adjacent area of the same arm where no serum has been previously injected.

There is little doubt that some individuals are allergic to common substances while others are not, and there seems to be an inherited allergic tendency. However, this may merely mean that what is inherited is susceptible tissues, so that individuals with such an inheritance are more easily sensitized than others. The actual mechanism causing an allergic reaction is probably the same as in anaphylaxis or immunity—an antigen-antibody reaction.

Coca has been so impressed by the differences in the two conditions that he has invented a new terminology. He uses the term *atopy* to indicate the allergic state, *atopen* to indicate the sensitizing substance or antigen, and *reagin* to indicate the antibody. There appears little reason to introduce a new nomenclature when an adequate one is already available, but the terms are mentioned here since they are frequently met with in the literature.

Allergy in man may manifest itself as an immediate or a delayed reaction.

IMMEDIATE REACTION—SKIN TESTS

In the immediate reaction the results of the test for allergy are seen within a few minutes. The tests commonly employed are:

Scratch Test

Scratches on the skin of the arm are made with a sharp needle, sufficient to break the upper layer of skin without causing bleeding. A solution of material to be tested is then rubbed into the scratch. A positive reaction is manifested by the development within a few minutes of a urticarial wheal at the site of test.

Intradermal Test

In using the intradermal method a small amount of the allergen to be tested (°.02 cubic centimeter) is injected intradermally. A positive reaction is shown, as with the scratch test.

Prausnitz-Küstner Test

Blood is drawn from the suspected individual, and the serum is separated. A nonallergic individual is used as the test person. Injections of 0.1 cubic centimeter of the serum are made intradermally on several sites of the arms. After 24 hours a different allergen is injected into each site, and the same allergen is injected intradermally into an adjacent site not previously prepared, as a control. A positive reaction is shown, as with the direct intradermal test.

Serum sickness is a form of the immediate type of allergy in man. This manifests itself in 6 to 10 days following the initial injection of a foreign serum. It may occur after the administration of large doses of diphtheria or tetanus antitoxin, since these are horse serums. The clinical symptoms of serum sickness are generalized urticaria with itching, edema of different parts of the body, enlarged lymph nodes, and pains in the joints. The mechanism of its occurrence is believed to be as follows: When the serum is first injected and absorption of antigen occurs, antibodies are formed in the cells and spill over into the circulation. Not all the serum is absorbed from the site of injection at one time. As absorption continues, some of the antigen reaches the sensitized cells, and a reaction occurs which is manifest as serum sickness. It will be noted that the mechanism of serum sickness is similar to that of anaphylaxis.

DELAYED REACTION—ADDITIONAL SKIN TESTS

In the tuberculin type, an extract of tubercle bacilli obtained from the medium in which the organisms have grown is, after proper dilution, applied by the scratch or intradermal method to the skin of an individual who has a tuberculous infection. The result is a local reaction characterized by redness and induration at the site of test. The reaction does not begin until some hours after the test and is seen at its height in about 48 hours. Thereafter, it gradually fades over a period of several days. If the individual tested has no tuberculosis infection, no reaction will occur.

Scratch or Pirquet Test

When the scratch test is used, the extract of tubercle bacilli is concentrated and applied in full strength (old tuberculin or O.T.) to a small scratch on the forearm.

Intradermal or Mantoux Test

If the intradermal method is used, the O.T. is diluted and 0.1 cubic centimeter of the diluted material is injected. To obviate a general reaction, the intradermal test is begun with a very weak dilution and, if the test is negative, a stronger dilution is used. As a routin two doses are used, 0.1 cubic centimeter of a 1:10,000 dilution which is equivalent to 0.01 milligram of old tuberculin, and 0.1 cubic centimeter of a 1:100 dilution, which is equivalent to 1 milligram of O.T. Tests may also be done with dilutions of a purified protein derivative of O.T. This is referred to as P.P.D.

Skin tests giving the delayed type of reaction are performed for diagnosis in other diseases than tuberculosis. They are used for diagnosis in brucellosis, tularemia, leprosy, histoplasmosis, coccidioidomycosis, lymphogranuloma venereum (Frei test), and mumps.

Patch Test

Another test giving the delayed form of reaction is the patch or contact test. This is commonly used in testing for sensitivity to drugs, chemicals, and other inorganic substances, but it has been used also with tuberculin. Its greatest use is in dermatological conditions resulting from contact with various substances. In performing the test a piece of gauze, 1/4 inch square, saturated with the material to be tested, is applied to the intact skin, covered with 1-inch square of Cellophane, and this covered with a piece of adhesive, 2 inches square. The patch is allowed to remain on the skin for 24 hours, and the test is read after another 24 hours. A positive reaction is indicated by erythema and a vesicular eruption at the site.

REFERENCES

1. Boyd, W. G.: *Fundamentals of Immunology*, 2d ed., Interscience Publishers, Inc., New York, 1947.
2. Dubos, R. J.: *Bacterial and Mycotic Infections of Man*, J. B. Lippincott Company, Philadelphia, 1948.
3. Ratner, B.: *Allergy, Anaphylaxis and Immunotherapy*, The Williams & Wilkins Company, Baltimore, 1943.
4. Wilson, G. S., and Miles, A. A.: *Topley and Wilson's Principles of Bacteriology and Immunity*, The Williams & Wilkins Company, Baltimore, 1946.

Chapter 5 TREATMENT OF COMMUNICABLE DISEASE

THE conquest of communicable disease has been proceeding along three lines: the control of environmental sanitation, immunization of susceptible hosts, and treatment of cases, carriers, and contacts with specific drugs. Treatment of the case also involves the use of nonspecific measures. While these may not act directly in reducing infectivity, they are of help in curing cases more rapidly and often in saving lives. A discussion of therapeutic measures commonly used in communicable disease is, therefore, desirable.

Sulfonamides

The ability of a specific substance to cure a specific disease has been known since ancient times. Cinchona bark was used in the treatment of malaria long before it was known what malaria was caused by, and even long before it was known that the essential principle in cinchona was quinine. However, the systematic experimentation with drugs for the treatment of certain diseases may be said to have originated with Ehrlich who, in 1910, after 606 trials, discovered salvarsan, a drug which could kill the spirochete of syphilis in the human body. When Domagk, in 1933, discovered that sulfanilamide, when taken by mouth, inhibited the growth of a number of microorganisms in the living body, a new principle was evolved. The drug was not directed at a specific germ. Rather, it modified the metabolic functions of the tissue cells, so that certain microorganisms could not grow and multiply. In rapid succession new sulfonamide drugs were synthesized, succeeding ones being more effective and less toxic than the earlier ones. The sulfonamide drug which is now considered the best for general use is sulfadiazine. It has a wide range of effect, not only against the gram-positive pneumococci, streptococci, and staphylococci, but also against the gram-negative meningococci and gonococci and against the gram-negative dysentery bacilli. It has also been used effectively in the treatment of chancroid, lymphogranuloma venereum, trachoma, and cholera. In some of the conditions mentioned, sulfadiazine has been largely supplanted by one or another of the antibiotics. It is still the drug of choice in meningococcus meningitis, bacillary dysentery, chancroid, and cholera.

Sulfadiazine is administered in tablets of 0.5 gram each. In children the dose is 0.2 gram per kilogram of body weight (1½ grains per pound) per day. In older children and adults the dose is 4 grams a day. The daily dose is divided into four and given at 6-hour intervals; or it may be divided into six and given at 4-hour intervals. Toxic effects of the drug are not common but may occur if the drug is taken for a long period of time. These consist of (1) fever, frequently associated with (2) a rash which resembles measles and is often itchy; (3) changes in the blood characterized chiefly by a rapid anemia and leukopenia; (4) hematuria, caused by the passage of crystals of the drug, which irritate the mucous lining of the genito-urinary tract; the crystals may be sufficiently large to obstruct the passage of urine and cause (5) anuria. If sufficient fluids are given and if alkalies are added, complications occur infrequently. If the drug has to be given for any length of time, a blood count and a urine examination should be performed once every 4 or 5 days.

Recently, a sulfonamide with a high degree of solubility and low toxicity has been introduced. This is Gantrisin. It is administered similarly to sulfadiazine except that an alkali need not be given, and, because of the solubility of the drug, large amounts of fluid need not be taken with it.

The antibiotics have largely supplanted the sulfonamides because they are less toxic. However, in some diseases, as mentioned above, the sulfonamides are still the drugs of choice. Furthermore, their cheapness makes them more available for large-scale treatment and for prophylactic use in institutions, schools, camps, or wherever large groups of individuals are exposed to infection by an organism that is sensitive to the drug.

Antibiotics

The antibiotics are chemical substances of biologic origin which inhibit the growth of, or destroy, certain microorganisms. Their wide use stems from the observation of Fleming, in 1928, that in a culture of staphylococci which had been contaminated by a mold, *Penicillium notatum,* the colonies of cocci immediately around the mold were dissolved. In 1938, Florey and Chain used penicillin, an extract of the mold, against a number of microorganisms, and proved its bacteriostatic effect. The manufacture of the antibiotic was rapidly stepped up, and by 1945 it came into general use.

Penicillin

This is the first of the antibiotics to be widely employed and still remains one of the most potent drugs known. As used originally, it was a crude mixture and was rapidly absorbed and eliminated. It was injected every 3 hours around the clock. At present the crystalline form of procaine penicillin G has supplanted most other forms. A cubic centimeter contains 300,000 units of penicillin, and an effective blood concentration can be maintained with one injection a day intramuscularly. In severe infections two injections a day are given. It is put up in both aqueous suspension and oil. In the former, it causes little discomfort when injected and can be given repeatedly over a number of days. In pediatric practice this is a great boon, since the comparative ease of administration does not cause the psychologic traumas that more painful injections do. When it is desired to have the effect of the injection persist for a long period of time, as in the treament of syphilis, the oily preparation is used, and several cubic centimeters may be injected as the initial dose. Penicillin is the most effective antibiotic in infections caused by gram-positive cocci. It is also the antibiotic of first choice in anthrax, syphilis and other spirochetal infections, gonorrhea, and actinomycosis. It is not effective in tuberculosis, or in infections caused by gram-negative organisms. Reactions to penicillin are uncommon. The one most frequently complained of is urticaria. It is treated with antihistamines. Penicillin has the disadvantage of being ineffective when taken by mouth unless doses five to ten times those usually recommended are given. Even then, they should be buffered and given on an empty stomach.

Streptomycin

The ineffectiveness of penicillin against infections caused by gram-negative microorganisms made the search for another antibiotic inevitable. In 1944 Waksman isolated streptomycin from a mold, *Streptomyces griseus,* and found it to be effective against a number of gram-negative and acid-fast organisms. It is the antibiotic of choice in tuberculosis, and has also been used effectively in influenzal meningitis, plague, tularemia, brucellosis, and granuloma inguinale. It is given in aqueous solution, intramuscularly, in a dose of 1 to 2 grams a day divided into four or six injections. It is ineffective when given by mouth. It is frequently given in combination with other drugs. Thus, in tuberculous meningitis, it is often given in combination with para-aminosalicylic acid (PAS), or with one of the sulfone drugs such as Promizole; and in plague and brucellosis it is given in combination with sulfadiazine.

One of the drawbacks to its use is its toxicity. It frequently causes disturbances in the function of the eighth cranial nerve, resulting in vertigo, loss of equilibrium, and loss or diminution of hearing. These disturbances may remain permanently. Attempts to obtain other forms of streptomycin, less toxic and more effective, have not met with success. Dihydrostreptomycin has been shown to be as toxic as the parent drug and no more effective. Neomycin is more toxic and has, therefore, not been released for general use.

Aureomycin—Chloramphenicol (Chloromycetin) —Terramycin

In 1948, Duggar described the antibiotic Aureomycin, derived from a soil fungus, *Streptomyces aureofaciens*. This was the first antibiotic which could be administered by mouth with effective results. Furthermore, it appeared to be active against both gram-positive and gram-negative organisms. It had the further virtue of being effective against the rickettsiae and the large viruses, such as those of the psittacosis–lymphogranuloma venereum group. In the same year Ehrlich and associates reported the production of chloramphenicol, or Chloromycetin, from a strain of *Streptomyces venezuelae*. This antibiotic, which can also be administered by mouth, has been synthesized, so that it can be produced in the laboratory without the growth of the organism in cultures. The latest of the antibiotics which are effective when taken orally is *Terramycin*, produced in the Pfizer laboratories from *Streptomyces rimosus*, and reported by Finlay and associates in 1950.

These three antibiotics are often referred to as broad-spectrum antibiotics, because they are effective against a large group of organisms. All are produced in crystalline form and are only slightly soluble in water. They are dispensed in capsules of 50, 100, and 250 milligrams. Their therapeutic properties are similar. In general, they are effective against gram-positive and gram-negative bacteria, against the rickettsiae, and against large viruses. For streptococcal, pneumococcal, meningococcal, gonococcal, and spirochetal infections, penicillin by intramuscular injection is the antibiotic of choice. For brucella, bacillus *coli* infections, influenza meningitis, pertussis, chancroid, granuloma inguinale, psittacosis, and lymphogranuloma venereum, the orally administered, broad-spectrum antibiotics are preferable. In typhoid fever chloramphenicol appears to be the most effective antibiotic. The dosage of Aureomycin and Terramycin is 20 to 30 milligrams per kilogram of body weight per day, in mild infections, and 50 to 60 milligrams in severe cases. The dose of chloramphenicol is twice that of either of the other two. The total daily dose is divided into four parts and given every 6 hours.

All three drugs may cause toxic symptoms. Among these are nausea and vomiting, diarrhea, itching of the skin, rash, an eczema-like eruption around the anus, and blacktongue. The toxic symptoms are said to be ameliorated by large doses of vitamin B. They disappear on withdrawal of the antibiotic. Chloromycetin may also cause serious hemolytic reactions.

No effective antibiotic has yet been found to combat the smaller viruses such as those of measles, chickenpox, mumps, encephalitis, or poliomyelitis. The use of antibiotics in some of these diseases may be warranted, however, in order to prevent complications and secondary invaders.

Blood Transfusion

A therapeutic measure of great value in the treatment of communicable disease is the transfusion of blood. This form of therapy, originally used only to replace blood lost as a result of hemorrhage, is now employed also in various forms of blood dyscrasias, in severe anemias of all types, and as a supportive measure in severe malnutrition, dehydration, shock, and infection. It may be life-saving in infants and small children who are anemic and undernourished and develop an exhausting disease like whooping cough.

Human beings are divided into four major blood groups known as O, A, B, and AB. Individuals belonging to the same blood group may exchange blood without the occurrence of a reaction. However, when blood of one group is mixed with blood of another group, a severe reaction may occur. This is due to the fact that the blood cells of one group are agglutinated by the serum of the other one. Group O blood contains red cells which are not agglutinated by the serums of any of the other blood groups. In an emergency such blood may be used without typing. For this reason, individuals in group O are sometimes referred to as universal donors. Such blood should not be used without typing when no emergency exists, since the serum of group O donors may agglutinate the cells of the recipient. In an emergency the blood is used without typing in the expectation that the serum of the donor's blood will be sufficiently diluted by the larger amount of blood present in the recipient so that little or no reaction will occur.

In recent years there has been considerable discussion of the Rh factor. This is an antigen which is present in about 85 per cent of individuals, irrespective of blood group, and is inherited. The significance of this factor may be observed when a man who has the factor (Rh positive) marries a woman who does not possess it (Rh negative). If the wife becomes pregnant, the fetus she is carrying may have Rh positive or Rh negative blood. In the latter case there is no risk. In the former, there is risk to the fetus due to iso-immunization reaction. There is exchange of antigens and antibodies between the mother's and baby's blood. Positive Rh antigens from the baby get into the mother's blood stream and stimulate the development of anti-Rh antibodies. These get into the baby's blood stream and tend to hemolyze the infant's red blood cells. As a result, the infant may be born dead or severely anemic and jaundiced. In the latter case the infant's life can be saved by immediate transfusions of Rh negative blood. An ensanguination transfusion is frequently resorted to in these conditions.

A similar iso-immunization reaction may occur if an Rh negative individual receives several transfusions of Rh positive blood. The first one or two transfusions will sensitize the individual and cause the development of anti-Rh antibodies. A later transfusion will cause a reaction between these antibodies and the injected Rh antigens, resulting in a hemolytic reaction. Whenever possible, persons requiring a transfusion should be tested for Rh as well as for type. If they are Rh negative they should receive blood from Rh negative donors only.

Convalescent Serum—Gamma Globulin—Antitoxin

With the increasing use of blood for therapeutic purposes, there has become available an increasing amount of blood products. In communicable diseases, the serums of patients convalescing from measles, scarlet fever, whooping cough, and mumps have been used for prophylaxis in children exposed intimately to these diseases. In scarlet fever and whooping cough, the serums have also been used in treatment of cases. The antibodies in serum are concentrated in the gamma globulin portion. By fractionation, it is possible to obtain gamma globulin from serum in a concentration of about twenty-five times. Instead of injecting 50 cubic centimeters of serum, it is necessary to inject only 2 cubic centimeters of gamma globulin. Gamma globulin from normal human serum for the prophylaxis of measles and gamma globulin from hyperimmunized pertussis serum for the prophylaxis and treatment of whooping cough are available.

Antitoxins are serums obtained from animals that have been injected with toxin or toxoid. Such serums are used prophylactically and therapeutically. Several serums are available on the market. The more commonly used ones are diphtheria and tetanus antitoxins. Others that are available are botulinus, gas gangrene, and anthrax antiserums.

Drugs

A variety of drugs, administered by mouth, by rectum, by instillation in the nose, by inunction, and by injection are employed in the treatment of communicable disease. Some of these are specific and are used for particular diseases only. Others are nonspecific and are employed to allay symptoms, as in noncommunicable disease. Among the former are such drugs as quinine and Atabrine in malaria, hexylresorcinol in helminthic diseases, carbarsone in amebiasis, and antihistamines in serum sickness. Among the latter are salicylates for joint pains, codeine for cough, morphine for severe pain, barbiturates for restlessness, and iron for anemia. The kind of drug and its method of administration are determined in the particular case by the attending physician.

Fluid Therapy

In diseases in which fever is a characteristic symptom, and this includes most of the communicable diseases, the patient may become dehydrated as a result of fluid loss by sweating, vomiting, or diarrhea, or on account of an insufficient intake owing to anorexia or nausea. This is a frequent occurrence in small babies. Dehydration results in a disturbance of the electrolyte balance in the body and, if maintained, will go on to acidosis, coma, and death. It must, therefore, be combated as soon as it is discovered. Since, in dehydration, fluid cannot usually be taken by mouth, it must be administered parenterally. It is usually given in the form of 5 per cent glucose solution in saline or as a buffered saline solution such as Hartmann's or Ringer's solution. The injection is given either intravenously or subcutaneously. In the latter case, hyaluronidase may be added to the solution to increase the rapidity of its absorption by the tissues.

Inhalation Therapy

Oxygen

The use of oxygen as a therapeutic measure in medicine began in the 1920's when it was employed in the treatment of pneumonia. Since then oxygen, in a 40 to 60 per cent concentration, has been

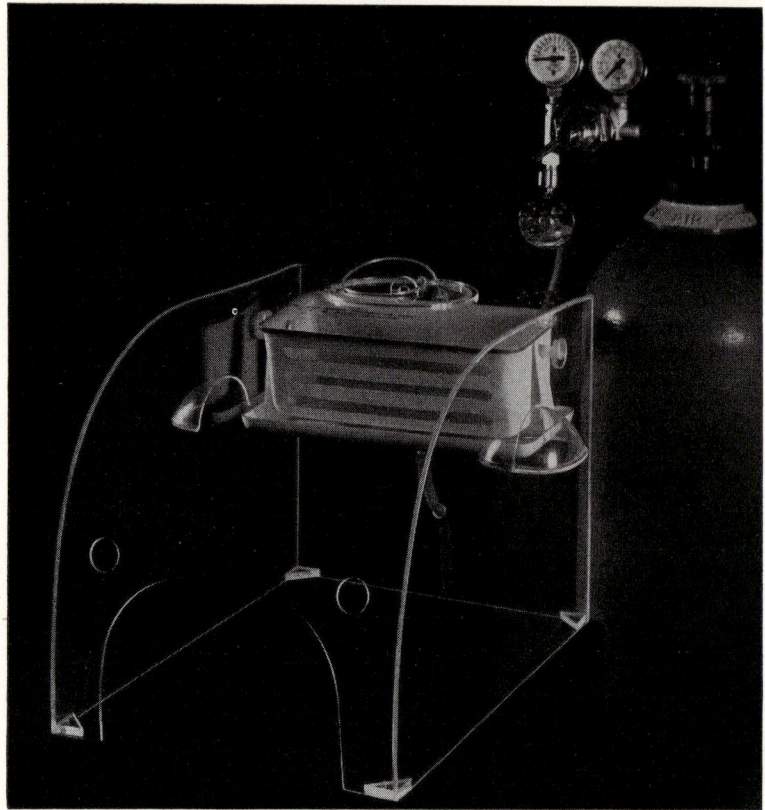

Fig. I. OXYGEN HEAD TENT FOR CHILDREN.

(Courtesy O.E.M. Corporation, East Norwalk, Conn.)

employed in a variety of conditions in which anoxia, or a reduced concentration of oxygen in the tissues, occurs. First among the communicable diseases requiring oxygen therapy is pneumonia. Since the advent of the antibiotics, patients are often cured before they develop anoxemia. However, there still are persons with severe cases of pneumonia who, in spite of antibiotic therapy, are cyanotic or have severe chest pains. Oxygen relieves their symptoms almost miraculously. Another disease in which oxygen is of considerable help is whooping cough, particularly in infants and young children. When such children are placed in an oxygen tent, their paroxysms decrease, their cough is less, and they appear more comfortable. In croup, from whatever cause, particularly if cyan-

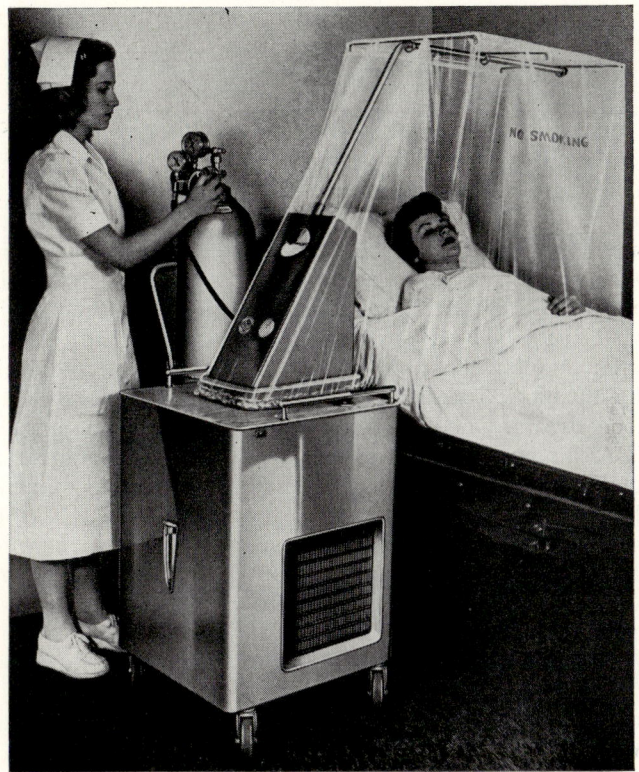

Fig. II. ELECTRIC OXYGEN TENT.

(Courtesy Ohio Chemical & Surgical Equipment Co., Madison, Wis.)

osis occurs, oxygen is indicated. In any communicable disease in which there are respiratory complications and cyanosis or dyspnea occurs, oxygen should be used in addition to other measures.

Oxygen may be administered by placing the patient in a complete or partial tent, by the use of a mask strapped over the patient's nose and mouth, or by nasal catheter. While the last two methods may be effective in adults, their use in infants and children is much resented. Oxygen tents are of three kinds: (1) a complete tent in which the patient's entire body fits, (2) a partial tent in which only the patient's head and shoulders are encased, and (3) a box with an open top. The first is the most efficient but also the most expensive. The last is the cheapest and easiest to use, but the concentration of oxygen cannot be accurately measured. The second method is a closed one and allows a good concentration of oxygen; at the same time, the child need not be taken out of the tent to be diapered or to receive parenteral therapy.

Aerosols

Aerosols are finely divided particulate matter which can be introduced into a local site by means of a spray. An example is the use of epinephrine, sprayed into the back of the mouth with a hand nebulizer to relieve an attack of asthma. With the introduction of the antibiotics, aerosols of penicillin were introduced. Apparatus were developed by means of which aerosols of penicillin or other drugs could be sprayed into the bronchial tree by the aid of oxygen under a pressure of 2 to 4 liters per minutes. In this way the antibiotic reaches the lungs rapidly and is absorbed into the blood stream. Good blood levels of penicillin can thus be obtained. Although it has been demonstrated that penumonia can be cured in this way, the intramuscular injection is so much simpler that there is no need to replace it in this disease. However, in certain cases of bronchitis, croup, or other local conditions where it is desired to have a drug come into contact with the tissues locally, aerosols can be used.

Steam—Water Spray

Infants and small children who have a respiratory illness are more comfortable and cough less when the atmosphere surrounding them has a high humidity. If they are in an oxygen tent, the air in it can be humidified. A reservoir of tap water is kept in the tent in a glass cylinder. This is connected by a tube with a nebulizer. Oxygen, at a pressure of 2 to 4 liters, from a separate tank is used as the motive power to blow the water spray into the tent. There is also on the market a tent in which the oxygen and water spray enter simultaneously. If the child does not require oxygen, a croup tent can be improvised by draping a blanket over the top and sides of the infant's crib. A water spray can then be blown into the tent by an apparatus, as described above, or by one using some other form of motive power.

When a child is suffering from croup, laryngitis, or tracheitis, steam inhalations aid in easing the pain and tightness of the cough, in quieting the child, and in making him more comfortable. A croup tent can be improvised by draping a blanket over the top, sides, and back of the head of the crib. This may be covered with a sheet. The croup kettle is placed on a chair or low table near the crib, and the steam is directed toward the covered part of the tent. It should be kept going continuously. Various drugs, such as tincture of benzoin, are often added to the water in the kettle. It is doubtful if they do more than give a medicinal odor to the atmosphere. The important part of the treatment is the steam. The old-fashioned kettle with a broad base and a wide spout is best, since it gives sufficient steam to humidify the air in the tent. In homes one frequently sees pint-sized glass containers in which the water is heated by an electric coil. The amount of steam issuing from the spout is so small as to make the apparatus a token steam kettle only.

In the case of older children who do not sleep in cribs with sides, and in the case of adults requiring steam inhalation, a tent can be constructed by placing a screen around the head of the bed and draping a blanket over the top, sides, and back. If a screen is not available, a tent can be improvised by opening up a man's umbrella on the bed. The patient lies in bed under the umbrella, much as he would on the beach in summer. A sheet, thrown over the umbrella, makes the tent more efficient. The arrangement of the steam kettle is similar to the one just described. If the patient is a child, an attendant should be in the room at all times to make sure that the child will not tamper with the steam kettle and cause a fire or a burn.

Occasionally, it is necessary to administer both oxygen and steam. This may happen in a case of croup, particularly if a tracheotomy has been done. In some hospitals, rooms have been constructed into which both steam and oxygen are piped. Where such conveniences are not available, the patient must be placed alternately in the oxygen tent and the steam tent, or in an oxygen and water-spray tent. An open flame or a lighted coil should never be permitted in a room where oxygen is used, because the danger of an explosion is great.

Physical Therapy

There are a number of physical measures that are used in the therapy of cases of communicable disease. They do not differ from similar measures used in other types of disease. One of the commonest is the alcohol sponge to keep excessive fever down. Children resent cold applications. It is therefore advisable to mix the alcohol with tepid water when sponging infants or young children. It should be pointed out that fever, per se, is not harmful. It is, as a matter of fact, nature's way of combating infection. No attempt should be made to bring down moderately high temperatures. It is only when the fever is excessive, so that the patient is very uncomfortable or there is danger that a convulsion may result, that attempts should be made to lower the body temperature. Dry heat, in the form of hot-water bags or electric heating pads, is used for the relief of muscle pains or abdominal cramps. Moist heat is used to relieve spasm. In the acute stage of paralytic poliomyelitis, woolen cloths wrung out of very hot water are applied to the spastic muscles. Cold applications are used to relieve the pain and discomfort resulting from fever or infection. Examples are the use of an ice bag to relieve headaches resulting from fever or an ice collar to ease the pain of a sore throat or inflamed cervical glands. Cloths wrung out of cold water are applied to inflamed tissue such as in cellulitis. The use of a cold tub bath in conditions of hyperpyrexia was common years ago. Such baths are not recommended today, because the shock caused by the immersion probably does harm, and the patient is made extremely uncomfortable.

Various forms of orthopedic appliances are used. The commonest is a wide board placed at the foot of the bed to prevent foot drop in cases where there is muscle weaknesses in the lower limbs. Rolled Turkish towels, sandbags, or pillows are used to assist in maintaining proper body alignment. More complicated apparatus may be necessary, such as various kinds of pulley arrangements and traction to keep a joint from becoming fixed in flexion, as in the case of arthritis complicating meningitis. Pillows or sandbags may be required to give support to the back in certain types of paralysis. In acute poliomyelitis, when there is paralysis of the respiratory muscles, it may be necessary to place the patient in a respirator for varying lengths of time.

In diphtheritic croup and in bulbar poliomyelitis, repeated suction may be necessary to dislodge and remove pieces of membrane or tenacious mucus from the throat in order to permit proper ingress of air. In laryngotracheobronchitis as well as in diphtheritic croup, there may be so much edema of the upper larynx that suction is of no assistance. In such cases a tracheotomy is necessary. Careful attention must be given to the tube to see that it does not get fouled up by secretions or membrane.

Nutrition

The body requires certain nutritional elements for growth and replacement of worn-out tissue, for the performance of normal functions, and for general well-being. The elements in food which serve these functions are proteins, which are essential for growth and replacement; carbohydrates and fats, which, together with proteins, are burned in the body to give energy, measured in terms of calories; and water, minerals, and vitamins, which are necessary for proper metabolism. Persistent lack of an adequate supply of proteins in the food will lead to stunting of growth. An insufficient intake of caloric requirements will cause a slowing of the body's activities and the symptoms which are associated with undernutrition and starvation.

There are a number of minerals necessary for the body's proper functioning. These include calcium, phosphorus, magnesium, sodium, potassium, sulfur, and chlorine. They are present in fairly large quantities. In addition, other minerals appear only as trace elements. Among these are iron, copper, iodine, manganese, and zinc.

The disturbances of metabolism resulting from a lack of some of these elements are known; for instance, an insufficient intake of iron results in hypochromic anemia; an insufficient intake of iodine results in goiter. In the case of some of the other minerals, the precise illnesses caused by their lack or absence are not known.

The deficiency diseases are caused by the lack of one or more vitamins in the diet. There have been a great many investigations of vitamins since Casimir Funk first used the term in 1912. Much has been learned, many of the diseases caused by the lack of certain vitamins have been identified, most common foods have been assayed for vitamin content, and many new vitamins have been discovered. Nevertheless, there is still much to learn.

Several well-known clinical entities result from the absence in the diet of certain vitamins; for example, scurvy due to lack of vitamin C, keratomalacia due to lack of A, and beriberi caused by lack of one of the B fractions. It has also been shown that slight deficiencies of vitamins in the diet may cause mild symptoms which are insufficient for clinical diagnosis. Such deficiencies, even though slight, have an adverse effect on body metabolism. The minimum daily requirements have been charted for many of the vitamins but not yet for all.

Water makes up 70 per cent of the total body mass. It is essential for proper nutrition. It transports nutritive elements and carries away waste products in the body. All chemical changes in the body take place only in the presence of water. By evaporation from the lungs and skin, water plays a major part in the regulation of body temperature. It is regularly lost to the body through exhaled air, sweat, urine, and feces. It must be replaced in liquids or in solid foods, all of which contain water. No person can survive many days without water. If the patient is comatose or if there is marked vomiting or diarrhea and fluids cannot be imbibed or retained, dehydration, acidosis, and death will follow unless fluids are given parenterally, either intravenously or subcutaneously. The fluids commonly used for this purpose are normal saline, 5 per cent glucose in saline, or certain buffered solutions like Ringer's or Hartmann's or Darrow's.

Children with acute communicable disease usually suffer from anorexia. As a result, their food intake is inadequate. This means, usually, a loss of weight, since the body burns food stored in the form of tissue. If the illness is of short duration, as in most of the acute communicable diseases, no harm is done, and no efforts should be made to stimulate the appetite. Soon after recovery the appetite increases, and the loss of weight is made up. What is important is to see that there is an adequate fluid intake. In young children especially, an inadequate fluid intake may result in acidosis. The type of fluid matters little. It may be plain water, weak tea, soda, ginger ale, or any of the cola drinks. Sweetened drinks have an added advantage in the sugar content, which is of some caloric value and which aids in combating acidosis. The intake should be 1 quart or more of fluid a day, if possible. Where all fluids are refused or where fluids cannot be retained because of vomiting or diarrhea, they should be given parenterally in the form of 5 per cent glucose solution or Ringer's or Hartmann's solutions.

If the illness is a long-term one, as in rheumatic fever or tuberculosis, attempts must be made, after the initial acute stage is over, to give the child a well-balanced diet. It should contain sufficient protein food to make up for tissue destruction caused by the illness and must be high enough in caloric value to equal the amount burned. The foods should be easily digestible. Usually, this means a diet high in protein and carbohydrate and low in fats. Vitamins must usually be added. Fortunately, there are concentrated forms of vitamins on the market, so that the total daily supply can be given in small bulk. Occasionally, anorexia is so marked that, in spite of all urging, no food is taken by mouth. It may be necessary under such circumstances to give solutions of amino acids or emulsions of fat intravenously to prevent depletion of the body stores.

Psychotherapy

Considerable attention has been paid in recent years to the emotional aspect of disease. More and more thought is being given to the psychologic effect on an individual of the sudden impingement of illness. Nurses and physicians are learning to treat patients as persons and not as cases. In the field of communicable disease, physicians and nurses must take into consideration the psychic trauma to a patient which results from the knowledge that he is suffering from an illness that has special, unhappy implications. Most illnesses cause anxieties in the patient on account of the pain and discomfort suffered and the fear of serious results. In illness caused by communicable disease, there is the additional anxiety engendered by special requirements such as isolation, sterilization of dishes, and other repetitive procedures.

It is important for the physician and the nurse to appraise the situation carefully and note its impact on the patient. The nurse should be sensitive to the patient's feelings and to his concern about himself and other members of the family. If she will take the time to listen to him, she may be able to get him to express his feelings and anxieties. She will then be better able to understand his problems. The reason for certain procedures, such as those involving medical asepsis or special treatment, should be explained in simple language. Questions about the nature and prognosis of the disease should be answered simply and cheerfully, and stress should be put on the good outlook and the short confinement generally required. The need of special assistance should be appraised. A conference with a social worker or spiritual adviser may be advisable.

The patient, especially if a child, suffers additional mental anguish if he is moved from the familiar atmosphere of his home to the strange and forbidding environment of a hospital. For this reason alone careful consideration should be given to home care. Most cases of communicable disease can be treated with little difficulty in the home. This holds true not only for the comparatively minor diseases such as chickenpox or mumps but for the more serious diseases such as diphtheria and poliomyelitis. Even a poorly equipped home is better for a young patient than a well-equipped hospital. A skillful nurse can organize the home so that the patient is adequately cared for, isolation is properly carried out, and the other members of the family are not overburdened. Not only are children spared the mental anguish of the sudden separation from home and parents, but hospital beds are made available for other more seriously ill patients who cannot be cared for at home.

Nursing

The nurse's function in the various therapeutic procedures outlined is a very important one. Some of the procedures, such as the administration of drugs, are carried out by her exclusively upon the doctor's orders. Others are initiated by the physician with her assistance. The responsibility of supervision is hers almost exclusively. She must have an understanding of the reason why a certain procedure has been put in motion, a clear concept of how it works, and a knowledge of the danger signals that indicate that it has ceased to function properly and that the patient is in danger. She must be continually attentive to details of treatment, alert to recognize symptoms of distress in the patient, and ready to call on the medical staff for assistance in matters beyond her competence. Another important function of nursing is to maintain adequate nutritional needs of the patient. It takes great skill, ingenuity, and patience to feed a person who is not hungry and who is ill and uncomfortable. The problem is a minor one in illnesses of short duration. In chronic illnesses a nurse needs to utilize the full resources at her command to make trays attractive. Palatable foods high in nutritive values may be served, even though the quantities are small.

REFERENCES

1. Barach, A. L.: "The Treatment of Anoxia in Clinical Medicine," *Bull. New York Acad. Med.*, **26**:370, 1950.
2. Block, M.: "Inhalation and Aerosol Treatment in Pneumonia," *Bull. New York Acad. Med.*, **26**:404, 1950.
3. Fischer, A. E.: "Inhalation Therapy of Acute Respiratory Infections, Measles, Whooping Cough and Pneumonia," *Bull. New York Acad. Med.*, **26**:468, 1950.
4. Fischer, A. E.: "The Present Status of Sulfonamide Therapy in Pediatrics," *New York State J. Med.*, **51**:228, 1951.
5. Funk, C.: "The Etiology of Deficiency Diseases," *J. State Med.*, **20**:341, 1912.
6. Greenberg, M.; Frant, S.; and Rutstein, D. D.: "Gamma Globulin and Placental Globulin," *J.A.M.A.*, **126**:944, 1944.
7. Jolliffe, N.; Tisdall, F. F.; and Cannon, P. R.: *Clinical Nutrition,* Paul B. Hoeber, Inc., New York, 1950.
8. Karelitz, S.: "Evaluation of Aureomycin, Chloromycetin and Other Newer Antibiotics," *New York State J. Med.*, **51**:234, 1951.
9. Landsteiner, K., and Wiener, A. S.: "An Agglutinable Factor in Human Blood Recognized by Immune Sera from Rhesus Blood," *Proc. Soc. Exper. Biol. & Med.*, **43**:223, 1940.
10. Levine, P.; Katzin, E. M.; and Burnham, L.: "Atypical Warm Isoagglutinins," *Proc. Soc. Exper. Biol. & Med.*, **45**:346, 1940.
11. McLester, J. S.: *Nutrition and Diet in Health and Disease,* W. B. Saunders Company, Philadelphia, 1949.
12. Soule, H. C.: "The Present Status of Penicillin and Streptomycin in Pediatrics," *New York State J. Med.*, **51**:228, 1951.
13. Stimson, P.: "Outline of Use of Respirators and of Oxygen in Poliomyelitis," *Bull. New York Acad. Med.*, **26**:495, 1950.

Chapter 6 MEDICAL ASEPSIS

THE commonest reservoirs of communicable disease are the patient and the carrier. The organisms causing the communicable disease are expelled by the patient or carrier and are dispersed into his environment. They may lodge in susceptible persons, causing them to become infected. The purpose of aseptic nursing is to prevent such dispersal and to reduce the total number of pathogens which may be disseminated to others. The principles underlying medical asepsis have been drawn from medicine, bacteriology, chemistry, and the allied sciences. They have been incorporated into measures and mechanical procedures which can be used in the hospital and home to prevent spread of disease and aid in its control.

Definitions

1. Communicable disease is a disease caused by a pathogenic organism, which can be transmitted from man or an animal to a susceptible person, directly or indirectly.

2. Infectious disease is a disease caused by the entry into the body of a pathogenic organism and its multiplication there. An infectious disease may or may not be communicable.

3. Contagious disease, strictly speaking, is a disease spread by contact. Most of the diseases to which this term has been applied are spread, however, in other ways, chiefly through the respiratory tract. There is a wide tendency to avoid ambiguous terms like "contagious" disease and to use the wider term "communicable" disease. The method of spread of a communicable disease can then be classified as being by direct contact, indirect contact, respiratory, intestinal, etc.

4. Isolation is the separation from other persons, during the period of communicability, of a person with a communicable disease. In some diseases, like measles, strict isolation is necessary. In other diseases, like meningitis, isolation is not the most important factor in limiting spread. Isolation may be carried out by confining the patient to a separate room, ward, or cubicle. The determination as to which of these forms to use depends on the type of illness.

Isolation by means of screening is occasionally used. It is not effective, interferes with the nurse's routine, and is psychologically unsound. It should be avoided whenever possible. Isolation serves two purposes. It prevents the spread of infection to susceptible persons and it protects the patient from secondary infections.

5. Quarantine is the restriction of movement placed on persons who have been exposed to a communicable disease, for a period of time equal to the incubation period of the disease, in order to prevent their contact with susceptible persons who have not been exposed. Such quarantine may be *complete,* in which case all persons exposed are restricted in their movements. More often the quarantine is *modified* so that there is selective limitation of movement. Certain individuals might be exempt, for instance, persons who are immune; or only certain persons might be quarantined, for instance, contacts to a case of typhoid who are food handlers.

6. Placarding is the posting of a notice on the door or entrance to a room, warning persons not to enter it because of the presence of a case of communicable disease. The practice of placarding has largely gone out of fashion. It has not helped in the control of communicable disease, it is difficult and time-consuming to enforce, it throws a scare into people who pass by, and it wastes nursing time which can be put to better advantage.

7. Aseptic techniques are procedures of cleanliness used to confine the organisms of disease to the source and to prevent their spread.

8. Contamination means the soiling of articles by contact with an infectious agent.

9. Fumigation is the destruction of small animals by the use of gases. In years gone by, fumigation was used after the termination of diseases like measles or scarlet fever. It is now used only when small animals, such as rodents or insects, are to be killed. Even for this purpose fumigation is not employed to any extent at present. To kill insects it is much more efficient to use an *insecticide,* which is a chemical substance applied as a powder or liquid, like DDT. To kill rodents it is common practice to use a *rodenticide,* which is a chemical substance usually ingested by the rodent. It is not necessary to fumigate a room occupied by a person suffering from one of the common communicable diseases, since most germs do not survive for long when they are outside the body of their host. Thorough cleaning of a room is superior to fumigation.

10. Sterilization means the killing of viable organisms. It is synonymous with disinfection, but the term is usually limited to destruction of microorganisms by the use of physical agents.

11. Disinfection is applied to the use of chemical agents. It is said to be *concurrent* or *terminal.* The former term is used to indi-

cate the destruction of pathogenic organisms as soon as possible after they leave the host's body and before they have come in contact with another person. The latter term is used to indicate the killing of pathogenic organisms in the patient's environment and on his clothing after he has recovered from the disease. It is much more important to carry out concurrent than terminal disinfection.

12. Bactericidal and bacteriostatic are two terms commonly used in connection with disinfection. The former means the destruction of bacteria; the latter means the inhibition of growth of bacteria. The two terms are frequently used in connection with the effect of antibiotics.

The use of disinfectants, as well as of aseptic technique, depends upon a knowledge of the fundamental principles of microbiology and epidemiology. Pathogenic microorganisms survive and multiply best in the body of a host. Some, like most viruses, cannot survive or multiply outside of living tissue. The virus of measles, for instance, dies quickly after it is expelled by a patient, unless it lodges in the respiratory tract of a susceptible host. Bacteria may live outside the host for variable periods of time, provided they have the proper moisture and environment. They vary, however, in this ability. The diphtheria bacillus does not survive long outside the human body, although it has been cultivated from the dust of patients' rooms. On the other hand, typhoid bacilli may persist for fairly long periods in water, milk, and food, and on flies.

Most microorganisms which are pathogenic for man do not infect animals. There are, however, certain organisms, like the salmonellae, which infect both man and the lower animals and which can easily be transferred from one to the other by contaminated food. Some organisms form spores. These are extremely resistant to destruction and may live in soil or on animal skins for months or even years. An example of such organisms is the anthrax bacillus.

It is important for a nurse to know the pathways by which pathogenic organisms enter and leave the body. It is obvious that there is no point in disinfecting the stools of a case of measles, since the virus passes out of the body only by way of the respiratory tract. On the other hand, there is no point in paying particular attention to respiratory discharges of a patient with malaria, since the *Plasmodium* does not escape that way. Indeed, in this disease a nurse would do much better to see that the windows are properly screened than to pay attention to the disinfection of body discharges.

In the solution of any nursing problem related to spread of communicable disease, the nurse must call upon her knowledge of the fundamental sciences and use her professional judgment and technical skill in the selection of those techniques which will assure safe care of the patient and eliminate the hazards of spread to others.

Sterilization

The measures used for the prevention and control of communicable disease are largely measures of cleanliness. However, microorganisms are being expelled by the patient, and these should be destroyed, when possible, by means which are convenient, practical, and inexpensive. A number of physical and chemical methods are used on hospital services and in the home.

Physical Agents

MOIST HEAT

This is the best method of sterilization when its use is practical. It kills all organisms, it is quick, and it penetrates. Even spores can be destroyed at 100° C. in a few minutes. It is the method of choice for sterilizing syringes, needles, and instruments. It requires no special equipment. A clean pot and some water and an adequate flame are all that are needed.

Sterilization by flowing steam is a method employed when it is desired to use moist heat but not to submerge the articles in water. A perforated tray above the level of the water in the sterilizer is used, and the articles are placed on the tray. The steam generated by the water below flows over the articles and sterilizes them. This method is the preferred one in terminal sterilization of equipment used in making babies' formulas. This method may also be used for *fractional sterilization* of mediums, if it is desired to make sure that all spores, which might accidentally have been present in the mediums, are destroyed. The mediums are sterilized by flowing steam, then stored at room temperature to give the spores a chance to germinate, and then resterilized once or twice. With the improvement and simplification in the manufacture of mediums, fractional sterilization is not used much today.

Pasteurization is a form of sterilization with moist heat. It is used to destroy pathogenic organisms at a temperature lower than boiling, so that the taste of the raw product will not be altered, as it is after boiling. Heating is kept up for 30 minutes at a temperature of 62° C. (143° F.). It is a method widely used in this country to sterilize milk.

A method of sterilization by flowing steam under pressure is widely used in hospitals and laboratories. The sterilizer used for this purpose is known as an "autoclave." The objects to be sterilized are exposed to steam, at a pressure of 15 pounds, for 20 to 30 minutes. The temperature rises to 120° C., enough to destroy spores and thermophilic bacteria. The modern autoclave is a double-jacketed drum. The objects to be sterilized are placed in the inner compartment, flowing steam is introduced and allowed to replace the air, and the door of the autoclave is securely shut. Steam continues to enter the compartment, is allowed to build up a pressure of 15 pounds, and is kept at this pressure for about ½ hour. The pressure is then released, and the steam is replaced by air which is kept hot by the steam jacket. This dries off the condensed steam, and the sterilized objects are dry when removed. This method of sterilization is excellent for gowns, caps, and masks, which must be dry before use. It is also of advantage in the sterilization of equipment used for intravenous treatment, since it destroys thermophilic bacteria and thus prevents reactions with fever after treatment.

Dry Heat

Dry-heat sterilization is not used to any great extent, since it ordinarily requires a higher temperature. For safe sterilization with dry heat, the temperature should be raised to 160° C. and kept there for 1 to 1½ hours. So high a temperature usually destroys fabrics. Its use is, therefore, limited to objects made of metal or glass. Even for such objects it is not commonly used, since autoclaving is just as good and much more convenient. A common use of dry heat is the flaming of a platinum loop in a Bunsen burner by bacteriologists, prior to using it in transferring colonies from one medium to another or to a slide. Another use of dry heat is *incineration,* which is a safe way to dispose of dressings, sputum cups, and paper tissues.

Drying

While drying has a tendency to destroy bacteria, exposure to air does not completely dry microorganisms. Most of them survive in dust for fairly long periods of time. As a matter of fact, the drying of organisms from the frozen state (lyophilization) is a method commonly used in the laboratory to preserve them alive for long periods of time. They must be kept at a very low temperature.

Sunlight

The destructive effect of sunlight on bacteria depends on its content of ultraviolet rays. Obviously, the more intense the sunlight the greater the germicidal effect. Since smoke, clouds, dust, and even glass screen out a good deal of the ultraviolet, and since the microorganisms in bodily discharges are protected by mucus or other organic material, the effect of the sun in sterilizing is not complete.

ULTRAVIOLET RAYS

Bacteria adequately exposed to ultraviolet rays will be destroyed. There are commercially available mercury-vapor lamps which act as a source of ultraviolet light. They are used in some laboratories to sterilize serums and vaccines. It is important to spread the fluid to be sterilized in a very thin layer so that there is complete and uniform exposure.

There has been a great deal of experimentation with the use of ultraviolet light for the sterilization of the air in classrooms, operating rooms, nurseries, and other places. Claims have been made that such irradiation reduces or abolishes air-borne infection. There are a number of conflicting reports on its efficacy. A final determination of its value in reducing air-borne infections cannot be made at present.

Chemical Agents

There is a greater variation in the reactions of microorganisms to chemical than to physical agents. The heat of boiling water will destroy all organisms, but a chemical may be lethal to one organism and not to another. Furthermore, in the use of chemical agents as disinfectants, a number of factors must be considered, such as the concentration of the chemical, the presence or absence of salts in the solution, the temperature, the acidity or alkalinity, and the presence or absence of pus or other organic material protecting the organisms from intimate contact with the chemical. Various methods have been introduced to determine the disinfecting power of chemicals, but, on account of the difficulty of controlling all the variables, none has been found satisfactory.

The introduction by Lister, in 1865, of a carbolic acid spray to sterilize infected wounds and the areas around them was followed by tremendous enthusiasm for antiseptic solutions and great confidence in their power of destroying germs. For many years later, even after the principles of asepsis had been demonstrated and accepted, people still sprayed Lysol and carbolic solutions in sickrooms, and hung up sheets soaked in an antiseptic solution to kill off the germs. Even today, the presence of a basin of Lysol solution on a ward or in a cubicle gives more confidence to many people than the presence of soap and running water. No antiseptic solution takes the place of cleanliness. A nurse who understands good housekeeping is far superior to one who has learned the phenol coefficient of various disinfectants.

METALS

One of the commonest metallic disinfectants in use is mercury. In the form of bichloride, it has been used for many years in a solution of 1:10,000 to 1:1,000. It is not bactericidal but bacteriostatic; it does not kill bacteria, but inhibits their growth. Various compounds of mercury, such as Mercurochrome and Metaphen, are more commonly used today. Like bichloride of mercury, they are bacteriostatic rather than bactericidal.

PHENOL

Phenol is one of the first disinfectants to be used. It kills most common bacteria. However, it is toxic to man, and does not destroy the viruses.

CRESOL

Cresol solutions, such as *Lysol,* are used more than the phenols today because they are less toxic, keep well, and are moderately priced. In a solution of about 1:200 they kill the common pathogens in 10 to 15 minutes. They do not, however, kill spores, nor are they effective against many of the viruses.

FORMALIN

Formalin is a solution of 37 per cent formaldehyde gas in water and methyl alcohol. It will kill the common bacteria in a 10 per cent solution and will even kill spores in a 5 per cent solution in about $1\frac{1}{2}$ hours. It is used to disinfect sputum of tuberculosis patients and is also recommended to disinfect shoes infected with the fungi of athlete's foot. Its effect on viruses has not been clearly defined.

ALCOHOL

In a concentration of 70 per cent, alcohol is a weak germicide against the common bacteria but is not effective against spores, nor is it very effective against the viruses. Absolute alcohol and solutions of less than 50 per cent are ineffective as germicides. The alcohol commonly used is grain or ethyl alcohol. Isopropyl alcohol is being used more and more. Used externally, it is nontoxic, about twice as germicidal as ethyl alcohol, and less corrosive for instruments. It should be used in full strength. Both ethyl and isopropyl alcohol are frequently used to disinfect thermometers after they have been cleaned. Alcohol evaporates and should be kept in a covered receptacle.

CHLORINE

One of the most widely used of chemical disinfectants, chlorine is employed chiefly for the purification of water and in the treatment of sewage. For common household or hospital disinfection, the gas is combined with lime to form chlorinated lime or bleaching powder. It is also sold as a solution. Chlorine is an excellent germicidal agent, even in high dilutions, and is effective against spores and viruses as well as vegetative bacteria. Unfortunately, both the dry powder and the solution deteriorate rapidly. The powder should be kept dry and stored in the cold. The liquid should be tightly stoppered and kept in a dark bottle. In the presence of organic matter the efficiency of chlorine as a germicide is depressed. Chlorine is used to a large extent on dairy farms and in pasteurizing plants to sterilize milking equipment after it has been washed.

IODINE

Iodine is a good disinfectant. Tincture of iodine is a 7 per cent solution of iodine in alcohol. It is the best skin disinfectant. However, it is irritating and stains the skin. Mild tincture of iodine is the commonly used iodine and is a solution of 2 per cent metallic iodine and 2½ per cent sodium iodide in 50 per cent alcohol. It is less irritating than the stronger solution but is nevertheless a good germicide for the skin.

SOAP

Soap is somewhat bactericidal. Its benefits are due to its cleansing properties and to the fact that bacteria are held in the lather until washed away.

SYNTHETIC DETERGENTS

Many synthetic detergents are on the market. They are generally effective against pathogenic organisms in high dilution, are fairly cheap, and nontoxic. Two detergents used widely are *Zephiran Chloride* and *Roccal*. Both are mixtures of alkyl-dimethyl-benzyl ammonium chlorides, the former more refined, the latter somewhat cruder. They can be used in dilutions of 1:20,000 to 1:40,000.

VAPORS

The use of germicidal vapors, in the form of a fine spray, as a sterilizing agent for air in rooms and wards has been experimented with for a number of years. There are many difficulties to overcome in its practical application. Sprays of *triethylene glycol* give the best results. However, the final word about its effectiveness has not been said.

Application of Aseptic Techniques

Medical aseptic techniques have been formulated for the purpose of limiting and controlling the spread of microorganisms from the infected patient to others around him. Not only should the measures be effective; they should be adaptable to the situation at hand as well as rational in application. They must be simple and easy to carry out and economical in time, materials, and costs. The techniques should be such as to prevent the spread of infection to other patients and to the nurse. They should also prevent other types of infection from reaching the patient.

The basic procedures that should be carried out are those relating to hand washing; use of gowns, masks, and caps; collection and disposal of bodily wastes; care of thermometers; care of linen, dishes, and equipment; and care of floors and furniture.

Hand Washing

In all nursing situations the importance of hand washing cannot be overemphasized. For proper hand-washing technique, it is essential to have running hot and cold water, towels, and sinks provided with foot or knee controls. In homes where sinks are provided with hand faucets only, paper squares may be used to turn the water on; or better still, the faucets may be turned on by hand and then soaped and washed while the nurse's hands are lathered.

Soap still seems to be the simplest and most economical detergent to use. A number of newer detergents are advertised for their disinfectant value. It must not be forgotten that the main reason for hand washing is to remove foreign matter mechanically and thoroughly.

Dispensers for either powdered or liquid soap appear suitable. In actual use they are hard to keep clean, require periodic refilling, and frequently become clogged. The use of the old-fashioned cake of soap is still considered the best method for hand washing.

The use of a hand brush is not advised. It irritates the skin by its scratching, it is difficult to keep clean, and it adds to expense without giving compensating advantages. In homes where running water is not available, washbasins occasionally must be used. Where hand-washing facilities are not easily accessible, it is preferable to walk through several rooms to reach a sink with running hot and cold water. In hospitals, washbasins should not be tolerated for hand washing.

TECHNIQUE OF HAND WASHING

If long sleeves are worn, roll up sleeves to the elbow. Remove watch and
    rings.
Standing away from the sink, turn on the faucets until the temperature of
    the water is comfortable.
Place hands under the running water and, firmly cupping the cake of soap,
    lather hands and arms up to the elbow.
Scrub hands, one with the other, using friction.
Rinse under running water from above down to the fingers.
Resoap hands and lather again, giving special attention to nails and areas
    between fingers.
Dry hands thoroughly. Apply hand lotion, if desired.
The minimum time required for proper hand washing is approximately
    1½ minutes.

GOWN TECHNIQUE

Discard method

If a gown is to be discarded after use, no special technique is necessary
for putting a clean gown on. The right side should be lapped over the
left side, the tapes of the belt crossed in back, brought together in front
and tied securely.

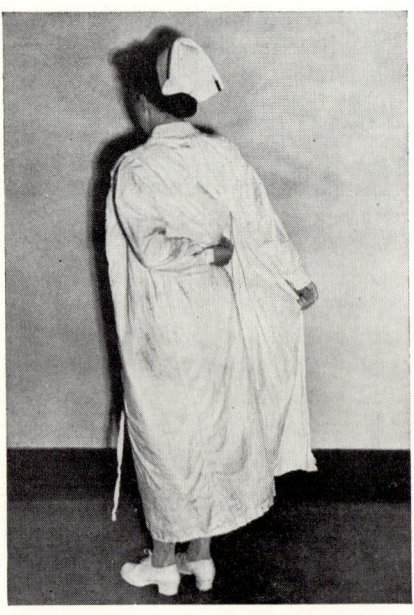

Fig. III. DISCARD GOWN TECH-
NIQUE: Putting the Clean Gown On.
There is no special method in putting
a clean gown on. The right side of
gown is lapped over the left side.

Fig. IV. DISCARD GOWN TECHNIQUE: Removing Gown.

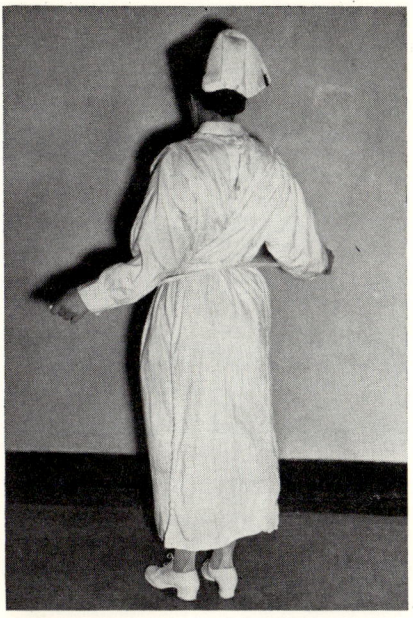

Step 1. Untying belt and bringing the ends forward.

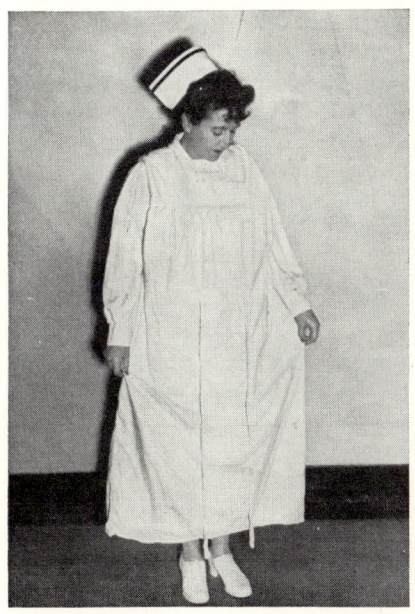

Step 2. Loosening the gown from the body.

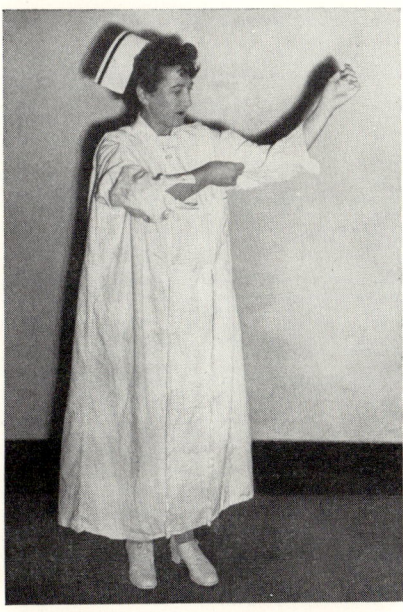

Step 3. Tucking the sleeve into uniform.

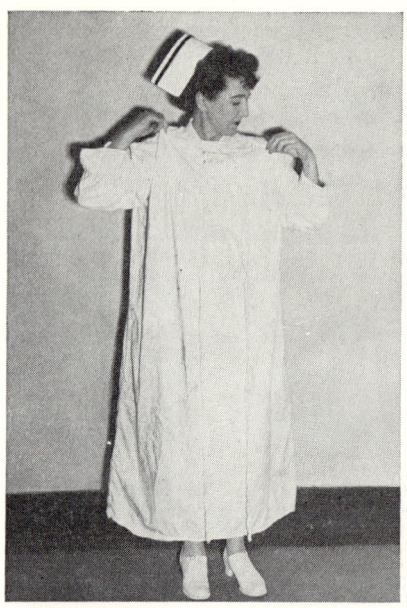

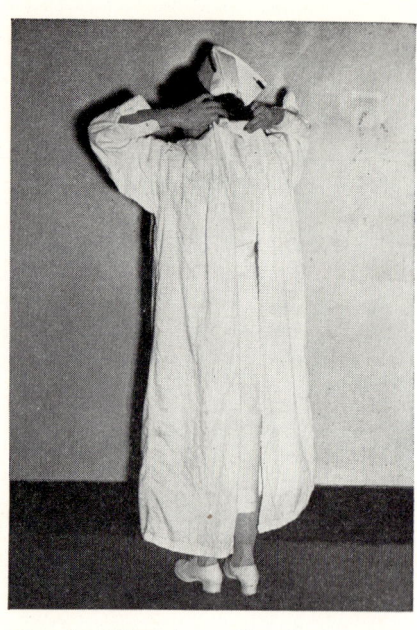

Step 4. Grasping the yoke of gown and working hands toward back of gown.

Step 5. Lifting the neckband away from the body and preparing to open gown.

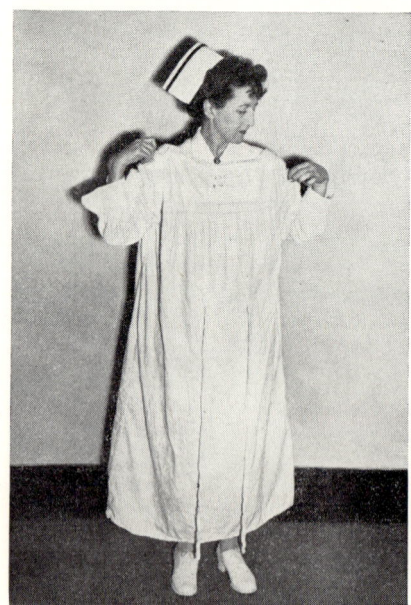

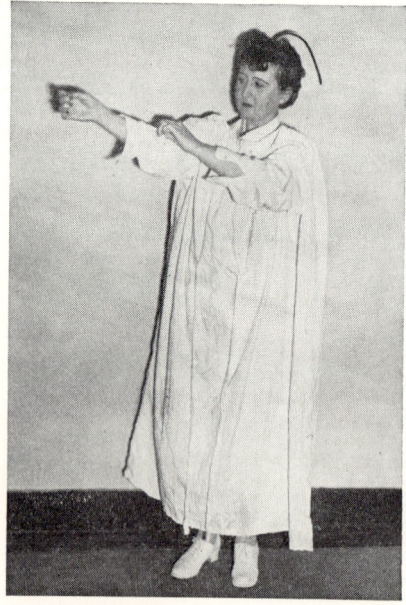

Step 6. Bringing the contaminated ends of the neckband toward the front of shoulders.

Step 7. Removing gown.

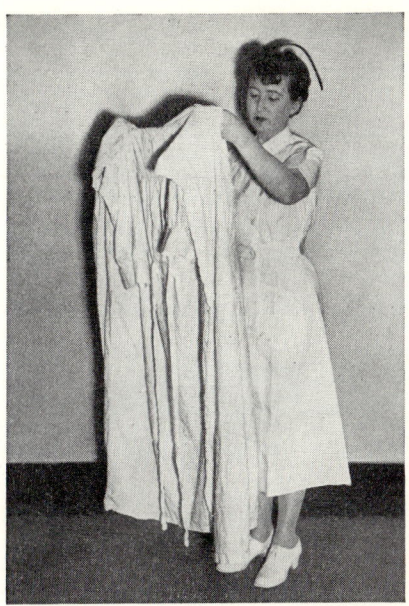

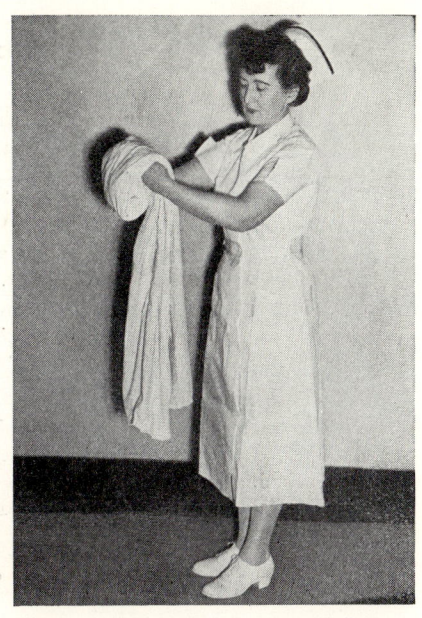

Step 8. Turning gown inside out, after removal and covering contaminated side.

Step 9. Rolling gown, keeping hands inside.

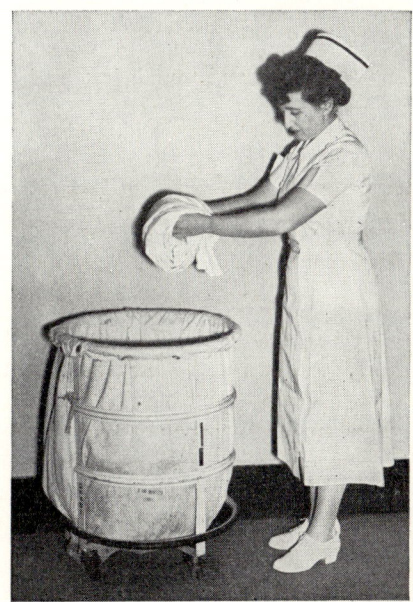

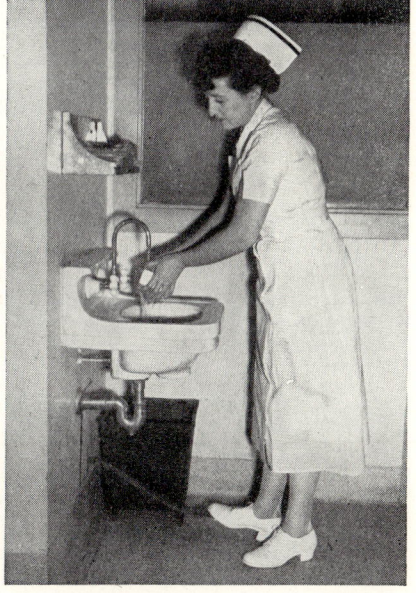

Step 10. Placing rolled gown in hamper.

Step 11. Washing hands for 1½ minutes after discarding gown.

Fig. IV. DISCARD GOWN TECHNIQUE. Removing Gown. (Continued)

Removing the gown

Untie belt in front of waist line and loop the ends under at each side.
Unbutton wrist band and push sleeves up to the elbow, tucking under
cuff of uniform.

Place fingers in center and below neckband and work around until
button hole or tapes are reached.

Unbutton or loosen tie tapes at neckband, and bring ends of neckband
forward to front of shoulders.

Lower arms. Slip out of gown, and turn inside out.

Roll and place in hamper designated for gowns.

Wash hands and forearms for 1½ minutes.

Unit gown method

The same gown can be used and left in the patient unit if a clean gown
is not possible for each contact with the patient and if the supply of gowns
is limited. Gowns should be changed whenever they become wet or soiled,
and at least twice a week, depending on the number of nurses using the
same gown.

Putting the contaminated gown on

Wash hands thoroughly.

Facing the patient in the unit, open gown at back of neckband with
palms of hands which are clasped together. Remove from hook. Separate gown by placing one hand in each armhole.

With index fingers at each armhole seam, support neckband at shoulder
seams.

Grasp the gown material firmly with the hands and thumb just below
neckband, and pull neckband into shape.

Grasping the inner side of left shoulder seam with right hand, pull over
left arm so that left side of gown fits comfortably over the shoulder.

Draw up right side of gown, elevate both arms and shake so that cuffs
drop below elbows.

Placing fingers inside center front of neckband, straighten and button.

Button cuffs—Fold wrist band holding securely with rubber band, twine
or bandage. If bandage or tape is used, loop at end. Place around cuff,
draw end through loop and tuck under.

Bring outer hem of back of gown together and extend away from body.

Transferring the edges to the left hand, roll gown with right hand from
waistline to hem.

Holding the roll in place with one hand, bring belt around waist crossing
in back and tie securely in front.

Removing the contaminated gown

Untie belt in front of gown, pull tapes and loop in front to prevent
touching floor.

Remove rubber bands or bandages and place on hook.

Unbutton cuff, raise hand immediately, turning open part of cuff away
from body.

Tuck sleeve under cuff of uniform to prevent slipping. Repeat procedure
for other sleeve.

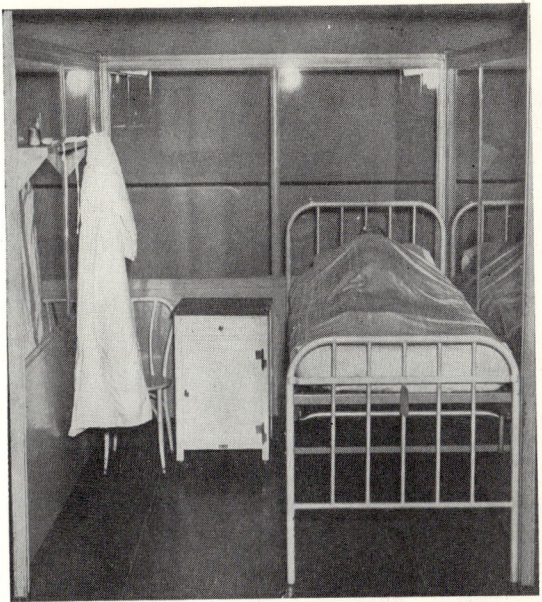

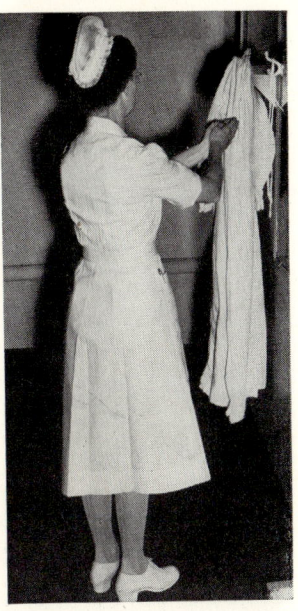

Fig. V. UNIT GOWN TECHNIQUE: Putting Contaminated Gown On.
Step. 1. Position of gown in unit.

Step 2. Preparing to grasp inner surface of gown at hook level, with palms of clean hands together.

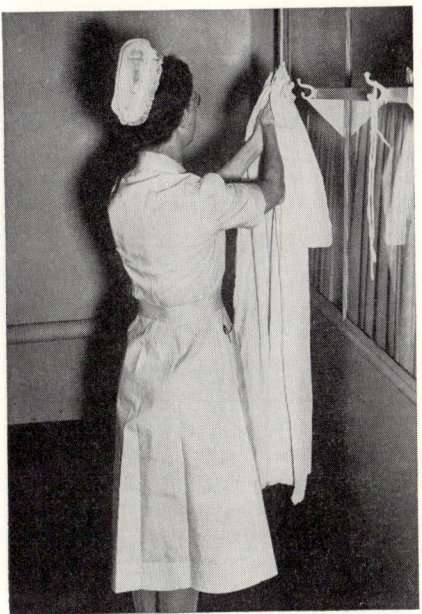

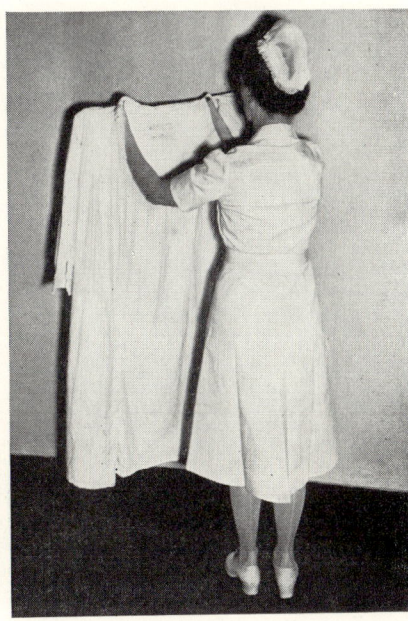

Step 3. Removing gown from hook.

Step 4. Spreading gown open, fingers extended in shoulder seam, thumb supporting neckband.

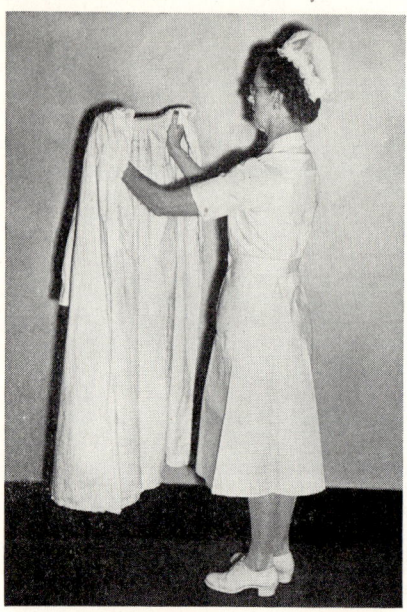

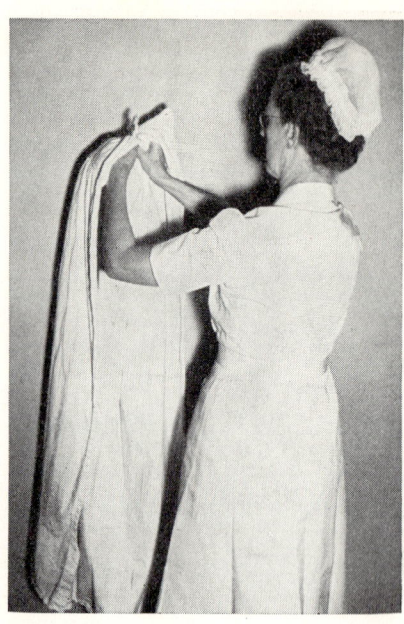

Step 5. Making fist along shoulder seams, thumbs supporting neckband, and stretching tightly.

Step 6. Bringing the gown together and preparing to draw on sleeve.

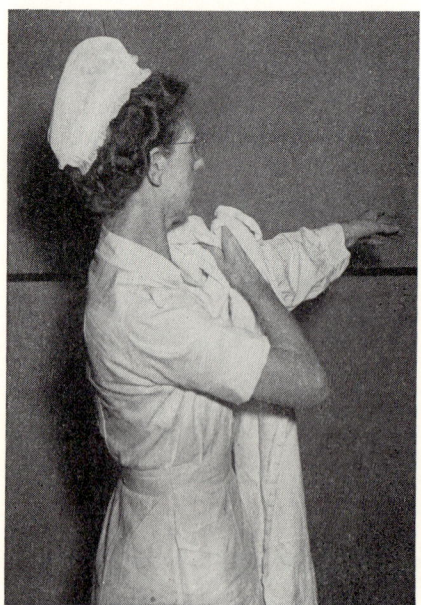

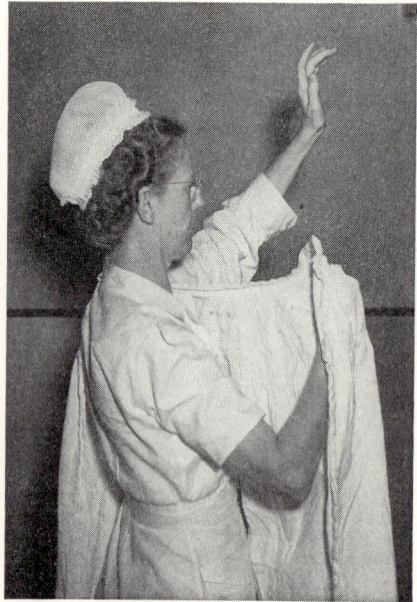

Step 7. Drawing left sleeve on shoulder.

Step 8. Shaking left sleeve to midforearm and preparing to put on right sleeve.

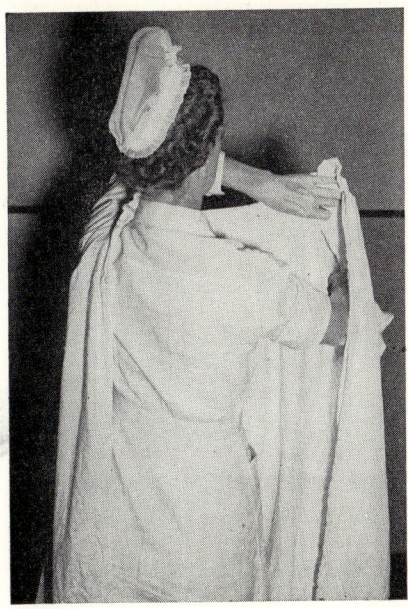

Step 9. Drawing right sleeve on.

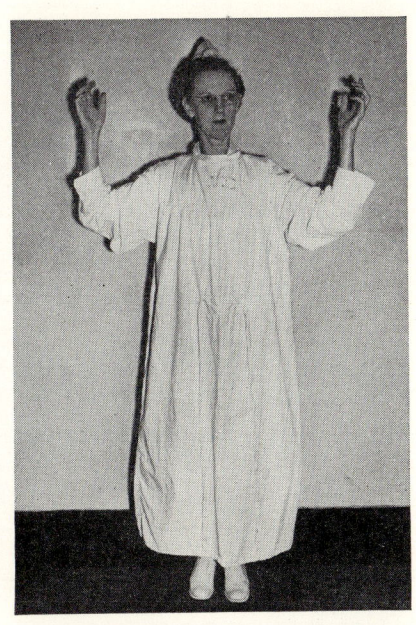

Step 10. Position of sleeves immediately before buttoning gown.

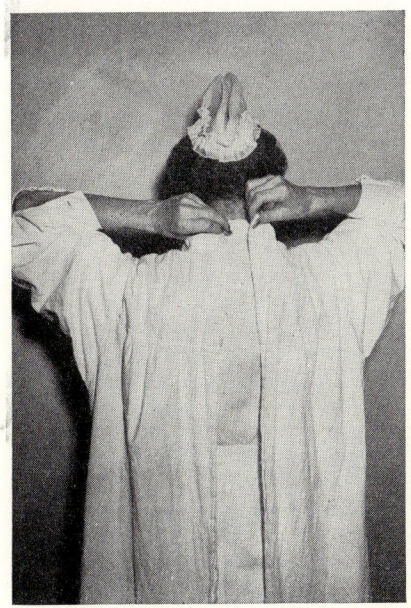

Step 11. Buttoning neckband.

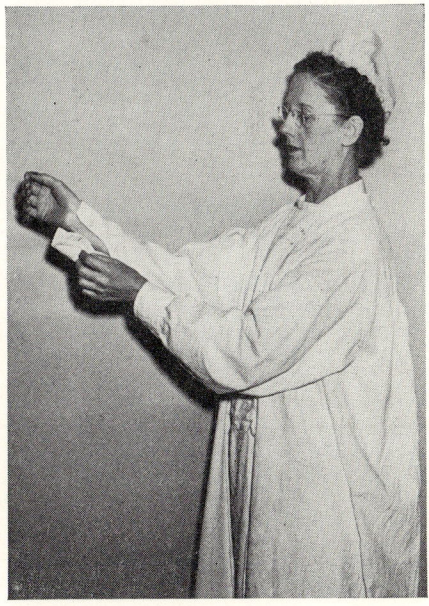

Step 12. Buttoning both cuffs.

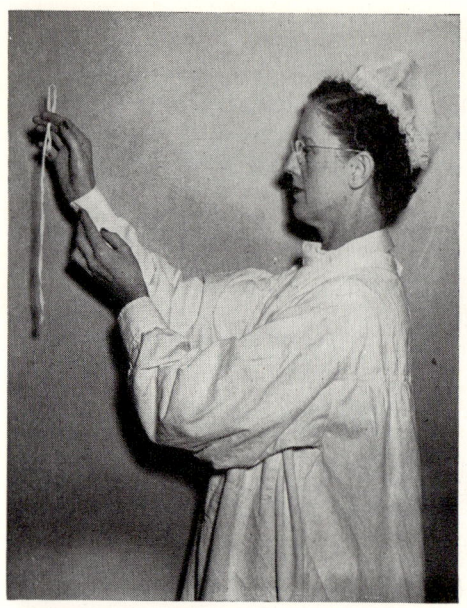

Step 13. Folding cuff to fit wrist and applying tape.

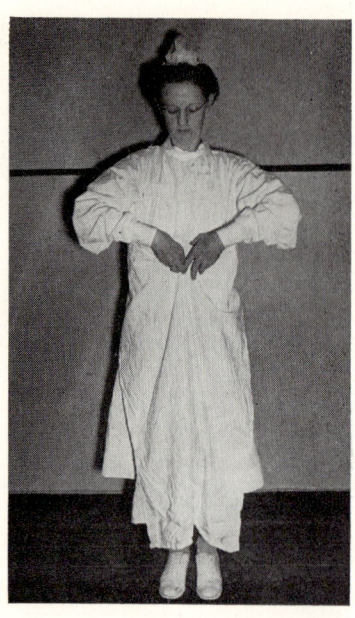

Step 14. Grasping gown at side seams and bringing to center front.

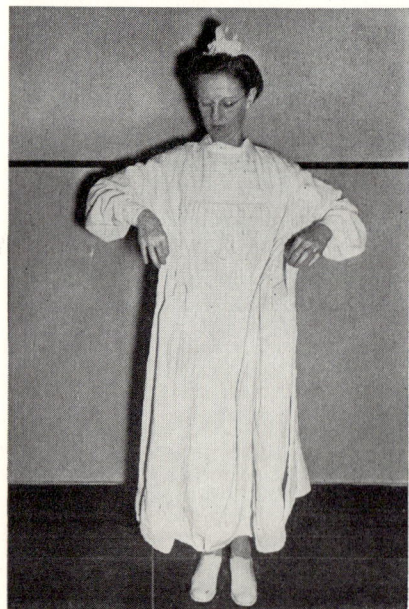

Step 15. Grasping outer contaminated edges of gown.

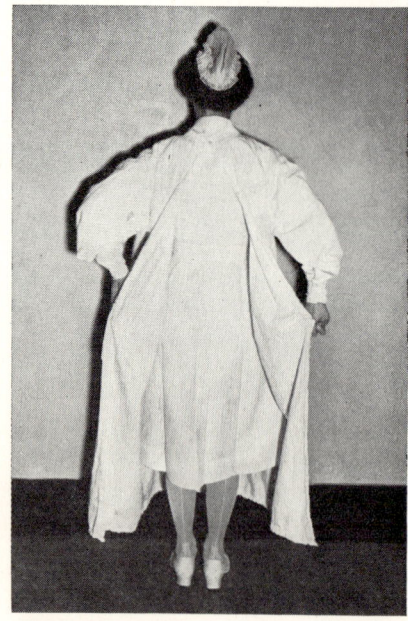

Step 16. Extending gown outward and bringing clean edges together.

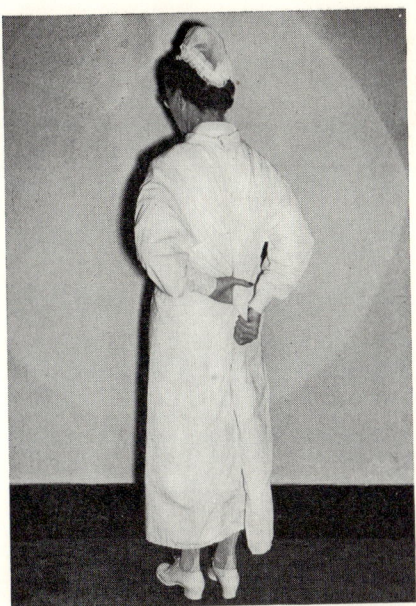

Step 17. Rolling the back of gown.

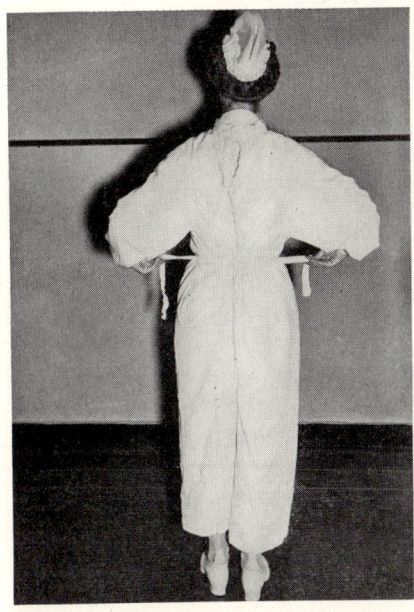

Step 18. Crossing belt ties in back to secure roll.

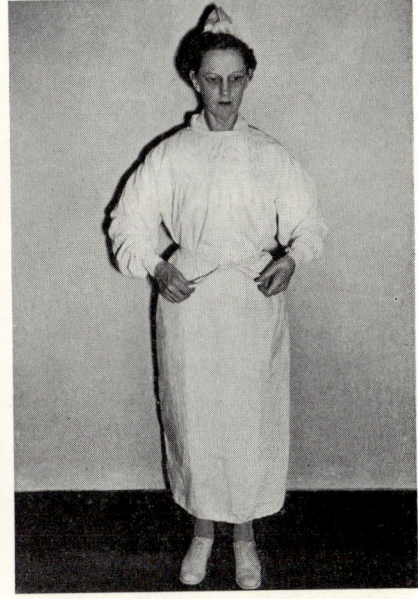

Step 19. Tying belt in front.

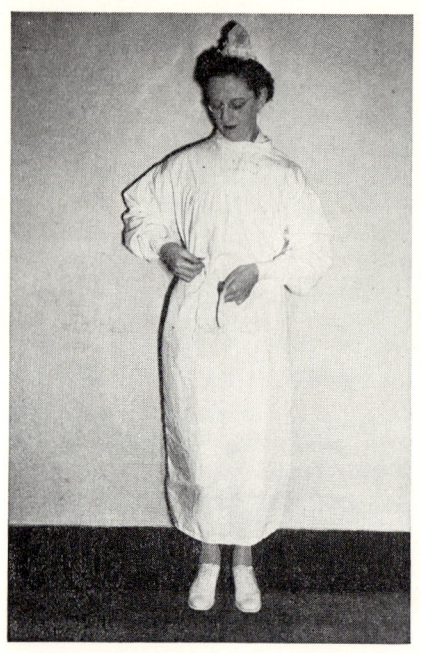

Fig. VI. UNIT GOWN TECHNIQUE: Removing Gown.
Step 1. Looping belt at sides.

Step 2. Removing wrist tapes.

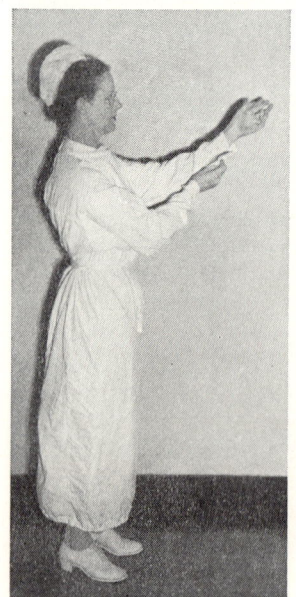

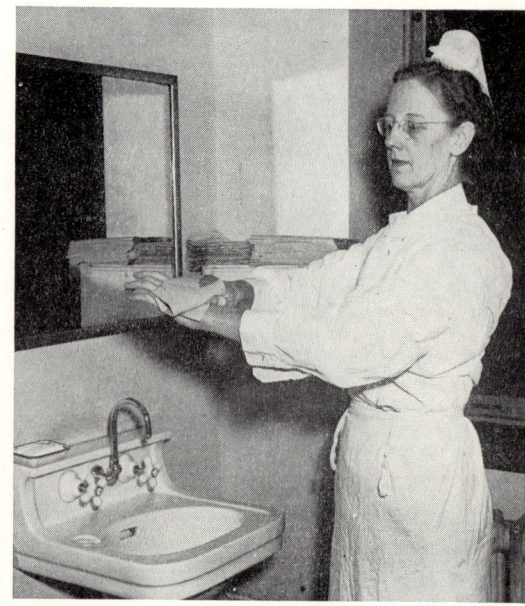

Step 3. Unbuttoning cuff.

Step 4. Drying hands after handwashing.

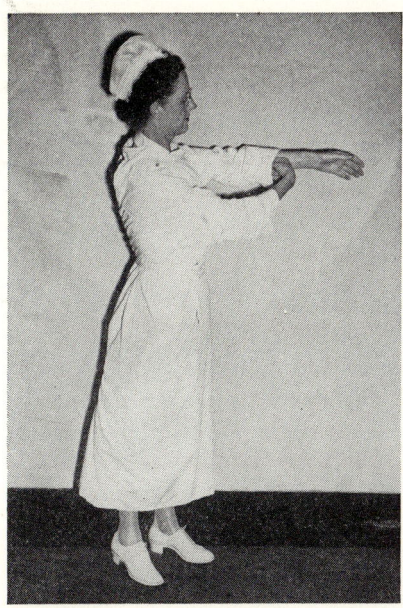

Step 5. Preparing to pull left sleeve down after neckband is unbuttoned.

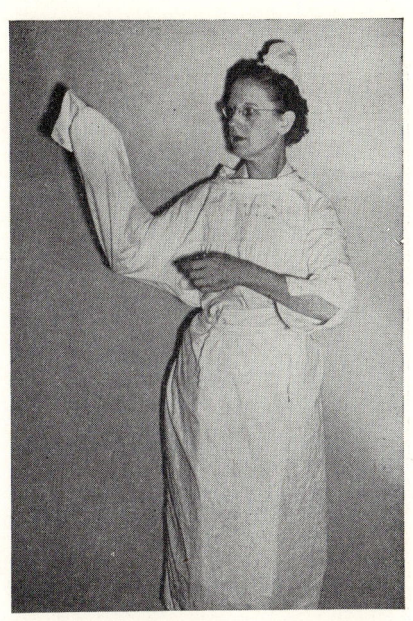

Step 6. Showing gown-covered hand.

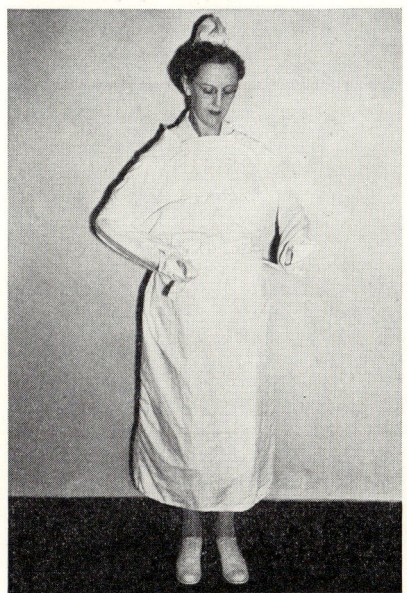

Step 7. Preparing to pull belt loops.

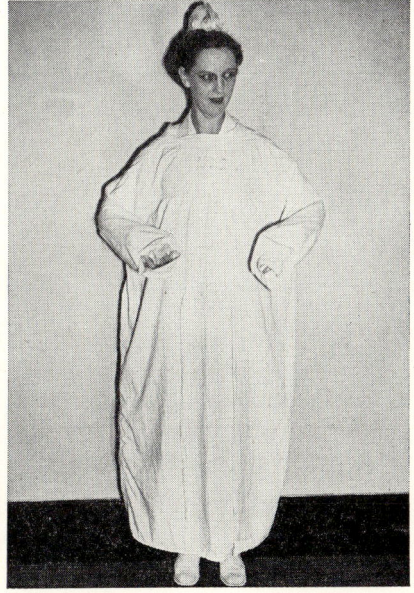

Step 8. Belt loosened.

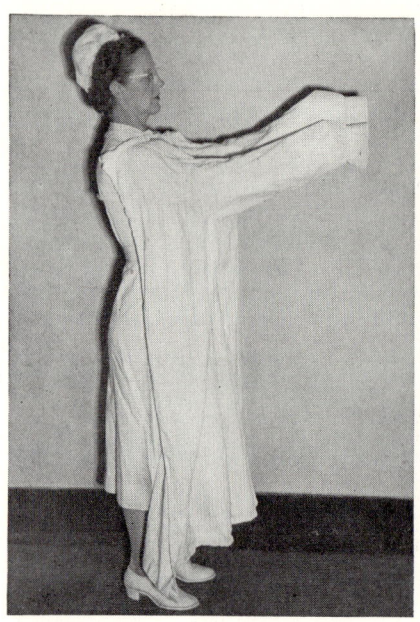

Step 9. Slipping out of gown.

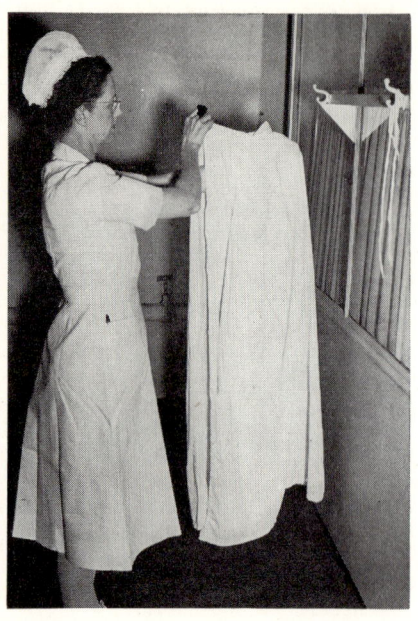

Step 10. Preparing to hang gown (a).

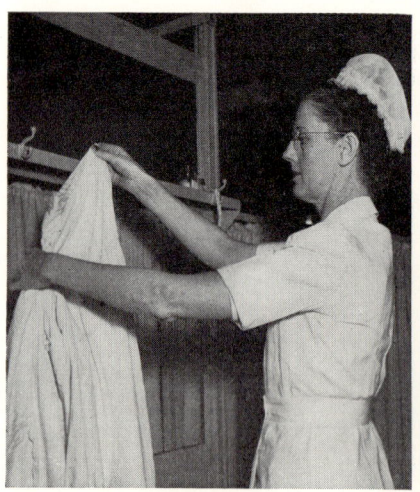

Step 11. Preparing to hang gown (b).

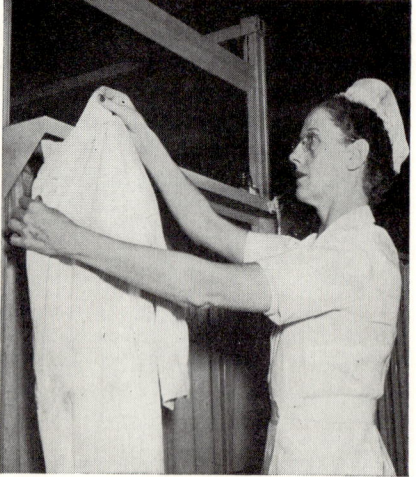

Step 12. Hanging gown on hook.

Wash hands approximately 1½ minutes.

Place the fingers of each hand inside center front of neckband and work around until button is reached. Unbutton or loosen tapes.

Place fingers of right hand inside of left sleeve below cuff, pull sleeve well over left hand so it is fully covered.

Release ends of belt allowing to drop in front. Pull right sleeve of gown forward and repeat, using covered right hand for pulling the left sleeve from shoulders.

Slip out of gown and place index fingers at each armhole seam.

Support neckband. Grasp material below with clenched fingers and thumb and pull into shape.

With neckband in upright position, and opening of gown facing entrance to the unit, bring the two inside edges together at the neckband.

Hold neckband at button hole, with one hand and insert other hand inside of gown along shoulder and armhole seams.

Cup armholes over hook at shoulder seams and adjust into proper position. The edges of the gown at back should be together and placed in position with opening away from patient. The neckband should be slanted at an angle.

Wash hands and forearms for 1½ minutes.*

In many homes or in some general hospital units hooks are not available. A standard may be used or the gown may be folded in reverse with contaminated side of the gown folded inside and placed in a large paper bag and left in the unit.

Masks

A mask that is carefully constructed and properly used probably serves as a protective measure for the nurse in caring for certain cases of respiratory disease. This is especially true if there is danger that she will inhale organisms of considerable virulence expelled by the patient in coughing or sneezing. The routine use of a mask is of doubtful benefit. Where a mask will protect a nurse from a patient's respiratory discharges, it may be more logical to have the patient rather than the nurse wear the mask while she is giving bedside care. A more extended discussion on masks will be found on pages 147-150.

If a mask is worn, it should cover the nose as well as the mouth and should be discarded after use. The practice of letting masks hang around the neck for a good part of the day, or of stuffing them into a pocket and then wearing them again, is a pernicious one. Masks, if worn, should be changed frequently, and especially after they have become wet.

An effective mask is made of gauze having 42 by 42 strands to the

* Adapted from Nursing Procedures, Kingston Avenue Hospital, Brooklyn, N.Y.

square inch. Two layers of gauze, 8 by 24 inches, are folded into 8 by 8 squares. They are stitched securely, and tapes are attached at each corner.

MASK TECHNIQUE

Putting the mask on. Masks with two sets of strings are more comfortable and secure than masks made with one set of strings.
Wash hands thoroughly.
Placing mask well over the nose and mouth, bring upper tapes over the ears and tie on top of head.
Bring lower tapes under the chin and tie at back of neck.
Removing the mask
Wash hands.
Unfasten tapes and hold mask by the tapes.
Drop in receptacle.
Wash hands thoroughly.

Caps

The wearing of caps contributes little to the protection of the nurse or patient, except in a few conditions, like pediculosis, where there is danger of transmission. If caps are worn, they should cover the hair completely. Ordinarily, a hair net is useful to keep short ends in place and eliminate the danger of brushing aside loose ends with contaminated hands. Caps are made of muslin or double thicknesses of gauze.

Collection and Disposal of Body Wastes

SECRETIONS FROM NOSE AND THROAT

Secretions from the nose and throat should be collected in paper tissues and placed in a paper bag pinned to the side of the bed. The bag can be collected at intervals, wrapped securely, and burned in an incinerator. It is important to teach patients, when coughing, to use tissues and to cover the nose and mouth. If the discharge is copious, two or more thicknesses should be used. If no facilities for burning are available, the tissues may be dropped into the toilet bowl and flushed away. The paper bag is then wrapped securely and disposed with the regular waste.

SPUTUM

Heavy waxed-paper cups with adjustable covers in metal ring holders should be provided for patients who are coughing and expectorating large amounts. Prior to collection, sawdust placed in the cup will help to absorb the liquid as well as prevent spilling. The cup should have the lid securely fastened before placing in a bag or other suitable receptacle for incineration. The metal holders should be washed with soap and water, and boiled at least once or twice a week.

In most hospitals the collection of the sputum cups is usually assigned to an attendant. In some hospitals the placing of the sputum cup in the paper bag is also done by the attendant, who then puts the bag on his collecting cart. A large cardboard box placed on the collecting cart may be substituted for the paper bag. The attendant then goes from bed to bed, collects the sputum cups, handling them with a paper towel or tissues, and places them directly in the cardboard box. When this is filled, the cover is put on and the box is incinerated.

In some hospitals the attendant is required to wear rubber gloves during the collection. In others, gloves are not worn, for fear that the attendant may have a false sense of security and not take proper precautions in the handling of the sputum cups.

VOMITUS

Vomitus may be emptied directly into the hopper or toilet, and the basin then washed and boiled.

URINE AND FECES

Urine and feces may be emptied directly into the hopper or toilet and the bedpan or urinal then washed and sterilized. The latter is effectively done in a combination washer and sterilizer. If the toilet is water-flushed and connected with a sewer or septic tank, all stools may be emptied into it. Where toilets are not so connected, infected stools, particularly those from patients with typhoid and paratyphoid A and B fevers, should be emptied into a covered can containing a disinfectant such as 5 per cent chlorinated lime or 2½ per cent cresol solution, allowed to stand for about 1 hour, and then emptied into the toilet. For stools from poliomyelitis and infectious hepatitis cases, the chlorinated lime solution is preferable. The stool should be well broken up with a wooden spatula or spoon so that the solution reaches all parts of it.

SOILED DRESSINGS

Soiled dressings, tongue depressors, and applicators should be placed in a paper bag or wrapped in newspaper. The wrapped newspaper or bag should be incinerated or disposed in waste cans.

Thermometers

After use, thermometers should be cleaned with two cotton pledgets moistened with soap, using friction. They should then be rinsed under cool running water, dried, and placed in a covered dish containing isopropyl alcohol, ethyl alcohol 70 per cent, Zephiran Chloride, 1:1,000 solution, or Lysol, 2½ per cent.

Linen

The nurse collects linen in a discarded pillowcase fastened over the back of a chair or crib. The fastened pillowcase is then placed in a special hamper which is brought to the door of the ward or room. If the hamper is kept in the utility room, the nurse takes the pillowcase there after she is through with her ward work and after she has washed her hands and removed her gown. After placing the filled pillowcase in the hamper, she washes her hands again.

Dishes

The tray is taken to the bedside of the patient by an attendant or the nurse and placed on the bedside table. No gown need be worn by the attendant or nurse. If the patient has to be fed, his tray is served last, and the nurse will wear a gown if it is indicated. When the tray is removed, it is taken to the common kitchen. There is no need for a special kitchen, though part of the general kitchen may be allocated for dishes from patients with communicable disease.

Equipment

Instruments commonly used in the examination of patients, such as a stethoscope, otoscope, ophthalmoscope, head mirror, flashlight, sphygmomanometer, and percussion hammer, should be kept on a special tray. After use, the instrument should be cleaned with soap and water, rinsed, and dried. The same procedures may be used for washable toys, rubber sheets, and bedsteads. Articles like books, mattresses, and pillows should be aired, preferably in the sun, for several hours.

Dust Suppression

The important consideration in the care of furniture and floors is to see that no dust is raised while they are being cleaned. Experiments in the control of air-borne infections indicate that droplets coming from the mouth or nose of an infected person may settle on blankets, floors, and furniture and later be swept up in the dust to become dispersed in the air and infect others. It is therefore essential that no dry dusting be allowed. Oiling of floors and furniture is much the best way of suppressing dust, since the dust adheres to the oiled surface. Such oiling of floors is now commonplace in many hospitals and large buildings, which use oiling machines. Only a thin film should adhere to the floor, so that it does not become slippery. The oil companies have developed special oils for this purpose; they give technical directions for the amounts to be used per unit of surface, and how frequently reoiling is necessary.

Oil is also used to impregnate blankets. This keeps dust from rising from the blankets when they are handled or touched. This quality is retained even after laundering.

Letters

There is little risk in transmitting disease through letters or signed documents even if these are not disinfected. Before writing the letters or signing the documents the patient should wash his hands.

Visitors

Visitors may be or become carriers of disease and thus transfer infection from the patient to others or from others to the patient. They should wear gowns and masks when these are indicated for nurses, and the visiting time should be limited.

REFERENCES

1. Dubos, R. J.: *Bacterial and Mycotic Infections of Man,* J. B. Lippincott Company, Philadelphia, 1948.
2. McCulloch, E. C.: *Disinfection and Sterilization,* Lea & Febiger, Philadelphia, 1945.
3. New York State Department of Health: *Guide for the Handling of Communicable Disease in General Hospitals,* 1950.
4. Winthrop-Stearns Inc.: *Zephiran Chloride,* New York, N.Y., March, 1951.

Chapter 7 HOSPITAL MANAGEMENT OF COMMUNICABLE DISEASE

THE management of communicable diseases in our modern hospitals has achieved such a measure of safety that the facilities of the special hospital are being utilized for other services. In former years special hospitals were established for a number of specific conditions, namely for skin diseases, eye, ear, nose, and throat diseases, and for crippled children. Similarly, hospitals were established for contagious diseases. The continuance of special-purpose hospitals appears illogical. The human organism is an entity. It is not made up of a group of dissociated tissues. For example, an abnormal condition of the skin or eye may be a symptom of a general body disorder. Individuals entering a hospital for a local condition should always receive a general physical examination and should be treated as persons and not as cases.

Historically, control of communicable disease was largely a matter of isolation and quarantine. With increased knowledge, the emphasis has been shifted to control of the environment, prophylactic immunization, and specific treatment with drugs or antibiotics. The need for isolation still exists, but the rigidity varies for different communicable diseases. General hospitals can arrange their facilities to provide strict isolation for certain cases and modified isolation for others. The physical layout should be specifically designated. It may comprise an organized unit in the medical and pediatric divisions, private rooms with adjoining bath, a section of the open wards, or a specially constructed unit with cubicles.

There are other reasons why the isolation hospital is no longer considered a necessity. Patients with communicable disease frequently require the services and facilities of the various specialties, just as do patients with other illnesses. These are not always available in a special hospital. Furthermore, the reduction in the number of patients admitted to special hospitals and the seasonal nature of many diseases creates uneven demands for space and service. In addition, the general cost of operating the hospital continues as usual.

Integration of communicable diseases into general hospital services has real educational value. Opportunities are provided for visiting physicians and medical and nursing students to learn about the care of patients suffering from these diseases. In addition, many other types of services are readily available so that patients can receive better and more complete medical and nursing care. Steps and procedures for effective follow-up of patients from hospital to home can also be more systematically instituted for continuous supervision.

In modern hospital management the lack of graduate professional nurses has become an accepted fact. More and more hospitals must make use of nurses' aides, practical nurses, and others who have had little or no training in giving care to patients. They are, however, able to perform certain ancillary duties which are assigned to them by graduate nurses. Their work must be skillfully directed, and they must be given a planned orientation in the simple techniques of medical asepsis. Only by employing such aids as part of a team, by clearly defining their duties, by properly supervising their work, and by evaluating relationships between all team members can a group work effectively and harmoniously.

Protective Health Measures

Upon entering a communicable-disease service, the nurse should be protected against diseases with which she may come in contact and against which adequate immunization procedures are available. These include vaccination against smallpox and inoculations against typhoid and paratyphoid fevers. If the nurse has a negative Schick test, she need not be immunized against diphtheria. If positive, and she has been previously immunized, she should receive a booster dose of diphtheria toxoid. In the event she has not received any previous immunization, she should receive a preliminary series, as outlined on pages 167–170.

Tuberculin tests should be performed on all nurses. Whether BCG vaccine should be administered to nurses having a negative tuberculin test is a debated question. Most authorities believe that it should be. Nurses with positive tuberculin tests need not be injected. However, all nurses should be X rayed for tuberculosis of least once a year, preferably every 6 months.

Some hospitals have Dick tests performed and immunize nurses with a positive test. Such immunization protects only against the rash of scarlet fever and not against infection with the hemolytic streptococcus. It is therefore of doubtful value and is not recommended.

The question arises whether interns and attendants on communicable-disease services should receive similar protection. There is little doubt that interns come into almost as close contact with patients as nurses do, and it is therefore reasonable to require the same sort of protection for them as for nurses. This holds true also for nurses' aides. Attendants vary in their contact with patients, depending on the work they do. If their contact with patients is a fairly close one, they too should be immunized in the same way as nurses. Gown, cap, mask, and hand-washing techniques should apply to doctors, aides, and attendants as they do to nurses.

A routine X ray of the lungs on admission of patients to the hospital is a recommended practice. Screening patients for tuberculosis is a protection to the medical and nursing staffs against exposure to active tuberculosis. Proper measures against disease spread can be taken and immediate treatment of the patient instituted when disease is discovered.

Educational programs for food handlers are practical and a precautionary measure against outbreaks of food-borne diseases in the hospital. Periodic examination of their stools will help to discover chronic carriers. The orientation should be consistent and planned in accordance with regulations of the local health department.

Communicable Disease Occurring on General Wards

Every hospital, particularly one that has children's wards, has been, at some time, in the embarrassing position of having one or more cases of communicable disease break out on its wards. The disposition of the case is not too difficult. If the disease is one that is highly communicable, the patient is either sent home, transferred to a communicable-disease hospital, or isolated in the general hospital, as outlined above. The question that is occasionally disturbing is what procedure to follow with the contacts in the ward. This depends on the nature of the disease and on the age of the contacts. Except in case of smallpox, nothing need be done if the patient with the communicable disease is on an adult ward. Most adults are immune to the highly communicable diseases— measles, chickenpox, whooping cough, mumps, German measles, and diphtheria. If smallpox occurs, all individuals in the hospital —patients, nurses, doctors, and other personnel—should be vaccinated, and all persons entering the hospital for any reason should be vaccinated until the case is no longer communicable.

If a highly communicable disease occurs on a children's ward, the procedure to be followed, after the case is isolated, will depend on the disease. If the case is measles, all contacts who have not had the disease should be injected with gamma globulin 0.1 cubic centimeter per pound of body weight. New patients may be admitted to the ward. If a secondary case develops, the procedure is repeated for all those who have not been previously injected or who were injected more than 3 weeks before.

No immunizations are available, at present, for children exposed to chickenpox, mumps, or German measles. If a case of one of these diseases occurs on a children's ward, it should be isolated and nothing further done. If two or more cases occur, the ward should be quarantined for a period of 14 days in the case of German measles and chickenpox, and 21 days in the case of mumps. If no further cases occur, quarantine may be lifted.

On most children's wards, Schick tests are performed on admission of all patients. It is therefore known which children are immune to diphtheria and which are not. If a case of diphtheria occurs on a ward, the susceptible children should receive a booster dose of diphtheria toxoid if they have been previously immunized. Otherwise, they should receive a prophylactic dose of diphtheria antitoxin. After the patient has been removed to isolation, all children on the ward should have nose and throat cultures taken. Those with positive cultures should be isolated until their status has been determined, and should not be permitted to return to the ward until two successive negative cultures, not less than 24 hours apart, are obtained from them.

Whooping cough is a serious disease among infants. If a case occurs on a general children's ward, it should be isolated. The remaining children should be given a booster dose of pertussis vaccine if they have been previously immunized. Otherwise, they should receive a prophylactic dose of convalescent pertussis serum or hyperimmune gamma globulin.

Carriers of disease should be isolated in the same manner as are cases of the same disease. Fortunately, carriers of disease germs, in most instances, are only temporary and cease to be carriers when they break contact with the case. There are few diseases in which carriers may exist for long periods of time. Typhoid fever is one of these.

Unit Arrangement

An important aspect in nursing care of the patient is the application of medical aseptic techniques. In order to carry out these procedures, it is necessary to determine in advance the clean areas and those that will be considered contaminated. The contaminated areas consist of the patient's room or cubicle or space sectioned off by screens, and all contents, as well as all sinks, hoppers, and floors.

The clean areas include nurses' offices, corridors, treatment rooms, kitchens, and utility rooms except sinks and hoppers.

Equipment

Each patient, whether in a private room, cubicle, or ward, should be provided with the following equipment:

Bedside table, containing washbasin, curved basin, mouthwash cup, soap and soap dish, comb and toilet articles
Chair
Pitcher and drinking glass for water
Towels and washcloth
Paper tissues and paper bag pinned to the bedside with safety pins

Other necessary supplies may be placed on a small tray and kept on the dresser if the patient is in a private room or on a shelf within the cubicle. Such supplies include clinical thermometer in container, lubricant or cold cream, and a jar of cotton for cleansing the thermometer. To prevent breakage of the bulb, the bottom of the glass container for the thermometer should be protected with cotton or gauze. In an open ward, individual thermometers are often kept in a test tube securely fastened with adhesive to the head or foot of the bed. Individual thermometers are not essential for ward use, providing sufficient thermometers are available for all patients. After temperatures are taken, each thermometer is cleansed with two soaped cotton pledgets, using friction, rinsed under cool running water, dried, and placed for a specified time in a receptacle containing disinfectant solution. After disinfection, they may be dried and stored in a clean container.

If a gown is used, it should be hung on a hook or clothes tree in the private room or cubicle. A standard may be substituted for use in a ward.

There are only a few diseases that are so highly communicable that strict isolation is required. Patients ill with these diseases can be isolated in a separate room or ward. Most of the communicable diseases can be cared for in a general open ward or in a ward with cubicle arrangement. All rooms and wards should have a minimum of furniture, should be clean, cheerful, and well ventilated. A sink with hot and cold running water operated by foot or knee controls should be located within the area.

Three types of units have been suggested for the care of patients with communicable disease: a separate room or ward, a cubicle arrangement, and an open ward. In the discussion which follows, the communicable diseases are listed according to their method of spread, and indications are given for their care in one or more of the three units. In all of the diseases, hand washing by the nurse before and after care of a patient is essential.

Respiratory Diseases

In caring for patients with respiratory disease, the nurse should wear a gown. The use of masks is discussed on pages 147–150. If worn, masks should be changed frequently and discarded when the nurse leaves the unit. Caps are not necessary.

The following diseases have a high rate of communicability and should be treated in a private room or in a ward limited to one disease.

Chickenpox
Diphtheria
German measles
Measles
Mumps
Smallpox
Whooping cough

The following diseases should also be treated in a private room, if possible. However, their communicability is not so great as those of the first group, and they may be treated with safety in permanently constructed cubicles in a general ward.

Common cold
Exanthem subitum (roseola infantum)
Hepatitis, infectious
Influenza
Meningococcus meningitis
Pneumonia
Poliomyelitis
Psittacosis
Streptococcal infection (including scarlet fever)
Tuberculosis, pulmonary

The three diseases listed below may be treated in an open ward. The first two are hardly ever transmitted from person to person. Rheumatic fever is believed to be related to, but not caused by, the hemolytic streptococcus. Its communicability is doubtful.

Coccidioidomycosis
Histoplasmosis
Rheumatic fever

Enteric Diseases

The diseases in this category are those in which spread is chiefly due to discharges from the enteric tract. None is air-borne, and it is doubtful that the use of gowns by nurses caring for patients is essential, except where the patients are extremely lax and contaminate their bodies or beds with excreta. Hand washing before and after caring for patients is even more important than in the other types of communicable disease. The use of masks and caps is not essential.

The only disease in the group that requires isolation in a separate room or ward is:

Epidemic diarrhea of the newborn

It has become common practice to establish isolation nurseries on maternity services. Epidemic diarrhea of the newborn is highly communicable in nurseries for newborns, and an infant developing this syndrome should be immediately isolated. The nurse in such an isolation room should wear a gown.

The three diseases listed below are preferably treated in cubicles.

Cholera
Typhoid fever
Dysentery, amebic and bacterial

Cholera rarely occurs in this country, and a discussion of its treatment is academic. Typhoid fever is frequently treated on open wards without causing spread. If possible, however, patients should be placed in cubicles.

The remainder of the enteric diseases, which follow, may be treated in an open ward.

Botulism
Brucellosis (undulant fever)
Helminthiasis
Leptospirosis

Contact Diseases

None of the diseases spread by contact or by discharges from mucous membranes requires isolation in a room. Gowns should be worn by the nurses when giving care, except in rabies and tetanus. Caps and masks need not be worn.

The following should be cared for preferably in a cubicle arrangement, although little risk will result from general ward care.

Anthrax
Impetigo contagiosa
Keratoconjunctivitis

Leprosy
Mycoses
Ophthalmia
Trachoma
Venereal diseases

The two diseases listed below are not transmitted from human to human and may be treated in an open ward without special precautions.

Rabies
Tetanus

Diseases Transmitted by Arthropods

In most of the diseases transmitted by insects and other arthropods there is an intermediate host. Transmission is by the arthropod from human to intermediate host to human. With a few exceptions, transmission from human to human does not occur. Patients suffering from these diseases, may, therefore, be treated in an open ward. No gowns, masks, or caps are necessary. Windows should be screened in warm weather.

Two of these diseases are transmitted by insects from human to human. These are:

Pediculosis
Scabies

Patients with these conditions should be isolated in cubicles. Nurses should wear gowns and be meticulous with hand-washing technique. Nurses caring for patients with pediculosis should protect their hair with a cap.

The other diseases, which may be treated in an open ward, are:

Encephalitis
Dengue
Malaria
Plague
Rickettsial diseases
Tularemia
Yellow fever

Outside Contacts

Visiting

Visiting on communicable disease units should be limited in order to avoid transmission of infection from patient to visitor and from visitor to patient. Gowns and masks should be worn by visitors when they are indicated for nurses. A capelike gown with opening for the head is frequently worn. It covers the entire clothing and does not permit freedom of the hands. After leaving the bedside, the cape or gown is removed, and the visitor washes his hands. Personal contact between the visitor and the patient should be avoided except when parents visit a child. In this case, the parent should be permitted to hold and fondle the child. The psychological trauma resulting from an attitude of apparent aloofness is greater than the possible danger of disease transmission. Visitors should not be permitted in nurseries for the newborn. They may see the babies in their cribs through a window or glass partition.

While planned educational programs for visitors in communicable-disease hospitals have been time-consuming and the results questionable, yet there are values in teaching large groups. However, the limitation of visitors' time and the fact that new visitors are always present do not permit continuity. Study and more experimentation are needed in this area, which is an excellent medium for teaching health promotion and protection.

Letters

There is no uniform method of dealing with outgoing letters from patients on communicable-disease services or with documents that must be signed by such patients. Some hospitals take elaborate precautions to sterilize the papers; others do little about them. As stated on page 109, there is very little risk of transmitting disease through letters. If patients are required to wash their hands before writing a letter or signing a document, and if the added precaution is taken of requiring them to wear a mask if they have a respiratory disease, nothing further needs to be done.

Admission and Discharge

Ambulance Technique

If ambulance service is provided by the hospital, the attendant should wear a gown for respiratory diseases and for the other diseases for which a gown has been recommended for nurses. He should also observe the hand-washing techniques outlined above. A sheet, blanket, hospital gown, or pajamas, and paper towels should accompany the attendant on ambulance calls. Time is saved if the materials which the attendant takes with him on ambulance calls are prepared in advance and kept in rolled bundles. Upon arrival at the home, the patient is dressed in a hospital gown or pajamas and covered with a blanket. The stretcher is draped with a clean sheet, the patient is lifted onto the sheet and is completely covered. The attendant then removes his gown, washes his hands, and dries them with paper towels.

When the patient arrives at the hospital, he is taken directly to the isolation unit. The attendant is responsible for washing the interior of the ambulance, using a suitable detergent in warm water, after which the ambulance is thoroughly aired.

Admitting Rooms

Admitting rooms in general hospitals should be prepared for the reception of patients with communicable disease. Each admit-

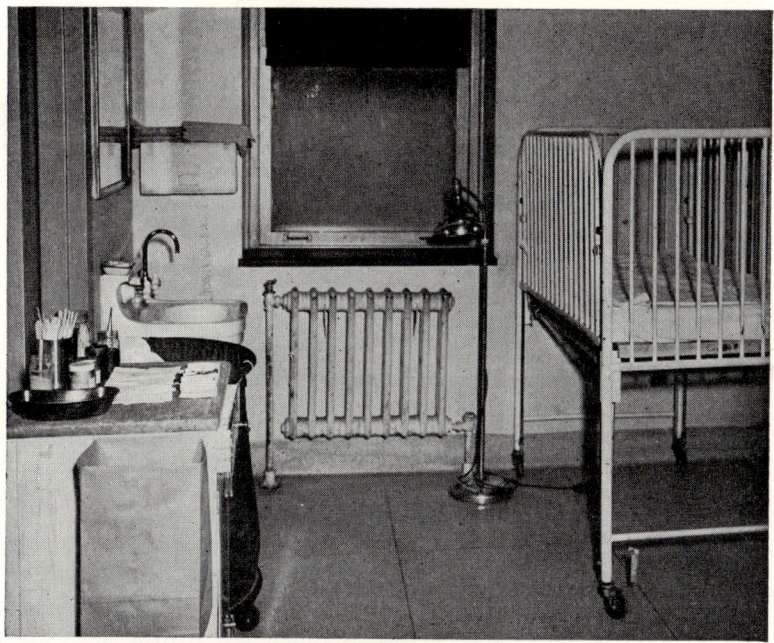

Fig. VII. ADMITTING UNIT AT KINGSTON AVENUE HOSPITAL, BROOKLYN, NEW YORK.

ting room should have running hot and cold water and a sink operated with foot or knee controls. A sufficient supply of paper towels should be on hand. A utility room for cleaning equipment, a sterilizer, and a small refrigerator for biologicals are essential as part of the unit. Among other required materials, the following supplies should be set up on a tray ready for use:

Clinical mouth and rectal thermometers in covered jars containing a disinfectant solution such as ethyl alcohol 70 per cent, Lysol 2½ per cent, or Zephiran Chloride 1:1,000

Sterile nose and throat culture tubes and applicators

Sterile Luer and tuberculin syringes

Sterile needles of different size for skin tests, and for subcutaneous and intramuscular injections

Cotton balls in a jar and cotton balls in alcohol in a jar

Alcohol cloth in a covered jar for cleansing equipment used by the physician

Necessary biologicals for skin testing and for injection should be readily available. They should be kept in a wire basket on a lower shelf of the refrigerator. Emergency drugs should also be available. These are usually kept in a cabinet which can be locked. The physician in charge of the admitting service should have the responsibility of drawing up a list of the necessary drugs and biologicals.

After a patient with a communicable disease has been removed to the isolation unit, the admitting room where he was examined should be aired, and contaminated equipment should be washed with a detergent and warm water. Linen used by the patient should be placed in a properly marked bag and sent to the laundry. Paper sheets may be used instead of linen. They can be discarded after use.

If the patient is accompanied by a member of the family, the patient's clothing may be placed in a paper bag, signed for by the family, and taken home to be laundered. Clothing that cannot be washed may be aired for several hours or dry-cleaned. Documents and money are placed in a large Manilla envelope and stored in the hospital safe if the patient does not wish to have them sent home.

Discharge of Patient

Upon recovery from a communicable disease the patient is bathed, dressed in his own clothing, and removed to a clean area. The room or cubicle is thoroughly cleaned with a detergent and warm water, and aired for several hours. The mattress is aired in the sun, and all equipment is sterilized by boiling.

Care of Body after Death

When a patient expires, the nurse preparing the body for the morgue wears a gown. The body is placed on a stretcher, covered with a clean sheet, and removed from the unit. Old sheets may be used for this purpose. The stretcher is cleaned with hot water and a detergent before being returned for general use.

Housekeeping Services

The work of the housekeeping staff needs to be closely co-ordinated with that of the nursing staff. When there is mutual understanding of functions and respect for the dignity of each person's job, co-operative relationships are possible.

Utility Rooms

If there is one utility room, a section of it should be designated for placing contaminated articles, linen, and equipment.

Waste Cans

Each waste can should be lined with a removable paper bag to receive soiled dressings and other wastes. This makes it easier to clean the cans and also is an aid in protecting the porter and sanitation personnel during the handling of the contaminated waste. To remove covers of clean cans, when the hands are contaminated, squares of tissue or newspaper should be used.

Cleaning

Maids should wear short-sleeved gowns and gloves when cleaning within the cubicle or in the room where a patient with a communicable disease is hospitalized. Furniture should be wiped with a damp cloth. If the furniture is polished, oil may be used. Doorknobs and window sills should be washed with warm water and soap. Floors should not be dry swept. Either a damp cloth should be used or, preferably, oil should be applied with a cloth or an oiling machine. If floors are washed, warm water and a detergent should be used, and the cloths or mops should then be placed in the sun or air to dry. Porters performing essential services on contaminated units should also wear gowns and be taught the importance of hand washing.

Kitchen

The kitchen is a clean area, and trays from patients with communicable disease should preferably be brought in after all the other dishes have been cared for. If contaminated trays must be collected at the same time, they may be placed on a special shelf in the kitchen. The shelf may be covered with newspapers; it should be cleaned with soap and water after the dishes have been washed.

Serving Trays

Trays may be carried to the bedside by attendants and placed on the patient's bedside table without becoming contaminated, providing the patient is able to feed himself. When patients need to be fed, their trays are served last. A gown is worn, and proper hand-washing techniques are observed when indicated.

Care of Dishes

If a mechanical dishwasher is available, no special precautions need be taken. The trays and dishes from cases of communicable disease are washed in the same manner as are those from other patients, except that they are washed after all the other dishes have been done.

If hand washing is used, a soap or other detergent and hot water are employed for washing. The dishes are then rinsed in boiling water and allowed to dry in the air. The trays are treated similarly. If paper cups and plates are used, these are discarded in the same manner as other disposable objects.

Glasses, dishes, and formula bottles taken into the kitchen between meals should be placed in a dishpan in the area designated for contaminated dishes, for proper cleaning later by the maid.

Disposal of Leftover Food

Solid food from the patient's tray should be scraped into a paper bag in the kitchen. It is wrapped securely in several thicknesses of newspaper, and placed in the regular garbage cans. Fluids and soft and pulpy foods may be emptied into a pitcher and then flushed into the toilet. The pitcher is then washed with hot water and a detergent and rinsed in boiling water.

Laundry

Linen at the bedside is collected by the nurse and placed in a discarded pillowcase which is fastened over the back of a chair or crib. After completion of nursing care, washing hands, and removing gown, the nurse may take the soiled linen to the utility room, being careful not to contaminate her uniform, and deposit it in the specially marked hamper. After this procedure, she should again wash her hands.

In general, laundry is collected into canvas or duck bags specially marked for contaminated linen. These bags are made with drawstrings and are pulled together before the laundry is sent through a chute or removed from the floor by the porter.

The most practical hamper is a metal frame which can be easily conveyed to wards. The canvas or duck bag fits into the metal frame. When used, a flap 6 inches or more long extends over the ring frame, and the drawstrings are pulled to fasten it securely to the frame. When two-thirds full, the flaps are folded over the linen, the drawstrings loosened, and the linen taken to the laundry by the porter.

The linen from the communicable-disease unit should not be sorted or counted until washed. No special treatment is necessary, since modern methods of laundering effectively sterilize it. It is customary for the linen from communicable-disease units to be laundered after the other linen, although this precaution is hardly necessary. All workers handling contaminated linen should wear gowns and practice hand washing.

In nurseries for the newborn, soiled diapers are placed in a metal can operated by a foot pedal. The can is kept outside the clean nursery. Special care should be taken in laundering linen and clothing for infants to keep them soft and fluffy.

After laundering, masks are autoclaved before being used.

REFERENCES

1. Bradley, Frank R.: "A Six-year Report on Care of Communicable Diseases," *Hospitals,* **24**:62–68, 1950.
2. Bugbee, George, *et al.*: "The General Hospital in the Poliomyelitis Program," *Hospitals,* **25**:37–60, 1951.
3. Bureau of Preventable Disease, New York City Department of Health: *Regulations Governing Quarantine of Wards in General Hospitals,* 1951.
4. Burgdorf, Alfred L.: "Hospitalization of Cases of Communicable Diseases together with Certain Consideration of the Isolation Techniques and Nursing Procedures Used," *Am. J. Pub. Health,* **39**:1289–1294, 1949.
5. Molnar, Joseph C.: "The Care of Polio Patients Is a Job for the General Hospital," *Mod. Hosp.,* **72**:56–58, 1949.
6. New York State Department of Health: *Guide for the Handling of Communicable Disease in General Hospitals,* 1950.

Chapter 8 NURSING PROBLEMS IN MANAGEMENT OF HOME CARE

THE presence of a communicable disease in the home is a disturbing element in any family situation. The upset may not be too great if the disease is of short duration. The inconveniences are temporary; the patient recovers and is able to return to his normal social and work activities. It is when the disease is complicated by sequelae, particularly physical distortion, or becomes chronic in nature that the psychosocial problems already present in the home are accentuated and threaten the equilibrium of the family. The tension in the home and the reaction of the ill person may affect all members and upset the balance of harmonious relationships. When the disease is long-term and chronic, it also imposes undue hardships and sacrifices upon all family members. All the resources within the family may have to be tapped to provide the patient with the best type of medical care.

The ultimate responsibility for nursing care rests with the family and is generally given by a family member or relative. It may, however, be shared by a private-duty or public health nurse. When nursing service is provided by a public health nursing agency, the policies for the types of cases to be visited, the services to be rendered, and the functions of the public health nurse may vary. In general, home visits to reported cases of communicable disease are made by public health nurses employed or designated by the health department. These differ in each community. The health officer decides which diseases shall be visited. Such decision depends upon the public health importance of the disease in that area and the availability of public health nurses. Home visits are sometimes made only if the patient is under a certain age, because mortality in that age group is high. Thus, in some communities, cases of whooping cough are visited if the patient is under 3 years of age. Regardless of the disease, the nurse's primary concern is recovery of the patient, prevention of disabilities, and control of spread of disease.

While it has been a stated policy of some health departments to limit the work of the public health nurse to instruction of the family in isolation procedures, it is becoming increasingly more important to demonstrate nursing care at the time of the first visit. When this is not possible, and another agency shares in the work, there should be mutual planning and sharing of responsibilities to avoid unnecessary conflicts. This eliminates confusion and duplication of service, and strengthens the nurse-patient relationship.

Structuring the Home Visit

There are common elements that are pertinent in the preparation of all home visits. This previsit planning includes organization of materials; review of agency policies and procedures; medical and nursing care in a particular disease or condition; administration, dosage, and reaction of certain drugs; and a review of the case record if the family is already known to the agency. If this is a first visit, information regarding source of referral and physician's orders regarding treatment are essential for making a satisfactory contact with the family.

In home visits to patients ill with communicable disease, an accurate knowledge of sanitary code regulations for isolation and quarantine is fundamental in controlling the spread of disease. The nurse's skill and ability to interpret these regulations in language that the family can understand determine how well they will be carried out. Other factors which affect the productiveness of these visits are time scheduling, family attitudes, and the nurse's own feelings toward communicable diseases.

Many families and patients are acutely sensitive about communicable diseases because of community attitudes and the restrictions imposed by sanitary code regulations. The facilities in the home may need to be completely rearranged to conform with these regulations. This may inconvenience other family members and necessitate readjustments in living. Recognition of these attitudes offers a rich opportunity to the nurse to allay fears and provide security, thereby enhancing effective relationships with the family.

When the home visit is not requested by the physician or family, emotional blocks in the nurse-patient-family relationship may arise. This is especially true when there is no apparent need for nursing service and the visit is not anticipated. The intrusion of a stranger to tell how things must be done may incur resentment. The physician can aid greatly by preparing and explaining to the family the purpose of the visit by a public health nurse. Prior to the visit, the public health nurse may find it helpful to confer with the physician by telephone. If necessary, conferences with the physician may be arranged at his office or in the home to discuss medical care plans.

The policies for home visits to patients with communicable disease vary. Some agencies give priority to communicable diseases over other visits planned by the nurse for the day, while others have a policy of postponing the visit until the end of the day. There is no reason why visits to patients with communicable diseases should be delayed if the nurse has a thorough understanding of the epidemiology of the disease and observes careful medical aseptic techniques. The danger of cross infection is negligible if these principles are understood. In addition, the patient is made more comfortable, the family is not kept in suspense waiting for the nurse, and sufficient time is available for the nurse to handle any problems which may have developed.

The time of day that is selected for making the initial home visit contributes to its effectiveness. An unannounced visit or one made at an inopportune time may cause annoyance to the family. It is sometimes possible and desirable to make a telephone call to the family and reach an agreement as to the most convenient time for visiting. The family is psychologically prepared and is receptive to instruction. It is also good practice to postpone a visit on the day the case has been reported if the patient has been removed to the hospital. Usually, the information to be obtained is not too important, and the family may not be at home. Moreover, a mother may be getting ready to visit her child at the hospital, and a visit by the nurse to get a list of detailed information may be very upsetting.

In most instances a public health nurse establishes a friendly relationship with the family at the very start and is able to get participation. Not only does the family accept her, but the various members also come to depend upon her for the solution of their difficulties. The alert nurse recognizes this relationship early and is able to direct them in assuming responsibility for solving their own problems.

Occasionally, a public health nurse may not be readily accepted by the family, and negative relationships may arise. These conflicts sometimes emanate from a misunderstanding of the nurse's role and the patient's concept of encroachment upon his individual rights. He may not want to accept the diagnosis either because of religious beliefs or lack of information, or because he associates the disease with filth and carelessness which seems to cast a reflection on him. Likewise, he may be reminded of a painful experience as a result of which he has built up antagonisms toward persons in authority. Consequently, he identifies the public health nurse as a figure representing authority. When such hostility arises, the nurse should listen attentively, note the difficulties with care, and interpret her functions, stating how she will help. In this way the confidence of the patient may be restored and his co-operation obtained.

An important factor in the nurse-patient relationship is the nurse's own feelings about communicable diseases. Since treatment requires participation, the nurse relates to the patient and he responds to her. If she lacks scientific information about these diseases, her security in the situation is threatened and impaired. Furthermore, the nurse's own anxieties and feelings are readily communicated to the patient and the family. These emotional factors have a definite effect upon the continuity in observing a patient's progress.

The confidential nature of some communicable diseases imposes upon the public health nurse strict observance of professional ethics at all times. When the nature of a patient's illness has been disclosed to relatives, neighbors, or others, resentment and dislike for the agency often develop. This is especially true where tuberculosis or venereal diseases are present. Similar reactions may occur when instructions to families regarding precautionary measures by different nurses appear conflicting. This misinterpretation may lead to indifference or may cause unnecessary anxieties and fears. Unfavorable impressions about an agency are often created and spread in a community in this way. These may influence public opinion against support of its service.

Community Resources

A knowledge of community resources for supplementing the social and health needs of families and the ability to work co-operatively with other community workers is desirable. If functions and relationships are clearly understood, there should be no conflict between nutritionists, social workers, physical therapists, clergy, and other nurses, as their special training and skills complement each other's work. It is a professional team relationship where collaboration in resolving complex problems may be necessary.

Protection of others in the community against the spread of disease is a responsibility of all nurses. Every nurse should be familiar with the current control practices in the community where she is employed. This information can be secured from the local health officer.

With the emphasis on positive and preventive health, many of the more serious diseases have decreased in incidence and virulence. As a result, community control regulations have been relaxed and are in continuous process of revision. Many timeworn practices once rigidly observed in the home have been discarded on the basis of new scientific facts. These changes occasionally create problems in a community, because people have become accustomed to certain law-enforcing measures by health departments and suddenly find that they have been discarded. Education of the public and explanations with supporting information are necessary to dispel fears and to avoid confusion. The present trend is being directed toward developing a co-operative sense of responsibility in the individual and family for protecting others against exposure to disease present in the household.

The responsibilities of the public health nurse in connection with diagnosed cases of communicable disease include: *

Reporting outbreaks of communicable disease in schools, industry, or in the community to the health officer

Giving or arranging for nursing care in the home as needed

Teaching general nursing care to family members, relatives, and attendants through demonstration and supervised practice

Teaching the family to carry out specific procedures and treatments

Aiding the physician and family in securing hospital care when necessary

Reporting other members of the family having symptoms of communicable disease to the attending physician

Observing and appraising home conditions to determine whether the patient can be properly cared for

Securing medical care when conditions demand such action

Taking nose and throat cultures from patient and contacts as required

Arranging for the collection of stool, blood, or sputum specimens

Giving instruction in concurrent and terminal disinfection

Arranging for immunization of the patient and his contacts in certain diseases

Excluding and readmitting patients and contacts to restricted occupations or school

Referring the family to the proper community agency as indicated by needs

Teaching citizen groups methods of care for communicable disease and the means available for preventing their spread

* Adapted from Bureau of Public Health Nursing, New York City Department of Health: *Nursing Procedures Relating to Acute Communicable Diseases,* New York, pp. 8–11, 1949.

Assisting with research studies by collecting and recording desired data

Assisting with epidemiological investigations under medical direction

Recording complete and accurate data on family service record

Pattern for Home Care

There is no formula or prescribed pattern for management of home care. The sociocultural setting varies in different situations and does not lend itself to a standardized method. The nursing procedures such as bathing, bedmaking, and mouth care are the same as in the hospital. However, certain modifications in medical aseptic techniques may be necessary for adaptation to the home environment. Many of these procedures need constant interpretation and require more time and patience on the part of the nurse. This is especially true where there are language barriers or where adjustments cannot be made easily.

In demonstrating nursing care of the patient to a family member, the public health nurse should direct her efforts toward measures which are readily understood. This requires general knowledge of disease processes, skill in improvising materials and equipment, and ability to teach on the family's level of comprehension. In considering plans for care, it is important to have an appreciation of and an insight into the social, emotional, and cultural factors which have a bearing on the family situation. An understanding of these factors is basic for intelligent planning and for guiding the family to action. If conditions in the home are inadequate for proper care of the patient, the nurse will need to confer with the physician regarding removal to the hospital.

In the past, considerable stress has been placed on isolation of the patient. While the importance of this cannot be minimized, conditions in the home are somewhat different from the hospital. By the time the doctor or nurse arrives, all members of the family have already been exposed. Isolation of the patient is emphasized to prevent further spread of the disease in the family and to guard the patient against the introduction of new pathogens which may cause sequelae.

While it is highly desirable for the patient to be in a separate room, this may not always be possible. Where such arrangement cannot be made, the patient should at least have his own bed, and the room may be shared with an adult member who is not susceptible to the disease. The surroundings should be quiet and pleasant. The furnishings should not be disturbed unless there is over-crowding.

While the wearing of a gown or coverall apron is recommended for the family member, the intricate method of putting the gown on and removing it as done in hospitals should be omitted. Its use is indicated for psychological reasons, and for protection of the nurse or family member. The explanation should be simple and one that can be readily understood.

The emphasis in the home situation should be on *frequent* and *meticulous hand washing and the proper disposal of secretions and discharges.* Hand-washing technique should be demonstrated by and carried out under the supervision of the public health nurse until its values are understood. The procedure should be carried out under running water, in the bathroom if possible. The use of basins should be avoided, as careful washing of the hands cannot be carried out safely, and cleanliness of basins is difficult to maintain.

Plans for Revisits

The number of home visits made by a public health nurse to a patient ill with a communicable disease will depend entirely upon the amount of help that is needed, the nature of the disease, the ability of the family to co-operate in carrying out nursing procedures, and other special problems.

The public health nurse often encounters other illnesses in a family. Besides giving instruction regarding nursing care, isolation, and prevention of the spread of the disease, she has the opportunity to observe other health problems and to aid in their solution. The instruction given to the family should be clear, reasonable, and adapted to the situation. When it is necessary to refer the family to a community agency, the public health nurse should be familiar with correct referral procedures and have accurate information about clinic hours. In addition, appointments made with patients for conferences at the office, clinic, or home should be kept at all times.

Procedures and Techniques *

Introduction

Prior to visiting the patient, the public health nurse secures from the attending physician recommendations and directions for nursing care.

* Adapted from Bureau of Public Health Nursing, New York City Department of Health: *Nursing Procedures Relating to Acute Communicable Diseases,* New York, pp. 8–11, 1949.

Upon arrival in the home, she leaves her hat, coat, and nursing bag outside the sick room. Before proceeding with nursing care, she observes and evaluates the home situation to determine facilities for isolation and nursing care of the patient. She instructs a member of the family to assemble all equipment needed for isolation and demonstration of nursing care. She removes from her nursing bag the usual hand-washing equipment plus extra towels for hand-washing unit (four paper towels plus an extra one for her watch).

Selection of the Room

A light, well-ventilated room not used by other members of the family and through which other members of the family do not pass is selected. The room should be as near to the bathroom as possible.

All windows of the sickroom should be screened during the fly season.

The patient's room should be cleaned daily and dust removed with a damp cloth. The atmosphere of the sickroom should be quiet and cheerful. Visitors and pets should be excluded.

Equipment for the Sickroom

A separate, comfortable bed
Necessary toilet articles assembled on a tray
Washbasin, soap, soap dish, bedpan or other receptacle, and
    toilet tissue
Glass pitcher, drinking glass, and tube
Clinical rectal or mouth thermometer and cotton for cleansing
Rubbing alcohol and dusting powder
Paper bags, newspapers, safety pins, paper tissues
Washable gown or coverall apron for attendant
Clean linen—towels, washcloth

Hand Washing

The hand-washing unit should be set up in or near the bath-
    room if possible
Remove rings and place watch on a paper towel
Place soap and extra towels on a paper towel
Wash hands thoroughly with soap and water before proceeding
    and after completion of nursing care
After last lathering, wash faucets and bowl with soap and run-
    ning water, using discarded paper towel

Use and Care of Gown

A butcher-type apron made of cotton material is worn when the public health nurse gives care to any patient with a communicable disease. If desirable, a paper apron may be substituted. After demonstration of nursing care to a family member, the paper apron is placed in a newspaper or paper bag and wrapped securely for burning or disposal with other waste. If care is not given, the apron may be used again. It is folded clean side out, placed in a large paper bag, and left in the patient's room. If a linen apron is used it is similarly folded and kept.

A coverall apron or gown is worn by the member of the family giving care to the patient. The outside surface of the gown or apron is considered soiled. The gown or apron is hung on a hook with the contaminated surface out. If no hook is available the gown is folded, clean side out, and placed in a large paper bag and kept in the room.

Care of Thermometer

If the nurse uses her own thermometer, it is cleansed with two cotton pledgets, moistened with soap, using friction, and then rinsed under cool running water. It is carried to the bedside on a towel, with a pledget of cotton. The temperature, pulse, and respiration are then taken. The same procedure for cleansing is followed after care is completed. The family should be encouraged to provide its own thermometer and taught how to take temperature.

Care of Patient

All articles are brought into the isolation unit at once.

The public health nurse takes the temperature, pulse, and respiration of the patient.

If a member of the family is to give nursing care, the nurse demonstrates and explains procedures in detail.

She proceeds with the bath, placing special emphasis on care of mouth and disposal of paper tissues for nose and throat secretions and other body discharges.

Disposal of Food

Solid food from the patient's tray is scraped and placed in a newspaper or bag, wrapped securely, and disposed with regular garbage. Fluids and soft and pulpy foods may be flushed into toilet.

Care of Dishes

The dishes and drinking utensils used by the patient are washed thoroughly with soap, rinsed under hot running water, and kept separate on a tray until the isolation period is over. They are then boiled for 5 minutes. If separate dishes are not kept, they must be boiled after each use.

Care of Linen

Personal and bed linen may be cared for with other family laundry.

Disposal of Body Secretions

NOSE AND THROAT SECRETIONS

All secretions from the nose and throat are collected in paper tissues or napkins and placed in a paper bag pinned at the patient's bedside. The bag and tissues are then wrapped securely and burned. If there are no facilities for burning, the tissues may be dropped into the toilet and flushed away, and the paper bag wrapped and disposed of with regular waste.

STOOLS

In infectious diarrheal diseases all stools may be emptied into water-flushed toilets connected with a sewer or a septic tank. The toilet and seat cover should be washed immediately with warm water and soap. Where toilets are not connected with a sewer or septic tank, stools are disinfected immediately with a 5 per cent solution of chloride of lime. The stool is broken up with a spatula or wooden spoon, 1 cup of disinfectant solution is poured over it, and the bedpan is tightly covered and allowed to stand for 1 hour. The bedpan is then emptied into the toilet, and the toilet seat is washed with soap and warm water. The bedpan should be boiled after the patient has recovered.

Disinfectant Solutions

Solutions used for disinfection are poisonous and require careful handling, particularly if there are young children in the family. Preparation of solutions possessing required strengths can be made at home.

Alcohol

Rubbing alcohol which is sold commercially is usually of 60 to 70 per cent strength. It may be used for disinfecting thermometers and instruments which cannot be boiled.

Chlorinated Lime

Use 3 tablespoons to 1 quart of water. This gives a 5 per cent solution. It is used for disinfection of feces.

Completion of Nursing Visit

When nursing care is completed, the hands are washed thoroughly, the apron is removed, and all articles are replaced in the nursing bag. All records are completed, and further instruction is given. When specimens for the laboratory are requested, the containers should be labeled in the home, and they should not be left with strangers.

Termination of Isolation and Quarantine

Upon recovery, the patient is bathed, the hair shampooed, and clean clothes are put on. Instructions regarding the need for a complete physical examination by the attending physician should be given to the family.

The sickroom is thoroughly cleaned and aired. All woodwork and floors are washed with warm water and soapsuds.

Mattress, blankets, and pillows are exposed to the sun, and all linen is sent to the laundry.

Toys are washed with warm water and soap. Books are exposed to the sun and air in an upright position with the pages fanned. Library books may be returned after airing and termination of isolation.

REFERENCES

1. Anderson, Gaylord, and Arnstein, Margaret: *Communicable Disease Control,* The Macmillan Company, New York, Chap. VI, 1948.
2. Berengarten, Sidney: "When Nurses Interview," *Am. J. Nursing,* **50**:13–15, 1950.
3. Bureau of Public Health Nursing, New York City Department of Health: *Nursing Procedures Relating to Acute Communicable Diseases,* New York, pp. 8–11, 1949.
4. Cantor, Nathaniel: "Understanding the Patient," *Pub. Health Nursing,* **38**:265–268, 1946.
5. Garrett, Annette: *Interviewing: Its Principles and Methods,* Family Welfare Association of America, New York, Chaps. I–VI, 1942.

6. Gilbert, Ruth: *The Public Health Nurse and Her Patient,* 2d Ed., Commonwealth Fund, New York, Chaps. II and III, 1951.
7. Gilbert, Ruth: "Nurse's Responsibility to Her Patient," *Pub. Health Nursing,* **39**:546–553, 1947.
8. Mann, James: "Human Relations in Public Health Nursing," *Pub. Health Nursing,* **40**:583–588, 1948.
9. Render, Helena Willis: *Nurse Patient Relationships in Psychiatry,* McGraw-Hill Book Company, Inc., New York, Chaps. I and III, 1947.
10. Seidenfeld, Morton A: *Psychological Aspects of Medical Care,* Publication No. 44, Charles C Thomas, Publisher, Springfield, Ill., 1949.
11. Shetland, Margaret: "Communicable Disease Nursing," *Pub. Health Nursing,* **40**:543–547, 1948.

Part II

THE SPECIFIC COMMUNICABLE DISEASES

A. Diseases Transmitted by Respiratory Discharges

B. Diseases Transmitted by Food and Water

C. Diseases Transmitted by Contact

D. Diseases Transmitted by Anthropods

Chapter 9 RESPIRATORY DISEASES

GENERAL DESCRIPTION

RESPIRATORY diseases may be caused by inanimate substances such as dusts, fumes, or pollen, or by microorganisms such as viruses, bacteria, or fungi. The substances may be either dissolved or suspended in air. Gases, carbon monoxide, for example, are usually in solution. Solids, such as dusts or other inorganic particles, and microorganisms are carried in suspension.

Transmission of infectious microorganisms may occur by (1) direct contact, as in kissing, or by (2) indirect contact, as in using another person's toothbrush. It may also occur by person-to-person transmission through the air in the form of (3) droplets. These are small particles of liquid enclosing bacteria, which are expelled from the mouth or nose in the course of sneezing, coughing, or talking. A sneeze may expel thousands of them. They are very small, many of them less than 1/250 inch. Fewer are expelled in coughing than in sneezing, but some may be expelled even in the pronunciation of a letter. The pronunciation of some letters causes a greater expulsion of droplets than the pronunciation of others. In pronouncing F, for instance, more droplets are expelled than in pronouncing D. Visual evidence of their expulsion has been obtained with a highspeed camera. Droplets usually travel only a few feet and fall to the floor because of their weight.

There is another method of transmitting infection to the respiratory tract and that is by (4) droplet nuclei, which are air-borne. These result from the evaporation of the liquid in droplets. The evaporation may occur in the course of the fall or after the droplet has sunk to the floor or settled on furniture. The nuclei are composed chiefly of microorganisms and are light enough to float in air. Those that have settled on furniture or the floor may be swept up in dust or in air currents and may keep afloat for long periods of time.

Until fairly recently, epidemiologists were convinced that respiratory infections were transmitted only by direct or indirect contact, including droplet infection. It was assumed that respiratory infection could be spread only if the infecting person were fairly close to the susceptible one. Experiments with animals, observations in laboratory outbreaks of disease, and the use of the air centrifuge in collecting and sampling specimens of air have convinced most modern investigators that respiratory infections may be transmitted even without contact with an infected individual. That many organisms may remain alive while suspended in air or dust has been amply proved. That they may cause illness in individuals breathing such air is a reasonable assumption on the basis of data obtained. It is still not clear how much of a part droplet nuclei play in the day-by-day transmission of respiratory infection.

The main factor influencing transmission of infection by droplets is distance, since the droplets are heavy and travel only a few feet. The factors which determine the dissemination of droplet nuclei, which are very light, are air currents, the temperature and humidity of the room, the amount and character of ventilation, and the washing of the air. Ordinary ventilation by means of an open window may cause several changes of air in 1 hour. In the winter, with windows closed, the overturn may be less than one per hour. Controlled ventilation by means of proper air conditioning may be extremely efficient in changing and washing the air in a sickroom, but such installations are expensive and space-consuming.

The disinfection of air in a room by ultraviolet irradiation or by the use of a disinfectant vapor is a comparatively recent trend. Irradiation of the air must be done carefully to prevent burns or injury to the eyes. The lamps are placed high up so that only the upper air is disinfected. Disinfectant vapors, like triethylene glycol, are cheap, odorless, and apparently nontoxic, and they have the advantage over ultraviolet light in that they permeate all parts of a room, but the air must be continuously saturated. Both methods are well suited for the sterilization of droplet nuclei, but they must still be considered as in the experimental stage.

The suppression of dust is still another method that is being used to prevent the spread of respiratory infections. This can be done effectively by oiling floors and woodwork and by impregnating blankets and bedding with oil. Methods have been evolved for the treatment of blankets so that a single oil impregnation may allow the dust-holding properties to be maintained for months, even after laundering.

THE CAUSATIVE AGENT

The incubation period varies with the agent. Some of the respiratory diseases, like the common cold, have short incubation periods, not more than 24 hours. Others, like measles and mumps, have incubation periods of 2 weeks or more.

The availability of the agent depends on the reservoir of infection. It may be a nonviable agent present in the air, as in carbon monoxide poisoning; or in dust and pollens, as in hay fever; or in emanations from the skins of animals, as in asthma. Infectious agents make up the bulk of respiratory diseases. They may be present in dust, as in coccidioidomycosis; or shed by animals, as in psittacosis; but mainly they come from the respiratory tract of humans.

The viability of the agent and its resistance to destruction are factors which influence the disease. Obviously, inanimate causes of disease cause damage only in the amounts absorbed. They do not multiply or persist in the respiratory system. An individual exposed to ragweed pollen who develops hay fever ceases to be affected as soon as he moves to an environment where pollen is not present in the air. This does not hold true for viable agents which multiply in the bodies of the patient. However, their viability is a factor. Some of the microorganisms have greater resistance than others and may persist alive outside the body. Poliomyelitis virus, for instance, remains alive in sewage and on the feet of flies; chickenpox virus, on the other hand, dies when not in contact with the human body. In the body, too, some viruses, like poliomyelitis, may remain alive for weeks, while others, like measles, die within a few days. The effect of physical factors, such as heat, moisture, and irradiation of air, have definite influence on the viability of droplet nuclei and may determine the survival or death of microorganisms in a room.

The pathogenicity of the agent of disease must be determined. An organism may resemble a pathogenic one in anatomic, staining, and cultural characteristics and yet be nonpathogenic. Thus, avirulent diphtheria bacilli cannot be distinguished from virulent bacilli unless tested on an animal or by a special culture technique. There are many examples of living microorganisms used in vaccines without causing damage to the vaccinated person. There are also bacilli resembling closely those active in human disease which are pathogenic for a certain animal but not pathogenic for man. An example of this is the avian tubercle bacillus which does not attack humans.

THE HOST

Personal Hygiene

An important factor in the dissemination of respiratory infections is personal hygiene in the individual with the disease. It is obvious, of course, that the more careful such a person is to cover his mouth and nose when sneezing or coughing and to refrain from spitting except into a handkerchief, the less opportunity will exist for the dissemination of microorganisms. The use of disposable paper tissues instead of linen handkerchiefs should be stressed. In the care of a patient at home or in the hospital, proper disposal of discharges from the respiratory tract is important.

Contact

The frequency of contact with an individual who has a respiratory infection frequently determines the probability of infection. This is well illustrated by the frequency with which normal infants born to actively tuberculous mothers develop miliary tuberculosis, or by the frequency with which bird handlers develop psittacosis.

Housing

Nowhere is intimacy closer than in the home. It is, therefore, not surprising that secondary attack rates of respiratory infections are higher in the home than elsewhere, even hospitals. The incidence will depend on how crowded the home is, how many people sleep in one room, what opportunities there are for adequate ventilation. In institutions, hospitals, barracks, and workrooms, too, the amount of crowding is an important factor in spread.

Allergy

Allergy to various substances is responsible for respiratory difficulty in a large number of individuals. The allergic state is a constitutional one, but those who are allergic do not show clinical evidence of illness unless exposed to a specific allergen. Pollens of grasses and weeds are common allergic incitants, and individuals sensitive to them may be able to move during the pollen season to locations where the plants do not grow. In the home it is often possible to dispense with allergenic substances. The frequency with which asthmatic children coming from a crowded home lose their asthma when they are put in a hospital ward where there are no animals, no hangings, no rugs, and no overstuffed furniture is an indication of the need of minimal, simple, easily washed furniture in the home of allergic individuals.

Chilling

Among the defense mechanisms of the host, those relating to constitutional factors such as age, sex, race, heredity, nutrition, etc., have already been discussed. The influence of fatigue and chilling in susceptibility to respiratory infections has not been thoroughly explored. It is universally accepted as a fact that chilling predisposes to respiratory infections. Many mothers have worn out their voices and their children's patience by constantly reminding them to put on their overcoats or their rubbers. At one time all male children were cautioned to put hats on before going out of doors. That custom has suffered the fate of atrophy from disuse in the United States, yet it is doubtful whether there has resulted an increase in respiratory infections in boys. It is not uncommon during the summer for people to plunge into cold water from a warm beach, yet they do not seem to become more susceptible to infections. In Switzerland and other places, extrapulmonary infections have been treated for a great many years by exposure to the sun all the year round, and, with snow covering the earth, children and adults play outdoors all day completely nude.

Fatigue

Similarly, the influence of fatigue on the incidence of respiratory infections has been taken for granted. Both physicians and lay people are too ready to explain the occurrence of a cold or pneumonia on the supposition that fatigue was an important predisposing cause. Yet one can recall instances of individuals who have been working under stress for long hours so that they are tired to death and still do not develop respiratory infections. It is interesting that in the reports of soldiers, sailors, and marines who bailed out of boats or airplanes and spent days on rafts with little clothing and food, respiratory infections apparently played a small part in their physical condition.

Immunity

Local factors, such as mucous secretions to wash out foreign material, eyelashes and hairs in the nose to keep them out, and cilia in the trachea and bronchi to sweep them back, play a part in the body's attempt to keep foreign substances out. When these fail, there are the lymph glands which act as a filtering mechanism. The final defense of the body consists of the extensive immune mechanism which it has built up.

Tonsillectomy

The tonsils and other lymphoid tissues in the throat are usually developed to the greatest extent in early childhood when growth is greatest and when acute infectious diseases are most common and serious. When an infection of the throat occurs, the tonsils usually become enlarged and swollen and then regress after the infection has subsided. Quite frequently the cervical lymph glands likewise enlarge, are tender during the infection, and subside later.

Furthermore, a number of studies indicate that lymphoid tissue takes part in the immune process. The question therefore arises whether, on theoretical grounds, there is justification for removal of tonsils in children.

There appears to be some evidence that when tonsils are removed after the fifth year of life in children who have previously had frequent attacks of tonsillitis or sore throat, such attacks diminish in frequency. Attacks of the common cold or of otitis media, on the other hand, are uninfluenced by tonsillectomy, and bronchitis and pneumonia are more frequent in children whose tonsils have been removed than in those in whom they remain intact. Allergic manifestations, such as hay fever, allergic sinusitis, bronchitis, and asthma are also unfavorably influenced by tonsillectomy.

A great deal of attention was riveted years ago on the relationship of tonsillar and throat infections to rheumatic fever, and the assumption was made that removal of tonsils might prevent the occurrence of rheumatic fever. When this was tested statistically, the facts did not corroborate the assumption. Removal of the tonsils does not signify that rheumatic fever will not occur, nor does it influence the number of recurrences.

Statements are occasionally made that removal of tonsils will improve a child's nutrition, development, or growth. No data have been presented to corroborate such beliefs, and many a mother has been disappointed to find that her child's status has not changed in spite of the miracles promised to her.

There is reason to believe that tonsillectomy in a child under 5 years of age offers even less benefit than in a child above that age. There is, furthermore, the child's psychological status to be taken into account. This is a very impressionable period in a child's life, when security is of great importance. Numerous studies have indicated the harmful results of separating a child from his mother at that tender age. A child, for no reason intelligible to him, suddenly finds himself snatched from the safe arms of his family to an absolutely strange environment peopled by persons he does not know, in a room he does not recognize, and is then wheeled into a more terrifying room with all kinds of instruments of torture. Here, someone clamps a mask on his face and chokes him. He struggles but is overcome and falls into unconsciousness. When he recovers he feels sick, he is nauseous, he vomits blood, and he has a fearful pain in his throat. There are few experiences more horrifying, and it is no wonder that many people carry the memory of such an experience into adult life.

The statement is occasionally made that tonsils should be removed when they are grossly enlarged, yet no one has seriously recommended the removal of large ears or noses. Size should certainly not be a criterion for removal. Physicians occasionally advise the removal of tonsils on the basis that they appear chronically diseased or infected. It is as difficult to make a diagnosis of chronic disease in a tonsil as in an appendix. It is problematic whether such a diagnosis can be made without removing the tonsils and examining them pathologically.

With the advent of antibiotics, a new factor has been introduced. The common infections of the throat and tonsils are now so readily cured by antibiotics that there is little fear of complications. Prolonged illnesses owing to throat infections have become rare, and there is less urgency to find a radical cure for recurrent sore throats.

The conclusion is inescapable that tonsillectomy should never be performed as a routine procedure, that it is rarely indicated in children under 5 years of age, and that in older children and adults it should be performed only when there are precise and definite indications.

Drugs

The discovery of the antibiotics has made a revolutionary change in the treatment of some of the respiratory infections. These include streptococcal sore throat, pneumonia, meningitis, and, to a lesser extent, whooping cough and diphtheria. The rapid recovery of patients and the bacteriostatic effect of the drugs on carriers have had a pronounced effect in reducing the incidence of cases and have offered the body an additional method of defense.

THE ENVIRONMENT

The physical environment determines to some extent the incidence of respiratory disease. It is a well-known fact that diseases like the common cold, pneumonia, influenza, and others are much more prevalent in cold than in warm weather. The exact reason is not clear. The presence or absence of certain animals in a community also plays a part in the determination. Q fever, for instance, is much more prevalent where cattle are kept or slaughtered, and the prevalence of psittacosis depends on the presence of psittacine birds. Furthermore, the accessibility and the population density are factors in spread. Diseases like measles and diphtheria are more prevalent in urban than in rural districts. There are isolated communities where some respiratory diseases have not occurred for years. This was true of the Faroe Islands, where measles had not occurred for 60 years. When it was introduced by a man who had been to the mainland, it spread rapidly until almost every inhabitant on the Islands came down with it.

Season

The season of the year influences the occurrence of respiratory diseases not only because of the differences in temperatures but also because in summer people are out of doors a great part of the time and escape the intimate contact of the home. Summer is also the season when pollens are present in the air and cause allergic respiratory symptoms in susceptible individuals. The amount of rain influences the concentration of pollens, so that a wet summer will bring much less hay fever than a dry one.

Social and Economic Environment

Social and economic factors play a similar role in respiratory as in other types of communicable diseases. The greater the density of a population, the greater the contact and the greater, therefore, the chance of exposure. Crowded homes allow frequent and prolonged contact with the agent of disease. The economic status of the family determines not alone the crowding in the home but the state of nutrition of the individuals in it, the amount of medical care received, and the educational status of the members of the family, which, in turn, determines the care exercised in personal hygiene.

Occupation

The occupation also plays a role in the possibility of exposure and in the spread of respiratory infections. While the intimacy of contact is not so great in the factory as in the home, it varies in different industries, being fairly close in some groups and fairly distant in others. The question of ventilation of the office or factory plays an obvious role. Then there are the specific hazards that attend working in certain industries. Nurses in a tuberculosis ward are exposed to a greater hazard than girls of the same age on a farm or in a factory. Slaughterhouse workers have a greater incidence of Q fever than workers in other industries.

The Community

As in other types of communicable disease, the wealth or poverty, the education or ignorance, the social awareness and the health consciousness of a community are important factors in the control of respiratory disease. Communities that are able and willing to support an active health department will have a better immunization program, better epidemiological control, and a greater availability of treatment centers than those that fail to support good public health measures.

MEDICAL ASEPTIC TECHNIQUES

Gowns

The wearing of gowns by nurses appears to be a reasonable precaution against the spread of respiratory diseases. It is not possible for a nurse to care for patients with these diseases without having infected droplets lodge on her person as a result of the patient's coughing and sneezing. A gown worn only in the room or on the ward where the patient is housed will catch such spray and will prevent spread outside. The gown should be sufficiently long to reach below the knees and should open the entire length down the back. It should be made of washable material and should have strings or tapes sewed on. Short-sleeved gowns have a considerable advantage over long-sleeved ones. They are more economical, easier to handle and sterilize, cooler and more comfortable, especially in hot weather, and have the added advantage that the cuffs do not get wet and soiled during work. In the operating room a long-sleeved gown is used in order to ensure sterility of the operating field. This is not needed or aimed for in the care of persons with communicable disease. What is desired is a reasonable precaution against spread. This is obtained as well with a short-sleeved as with a long-sleeved gown, if the nurse takes pains to wash her hands and arms thoroughly with soap and water before leaving the infected room or ward.

Caps

The use of caps by nurses when caring for cases of respiratory communicable disease does not have as good a justification as the use of gowns. The cap that should be worn on a communicable-disease ward should be large enough to cover the hair completely and should be made of washable material. With a little ingenuity a simple, large, washable kerchief can be used to fashion such a cap.

Masks

The use of masks by patients with respiratory disease in a hospital ward is probably not feasible. The use of masks by nurses in various fields of hospital activity has been accepted as a worthwhile procedure. A study of the problem indicates, however, that there has been an insufficient amount of clinical investigation to determine their need and usefulness. There are two general types of mask in use: (1) a filtering mask, which filters bacteria and is permeable to air, and (2) a deflector mask, which is made of an impermeable substance and which does not allow air to pass through. The latter type of mask is used very little. First, it must have a rigid frame to which the impermeable material is attached. Second, since it does not allow air to pass through, it does not act as a filter. The air is deflected around and under the mask. While it may prevent direct infection from person to person, it has no effect on infection by droplet nuclei or by dust; in other words, it is no protection against air-borne infection. Not a great deal of experimentation has been done with masks, and much of it has been crude and not applicable to everyday conditions in a hospital. Some of the early experiments consisted in covering sterile agar Petri dishes with filtering masks and spraying, from various distances, bacterial suspensions over them and over uncovered dishes. Fair protective results were obtained by some investigators and not such good results by others. Other experiments were made in wards of contagious-disease hospitals by masking nurses for certain periods and leaving them unmasked for other periods and determining the incidence of certain respiratory infections among them. The controls were poor, and other methods of spread could not be excluded, so that the findings are not of great value.

Recent experiments have been planned to simulate conditions in a room or ward. In one such experiment a specially built chamber was sprayed with a suspension of bacteria, and after a few seconds a vacuum pump was used to draw the air in the chamber through two funnels, one of which was covered over its wide end with a mask. Petri dishes of nutrient agar were exposed at the end of the funnels. The filtering efficiency of the mask was judged by the colonial growth on the Petri dish, and the resistance was measured by a water manometer. The materials showing the best results were (1) gauze, 42 by 42 strands to the square inch, six layers, washed twenty times, (2) gauze, 42 by 42 strands to the square inch, two layers with a layer of thick absorbent cotton between, washed twenty times, and (3) cellucotton, eight layers. Commercial masks gave a high resistance to air flow, which increased after washing. Cellucotton masks were torn too easily. Gauze masks shrank after much laundering, and if they were stretched to cover the mouth and nose the filtering efficiency was diminished.

Another investigator exposed rabbits in a chamber in which bovine tubercle bacilli were nebulized. The infected air was then drawn over the heads of rabbits which had close-fitting six-layer gauze masks covering their heads. Control rabbits were exposed simultaneously. About 60 per cent of the masked rabbits were completely protected, whereas all the uncovered rabbits were infected with tuberculosis.

Neither of these experiments simulated actual conditions in a hospital. In both experiments the concentration of organisms in the chamber was far beyond what is found in a ward. In both the air was drawn by suction over the mask, and in both the masks were held rigidly in one position, while a nurse on a ward constantly moves about. It would be unwise to apply the results of such experiments rigidly to conditions in actual life, and experiments with animals should not be accepted as always applicable to man.

A field experiment with conditions as they occur on a ward was carried on at the Herman Kiefer Hospital. Two nurses were masked with six-layer gauze masks, 42 by 42 strands to the square inch, and were given routine work on a tuberculosis ward in which there were eight patients with positive sputum. Glass slides with glycerin-coated centers were attached to their clothing, three on the cap, three on the mask, and four on the gown of each. Acid-fast bacilli were found on five slides attached to the cap and to the mask. In another experiment in which the central portions of masks worn by the two nurses were placed in solutions which were cultured for tubercle bacilli, organisms were found in 3 of 600 cultures.

There is need for further experimentation under actual working conditions in rooms and wards. Various factors should be considered, such as the comfort of the nurse, the periods of time that she wears the mask, the effect of getting the mask moistened with saliva, and other variables. In evaluating results, two factors must be considered. What protection does the masking of the nurse give to the patient, and what protection does it give the nurse? It is doubtful whether patients get much protection from this procedure, except from possible contact infection. There is much greater danger of air-borne infection from other patients in the ward, from bedding, drapes, and dust, and attempts should be made to minimize the effects of these. Dangers to the nurse will also be minimized by proper sanitary procedures, by immunizing her against those diseases for which immunizing procedures are available, and by carrying out good nursing techniques. In operating and delivery rooms it appears reasonable to have all personnel masked, since in this way contact and droplet infections may be prevented from reaching the raw surfaces of the patient. The mask may have some benefit in certain other localized spheres of activity. For general use in wards, nurseries, and rooms, it does not appear to have any advantage. It gives a false sense of security and, particu-

larly on hot days, is a source of annoyance and discomfort to the
wearer.

Hand Washing

This is probably one of the most important measures in nursing technique for the care of communicable disease. Hand washing
should be practiced before and after care of each patient. The
nurse should take the time to do it thoroughly and properly. Dipping the fingers in Lysol solution or using a light spray of alcohol
is not a substitute for an old-fashioned soap-and-water scrub. The
addition of antiseptics to the water is of questionable value. What
is needed is a physical cleansing agent which will adequately
remove foreign material from the hands and arms. Warm water
and a detergent, like soap, are ideally suited for this purpose. It
should be remembered that the aim in hand washing is not to
make the hands sterile but to make them clean.

Concurrent Disinfection

The need of proper sterilization of utensils used in giving nursing care and treatment requires no discussion. Nasopharyngeal
discharges from the patient should be collected in paper tissues
and deposited in a paper bag securely fastened to the bedside and
within easy reach of the patient. These should be burned, if possible. If facilities are not available, the tissues may be flushed into
the toilet and the paper bag wrapped securely in newspapers for
disposal with other waste.

Terminal Disinfection

After termination of isolation or after discharge of the patient,
the room or unit is thoroughly aired and the mattress exposed to
the sun and air. All equipment is washed with soap and hot water.
All metalware is sterilized, and blankets are laundered or dry
cleaned.

GENERAL REFERENCES

1. Anderson, G. W., and Arnstein, M. G.: *Communicable Disease Control,* 2d
   ed., The Macmillan Company, New York, 1948.
2. Bower, A. G., and Pilant, E. B.: *Communicable Diseases for Nurses,* 6th ed.,
   W. B. Saunders Company, Philadelphia, 1948.
3. Boyd, M. F.: *Preventive Medicine,* 7th ed., W. B. Saunders Company, Philadelphia, 1945.
4. Cecil, R. L.: *A Textbook of Medicine,* 7th ed., W. B. Saunders Company,
   Philadelphia, 1947.
5. Dubos, R. J.: *Bacterial and Mycotic Infections of Man,* J. B. Lippincott Company, Philadelphia, 1948.

6. Harrison, T. R.: *Principles of Internal Medicine,* The Blakiston Company, Philadelphia, 1950.
7. McQuarrie, I.: *Brennemann's Practice of Pediatrics,* W. F. Prior Company, Hagerstown, Md., 1949.
8. Pullen, R. L.: *Communicable Diseases,* Lea & Febiger, Philadelphia, 1950.
9. Rivers, T. M.: *Viral and Rickettsial Diseases of Man,* J. B. Lippincott Company, Philadelphia, 1948.
10. Stimson, P. M.: *Manual of Common Contagious Diseases,* 4th ed., Lea & Febiger, Philadelphia, 1947.

Chapter 10 CHICKENPOX (VARICELLA)

GENERAL DESCRIPTION

GENERAL DESCRIPTION

VARICELLA is an acute communicable disease occuring chiefly in children, caused by a virus and characterized by mild constitutional symptoms and a vesicular eruption.

THE CAUSATIVE AGENT

The causative agent is a large virus and is found in the fluid of the vesicles and in the upper respiratory tract. Eosinophilic inclusion bodies can be seen early in the nuclei and later in the cytoplasm of infected cells. The disease does not occur in any animal other than man, nor can it be transmitted to any other animal. It does not grow in tissue culture or on chick embryo.

THE HOST

Symptoms

The incubation period is 14 to 16 days. There is a rise in temperature, usually not very high, and the appearance of pink-colored papules on the trunk. They rapidly change into vesicles, which are superficial in appearance and break readily on pressure. Successive crops of lesions appear in different parts of the body for several days. After 24 to 48 hours they begin to dry, first in the center, giving an umbilicated appearance. After 1 or 2 more days the vesicle is replaced by a scab, which remains attached for several days to 1 week, after which it falls off without leaving a scar. Since the lesions erupt at different times and each goes through the same process of maturation, it is usual to see at the same time lesions of different ages from vesicle to crust.

The lesions of varicella are more abundant on the trunk than on the face or extremities. On the latter they are more common on the dorsal than on the ventral surfaces. They are seen quite regularly on the scalp and on the mucous membranes of the mouth.

The constitutional symptoms of chickenpox are usually very mild. Often the rash is the only sign of the disease. However, cases occasionally occur in which there are high fever, a profuse erup-

tion, and constitutional symptoms. It is in this type that differentiation from smallpox becomes a diagnostic problem.

Complications are not common. Occasionally, vesicles are infected as a result of scratching or rubbing. Postinfectious encephalitis may follow chickenpox, as it sometimes follows measles or
vaccinia.

Diagnosis

Severe cases of chickenpox must be distinguished from smallpox.
In chickenpox there are no premonitory symptoms, the vesicles are
superficial, they are commoner on the covered surfaces than on the
face or hands, and the lesions are in different stages of development. The virus of chickenpox does not grow on chick embryos,
whereas that of smallpox does.

Immunity

One attack of chickenpox usually confers immunity for life.
Carriers are not known. There are no known procedures for active
or passive immunization.

THE ENVIRONMENT

Chickenpox was not recognized as a clinical entity prior to the
seventeenth century. Even after, it was confused with smallpox
until the nineteenth century. It occurs in all climates, among all
races, and in both sexes. It is seen chiefly in childhood, where it
commonly occurs in epidemic form. Unlike measles, it may occur
in very young infants. By adult life, more than three quarters of
the population has had the disease. On this continent it is commonest in the winter and spring but may occur in other seasons.
It is highly contagious. The virus is present in the respiratory tract
and in the vesicles and is spread from person to person by discharges
from these two sources. Since there are no carriers, spread through
an intermediary does not occur. The period of communicability begins about 1 day before the lesions appear and continues until the
scabs have dried. Unlike smallpox, the dried scabs are not infectious.

More than half a century ago von Bokay called attention to the
relationship between chickenpox and herpes zoster. Since then a
number of other investigators have called attention to the relationship. Epidemics of chickenpox have been described following exposure to herpes zoster, and cases of herpes zoster have occurred in
adults who were in contact with cases of chickenpox. On the other
hand, herpes zoster is known to occur in individuals who have had
chickenpox, whereas second attacks of chickenpox are extremely
rare, indicating that chickenpox does not confer immunity against

zoster whereas it does to its own virus. At present there is no convincing evidence either in favor or against the theory that the two diseases are caused by the same virus. Proof will probably have to wait for the discovery of methods of cultivation.

Control

Patients should be isolated for a period of 7 days from the appearance of the vesicles, by which time the scabs will have dried. Contacts need not be quarantined. If chickenpox occurs in individuals above the age of 15, great care should be exercised to make sure that the disease is not smallpox.

If the disease is cared for in a hospital, rigid isolation procedures should be observed, since the communicability is great. Patients should be isolated in a separate room, ward, or isolation unit. If the patient remains at home he should be isolated in a separate room, and susceptible contacts should be excluded.

MEDICAL CARE PLANS

Treatment

There is no specific treatment for the disease. The patient should be kept in bed if he has fever. The antibiotics are of no value except in the treatment of secondary infections if these should occur. General cleanliness and the use of antipruritic measures are all that are necessary. Children do not, as a rule, scratch the lesions. If discomfort is excessive, mild sedatives may be used.

Diet

A liquid or semisolid diet is given during the febrile period. A full diet is permitted if there is no fever.

Supportive Nursing Care

Nursing care consists mainly in keeping the patient clean and comfortable. Cleanliness is maintained by sponge baths if there is fever, or by tub or shower baths if there is no fever. The skin should be dried gently with a soft towel and without rubbing so as to avoid breaking the vesicles. Clothing should be clean, light, and worn loosely to prevent irritation of vesicles. The fingernails should be kept trimmed and scrupulously clean.

Since chickenpox attacks large numbers of children in nursery and school groups, it frequently comes to the attention of the public health nurse. These children should be isolated until called for by their parents or taken home by a responsible member of the school staff. Routine home visits by public health nurses are not indicated, since the disease is usually mild. When a case is discovered during the course of home visiting, the public health nurse should instruct the family in isolation and nursing care.

Chapter 11 COCCIDIOIDOMYCOSIS (VALLEY FEVER OR DESERT FEVER)

GENERAL DESCRIPTION

COCCIDIOIDOMYCOSIS is an infectious disease caused by a fungus, *Coccidioides immitis,* which manifests itself as a disease of the lungs or as a progressive granulomatous disease.

THE CAUSATIVE AGENT

Coccidioides immitis is a fungus which grows well on all usual mediums. On Sabouraud's medium it grows at room temperature as a fluffy, white, cottony colony. With age, the growth becomes brown and powdery. Under the microscope there are visible rectangular spores separated by clear spaces between hyphae.

THE HOST

The disease may manifest itself in one of several forms:
1. As an acute pulmonary infection resembling influenza, with rapid recovery
2. As an inapparent infection resembling primary tuberculosis
3. As a chronic pulmonary infection resembling tuberculosis
4. As a rapidly fatal acute infection involving the lungs and other organs, simulating fulminating tuberculosis infection
5. As a skin lesion

Symptoms

When the disease occurs as a benign pulmonary infection, the incubation period is 1 to 3 weeks. The symptoms resemble those of influenza or a mild pneumonia. Anorexia and malaise are common, and so is pain in the chest. There are low-grade fever and a non-productive cough. There may be chills and sweats, and there is usually a loss of weight. The physical signs are minimal; occasionally, a few rales can be heard. In about 5 per cent of cases, erythema nodosum occurs. The entire acute illness lasts from 1 to 3 weeks, and recovery follows, as a rule.

From one half to two thirds of individuals infected with *Coccidioides immitis* develop no clinical symptoms. Occasionally, however, they may develop erythema nodosum.

156

Occasionally, individuals with acute symptoms of the disease, as described above, do not clear up but go into a chronic course resembling pulmonary tuberculosis. Cavitation of the lung is not uncommon, pain in the chest is often complained of, and hemoptysis may occur. Cough is a frequent symptom in these patients.

Again as in tuberculosis, the initial infection, instead of healing, progresses and not only involves the lungs but spreads to the rest of the body. It may localize in the skin, bones, lymph nodes, or meninges. It gives symptoms similar to those of miliary tuberculosis.

Coccidioidomycosis may occur as a skin lesion, usually as a nodule which is pinkish in color. It ulcerates and discharges a thick pus, from which the organisms may be obtained. The lesion is chronic but may eventually heal or may spread. Sometimes the granuloma occurs in the subcutaneous tissue, or it may localize in the superficial lymph nodes, particularly those of the neck. These may ulcerate and result in draining sinuses, much like in tuberculosis.

Diagnosis

The disease must be differentiated from influenza and pneumonia in its acute stage and from tuberculosis in all its stages. The blood count usually shows a slight leukocytosis.

X rays—The X rays of the lungs may be negative or resemble atypical pneumonia or primary tuberculosis, in the early acute form. In the chronic form they may resemble tuberculosis.

Recovery or fungus—Pus and sputum should be examined fresh under the microscope. Pleural fluid and gastric contents should be centrifuged, and the sediment should be examined. Preliminary treatment with cupric sulfate will kill bacteria except tubercle bacilli and will not destroy the fungus. The infected material can be cultured on Sabouraud's medium and also inoculated intraperitoneally in mice. The finding of the fungus is presumptive evidence of infection.

Skin test—In from 1 to 3 weeks after infection, patients develop a positive skin test to coccidioidin, which is the product of a filtered culture of *Coccidioides immitis*. The test is performed intradermally with a 1:100 dilution, similar to the tuberculin test. The reaction is read in 24 to 48 hours. A positive test shows erythema and induration and indicates an infection with the fungus but does not indicate when the infection took place or its extent.

Serologic tests—The blood of patients develops complement-fixing and precipitin antibodies. These can be demonstrated with the use of a proper antigen. The complement-fixation test is of some prognostic value. As in syphilis, the higher the titer the more severe the infection.

Immunity

The development of immune bodies in the patient has already been discussed. An inapparent or primary infection appears to confer immunity against more severe infection. There is no available method for active or passive immunization.

THE ENVIRONMENT

The disease was first reported from Argentina in 1892. A few years later a case was reported in California. These were in patients with skin lesions. Only in the past 15 years has the benign, pulmonary type been recognized. The disease is found chiefly in the United States, although cases have been reported from Argentina, Mexico, Hawaii, and Southern Europe. In this country it is endemic in the arid regions of the West and Southwest, and infects not only man but also cattle, sheep, dogs, and rodents.

There is a seasonal distribution. This depends on the amount of rain, since the spores are spread in dust and so are disseminated in dry, arid weather but suppressed in rainy periods.

Like tuberculosis, coccidioidomycosis spreads more rapidly in Negroes than in whites, and the mortality is higher among them. Males are more commonly affected than females, but this is probably due to greater exposure.

The disease is spread by dust from which it has been cultured. The fungus, when obtained from infected humans, is in the sporangial or spherule form and is not readily transmissible. The spores in dust are, however, readily spread and inhaled. For this reason a considerable number of individuals living in endemic regions are infected, but usually with the inapparent or benign form. Laboratories working with cultures of the fungus must exercise great care, since the spores are readily spread from cultures, particularly if these are old and dry.

Control

The patient need not be isolated, since he is not the source of infection. For the same reason, contacts need not be quarantined. Control of the disease in endemic areas is largely a question of dust suppression. This includes paving of roads, planting of shrubs and lawns, and oiling of large fields such as tennis courts, sports stadia, etc.

Medical Care Plans

Treatment

There is no specific treatment. Fortunately, most patients with inapparent or early infections clear up spontaneously. The difficulty arises in treating chronic cases and the rapidly spreading ones. Various drugs have been used without benefit. Penicillin and streptomycin are not effective. General supportive measures and symptomatic treatment are used. These are similar to the measures used in tuberculosis. Bed rest is essential in the acute phase. Salicylates are used to relieve discomfort, and sedatives are given for cough. As the patient improves, he is permitted to be up and about for longer periods.

Diet

As in tuberculosis, the nutrition of the patient is often a problem since the appetite is poor. There are no dietary restrictions. The diet should be high in caloric and protein intake and should be supplemented with vitamins.

Supportive Nursing Care

In endemic areas the public health nurse assists in case finding and in demonstrating nursing care procedures to the family. Since the illness may be prolonged, the family may require help with social and other health problems.

REFERENCES

1. Berke, R.: "Contagiousness of Coccidioidomycosis," *Am. Rev. Tuberc.*, **61**:44, 1950.
2. Emmons, C. W.: "Isolation of Coccidioides from Soil and Rodents," *Pub. Health Rep.*, **57**:109, 1942.
3. Rosenthal, S. R., and Elmore, F. H.: "Studies on the Contagiousness of Coccidioidomycosis," *Am. Rev. Tuberc.*, **61**:106–114, 1950.
4. Smith, C. E.: "Epidemiology of Acute Coccidioidomycosis, with Erythema Nodosum ('San Joaquin' or 'Valley Fever')," *Am. J. Pub. Health*, **30**:600, 1940.
5. ——— "Coccidioidomycosis," *M. Clin. North America*, **27**:790, 1943.

Chapter 12 COMMON COLD

GENERAL DESCRIPTION

THE common cold is a clinical syndrome of short duration characterized by sneezing, nasal discharge, chilliness, general malaise, and fever.

THE CAUSATIVE AGENT

The etiologic agent is unknown. Successful transmission from man to man and to chimpanzees has been described, as well as successful growth on chick embryos. It is therefore believed that the causative agent is a virus. Its cultivation and identification are still, however, in the experimental stage. Experimental transmission to the lower animals has not met with success.

THE HOST

Symptoms

The incubation period is short. It may be only a few hours or 1 to 2 days. At the onset there are usually feelings of general malaise, headache, backache, and discomfort in the upper respiratory passages. Sneezing and a thin nasal discharge follow. The latter may be copious and almost continuous, so that constant resort to a handkerchief or nasal tissue is needed. Fever is usually low grade. The conjunctivae may be injected and the mucous membrane of the nose and pharynx reddened and congested. The cervical glands are usually enlarged and slightly tender. After 1 or 2 days the nasal discharge thickens and may then become mucopurulent. After a few more days the symptoms abate, and recovery sets in. During the first few days however, the patient looks and feels much more miserable than the outcome warrants. Secondary bacterial infection is fairly common, causing otitis media, sinusitis, bronchitis, and even pneumonia. The mortality from the uncomplicated disease is practically nil.

Diagnosis

There is no laboratory procedure to assist in the diagnosis.

Immunity

Immunity apparently does not follow an attack. No antibodies have been demonstrated following the disease. The recurrence of colds several times a season is not an unusual phenomenon. There is no available vaccine for immunization, although experimental work toward that achievement is in process in some laboratories.

THE ENVIRONMENT

No place and no climate are immune to the common cold. Seasonal incidences do occur, particularly in temperate climates, but an adequate explanation for the more frequent occurrence of colds in cold weather has not been given. Children from 2 to 6 appear to be more susceptible than infants or adults. Transmission appears to be by direct contact or by infected droplet nuclei in the air.

Control

Persons suffering from the common cold should be isolated during the acute stage. They should be taught to cover the nose and mouth when sneezing or coughing and to use paper tissues for the collection of discharges. The tissues should be deposited in a paper bag at the bedside and burned or flushed into the toilet. Toys and books used by children with a cold should not be shared with others during the acute stage. Hands should be washed before meals and at other times when soiled with nasal discharge. Contacts need not be quarantined.

MEDICAL CARE PLANS

Treatment

No specific treatment is available. Rest in bed during the catarrhal stage should be encouraged. The temperature of the room should be warm and free from draughts. Infants and young children should be dressed comfortably.

The discomforts which accompany a cold are due to general symptoms such as headache and body aches and to local symptoms such as nasal obstruction or discharge. For the former, antipyretic drugs such as acetylsalicylic acid are commonly employed. For the latter, nose drops containing ephedrine or Epinephrine are frequently prescribed for their decongestive effect. The use of nose drops containing oil is discouraged on account of the possibility of a resulting lipoid pneumonia. The nurse should teach adult patients the correct procedure in the instillation of nose drops. If ambulatory, the patient should tilt his head backward and instill the drops with a medicine dropper into the nares. If in bed, the patient should lie in supine position with the head lowered to one side. When the nasal discharge is profuse, it frequently irritates the upper lip and nares. The application of cold cream or a mild ointment is soothing and may prevent crusting or superimposed skin infection.

The complications of the common cold are acute otitis media, cervical adenitis, tracheitis, bronchitis, and pneumonia. The use of antibiotics has reduced these complications considerably. When cough is persistent, it may be necessary to prescribe a soothing sirup or small dose of codeine. For dry, irritating coughs, steam inhalations are usually comforting. The use of counterirritants such as medicated ointments or mustard plasters is of questionable benefit, but some physicians consider such measures of distinct help. In recent years antihistamines have been widely advertised as effective preventives of colds if taken early. The literature contains some reports which are favorable and others indicating no benefit from such treatment. The consensus is that the value of antihistamines in the treatment of colds has not been proved.

Diet

Appetite for food is frequently lost during a cold as during other acute infectious conditions. Parents should be instructed not to force food to children. Since recovery usually occurs in a few days, no harm is done if the normal amount of food is not taken. Liquids should be offered in usual quantities.

Supportive Nursing Care

Nursing care is essentially directed toward relieving discomfort.

The public health nurse plays an important role in the education of the community during epidemics of colds and during their seasonal occurrence. Teachers should be instructed to refer the children with early symptoms of a cold to the school nurse. In industry, in hospital clinics, and in contacts with families in their homes, the nurse has the opportunity to teach sound principles of personal hygiene, maintenance of good nutrition, and importance of keeping away from personal contact with individuals who have colds. She should stress the need for medical care if symptoms do not subside in a few days.

REFERENCES

1. Dochez, A. R.; Mills, K. C.; and Kneeland, Y., Jr.: "Study of Virus of Common Cold and Its Cultivation in Tissue Medium," *Proc. Soc. Exper. Biol. & Med.,* 28:513, 1931.

2. Jordan, W. S.: "Acute Upper Respiratory Infections," *Am. J. Nursing,* **50**:39, 1950.

3. Paul, J. H., and Freese, H. L.: "Epidemiological and Bacteriological Study of the Common Cold in Isolated Arctic Community," *Am. J. Hyg.,* **17**:517, 1933.

4. Ward, T. G., and Proctor, D. F.: "Isolation of a Common Cold Virus in Chick Embryos and the Clinical Manifestations It Produces in Human Volunteers," *Am. J. Hyg.,* **52**:91, 1950.

Chapter 13 DIPHTHERIA

GENERAL DESCRIPTION

DIPHTHERIA is an acute infectious disease caused by the diphtheria bacillus and characterized by involvement of the upper respiratory passages with the production of a membrane and of generalized toxic symptoms.

THE CAUSATIVE AGENT

The diphtheria bacillus is officially known as *Corynebacterium diphtheriae,* and is sometimes referred to as the Klebs-Löffler bacillus. It is a gram-positive rod which is nonmotile, does not form spores, and stains irregularly. The poles of the bacillus have club-like swellings known as "polar bodies," which stain deeply. In a smear the bacilli are usually seen at sharp angles to each other. *Corynebacterium diphtheriae* is destroyed by a temperature of 60° C. but survives freezing and drying.

The diphtheria bacillus grows well on the usual laboratory mediums. Löffler's medium is commonly employed because the organism grows readily on it, whereas the streptococci and staphylococci do not. By the use of the tellurite medium the bacillus has been classified into three types, *gravis, mitis,* and *intermedius.* It was believed at first, that the *gravis* type was the cause of severe infections, the *mitis* type of mild, and the intermediate type of moderately severe infections. In this country such a correspondence between bacterial types and clinical infection has not been proved.

Diphtheria bacilli may be virulent or nonvirulent, depending on whether they produce an exogenous toxin or not. It is this toxin which is responsible for most of the symptoms and deaths in diphtheria. To test for virulence 0.1 to 0.2 cubic centimeter of a suspension of the bacilli from a culture is injected intradermally on the shaved skin of each of two guinea pigs one of which was immunized the day before with 500 units of diphtheria antitoxin intraperitoneally. An inflammatory lesion at the site of injection of virulent strains develops in 24 to 72 hours in the nonprotected guinea pig, while no reaction occurs in the protected one. Nonvirulent strains

164

cause no reaction in either pig. The toxin is readily destroyed by heat and chemical agents.

Diphtheria occurs naturally in man only. However, many experimental animals are susceptible to the toxin of diphtheria bacilli. In human infection the organisms are found localized in the mucous membranes of the upper respiratory tract, where they produce diphtheria toxin which is absorbed and causes damage to the tissues.

THE HOST

Symptoms

The incubation period is generally from 2 to 5 days but may be longer. In pharyngeal diphtheria the onset is usually gradual, with a sore throat, general malaise, and fever of 100° to 102° F. If the throat is examined, an exudate is seen on one or both tonsils. If not treated, the exudate spreads to adjacent tissues, and in severe cases will cover the faucial pillars, uvula, pharynx, nasopharynx, and even larynx. The patient will now look very sick and toxic. His fever is high, and he appears listless and prostrated. The pulse becomes rapid, and the heart sounds are weak. There is a thick, mucoid discharge from the mouth and throat, and there is swelling of the palate and faucial tissues. The membrane may cause obstruction to breathing, so that the mouth is kept open. The breath is foul. The glands of the neck enlarge, sometimes to such an extent as to give an appearance of a bull neck. The membrane is grayish in color, sometimes dirty gray, and is adherent to the mucous membranes so that it is not readily wiped off, and if it is wiped off, bleeding points remain.

The laryngeal form, known as diphtheritic croup, a dreaded disease years ago, is now seen much less frequently than before. It may result from extension of pharyngeal diphtheria or may occur as a primary disease. The symptoms do not vary from other types of croup. At first the voice is hoarse, and there may be a dry, slightly metallic cough. Soon, difficulty in respiration is noted, and if this is not relieved, signs of asphyxia result. The child is restless and anxious, and his breath is pulled in with difficulty, giving a crowing sound. He works with his accessory muscles of respiration. There are dilatation of his alae nasi and retraction of his chest wall. The temperature, which was low grade, begins to mount, and the pulse gets rapid. He becomes cyanotic, tosses around, gasps for air, goes into a stupor, and then into coma. If he gets no mechanical relief to the obstruction, he chokes to death.

In nasal diphtheria there is frequently no membrane formed. The infected person does not feel or act sick. The only manifestation may be a persistent nasal discharge, often unilateral, frequently admixed with blood. Examination will reveal excoriation of the nares.

Less commonly, diphtheritic infections may occur in the skin or the ear or eye. Usually, they are the result of inoculatin of the tissues at the site of some injury, often minor. An ulcer results, covered with a dirty gray membrane and showing little disposition to heal.

Complications are not common in mild cases or where diphtheria antitoxin is promptly used. In severe and untreated cases, complications are not unusual. Myocarditis is one of the more serious complications and is often first recognized by the pulse, which is weak and rapid. It may cause death. Peripheral neuritis is another common complication. It is first suspected when the patient develops a nasal voice. Examination of the palate and uvula while the patient vocalizes indicates that they are immobile. Strabismus may result from paralysis of one of the extrinsic eye muscles.

Paralysis of the muscles of the limbs may also occur. Usually, complete recovery follows. If the intercostal muscles become paralyzed, there is interference with respiration. This type of paralysis is serious and requires prompt treatment in a respirator. In laryngeal diphtheria relief to breathing must be given by sucking out the obstructing membrane or performing an intubation or a tracheotomy.

Diagnosis

The appearance of the throat in a severe case is quite characteristic. Mild cases may be mistaken for tonsillitis. All cases of throat infection showing an exudate should be cultured on Löffler's medium, and the organisms should be stained with Löffler's methylene blue. Diagnosis by the examination of a direct smear is unreliable.

Immunity

An attack of diphtheria usually confers immunity on the patient. Such immunity is however, not so solid as in measles or chickenpox, so that second attacks are not rare. In a population where diphtheria is endemic, the adult population is usually found to have considerable immunity. This is probably due to subclinical infections which are constantly occurring. It is possible that the prevalence of nonvirulent diphtheria bacilli may also contribute to the immunization of a population. The immunity obtained by a woman is passively transferred to her child, which is born immune and which remains so for the first half year of its life, the immunity gradually receding thereafter. In children, susceptibility to diphtheria is very high.

Active Immunization

Several antigens are available for active immunization against diphtheria. The first to be used was *toxin-antitoxin,* a mixture of toxin and antitoxin with a slight preponderance of the former. Although it is an effective immunizing agent, it has several disadvantages: (1) Only about 85 per cent of those injected were immunized; (2) the immunity took from 1 to several months to develop; (3) the presence of antitoxin, which is a horse serum, in the mixture permitted sensitization or the development of a reaction in sensitized persons; and (4) certain physical conditions, like freezing, allowed the mixture to dissociate and cause severe toxic manifestations. It was administered in three doses, of 1 cubic centimeter each, at intervals of 1 to 2 weeks.

Fluid toxoid, or *anatoxin* as it was originally called by Ramon, who introduced it, is toxin modified by the addition of Formalin and heat until the toxicity is lost. The antigenic potency, however, remains. It is usually administered in three doses of 1 cubic centimeter or 0.5 cubic centimeter each at intervals of about 1 month. The number of injected children that are immunized is higher than 90 per cent, and the other disadvantages of toxin-antitoxin are eliminated.

Alum-precipitated toxoid was the last antigen to be introduced. It consists of fluid toxoid to which alum has been added. The alum holds the toxoid as a repository in the tissues at the point of injection and allows for slow absorption of toxoid and increased antigenicity. Two doses of 1 cubic centimeter each are given at an interval of about 1 month. The number of immunized individuals rises to between 95 and 98 per cent with the use of this antigen. It is somewhat more irritating than fluid toxoid and occasionally causes a swelling, the so-called "sterile abscess," at the site of inoculation, which may persist for several weeks.

Several modifications of toxoid have been experimented with, chiefly in order to eliminate reactions. In England, a mixture of toxoid and antitoxin, known as T. A. F. (toxoid-antitoxin floccules) is fairly popular, but it is not used in this country. The chief immunizing agents used in this country are alum-precipitated toxoid and fluid toxoid, in that order.

There has been considerable discussion as to the age when immunizaton against diphtheria should be begun. There are two disadvantages to giving it too early in the child's life. One is that very young infants do not seem to have as good an antibody-production mechanism as older infants and children. The second objection is that the antitoxin present in the young infant's blood tends to fix the injected toxoid and prevents it from reaching the cells where the stimulation of the antibody-forming mechanism takes place. If diphtheria immunization alone is used, a good age to begin is from 6 to 9 months.

The use of combined antigens for the immunization against diphtheria and tetanus or diphtheria and whooping cough or all three has been increasing in popularity. Such mixtures, as well as the time of administration and the dosages, are discussed on pages 304–305.

There have been several reports on the duration of immunization after the primary series. There is evidence that loss of antitoxin titer begins fairly soon and decreases very gradually. However, more than 95 per cent are still immune at the end of 2 years, and a considerable percentage of the immunized group continues to be immune for as long as 5 or 6 years.

Experiments indicate that when an individual has been immunized against diphtheria and the titer of antitoxin in his blood has diminished after some years even to a point where it is not measurable, the injection of a small amount of the immunizing agent will raise the titer of the immunity to its original level, or even higher, in 5 to 10 days. Such an injection is known as a *booster* or *reactivating* or *recall* dose. Only a very small amount need be injected. Even the performance of a Schick test may introduce enough antigen to raise the titer. In practice, the dose used is 0.1 to 0.2 cubic centimeter. It is considered good public health practice to give a booster dose of fluid diphtheria toxoid every 3 years after the primary series until the child is 10 years old.

Primary immunization with diphtheria toxoid of individuals above the age of 10 years is often accompanied by severe reactions. Although such reactions have not been known to cause death, they cause symptoms which are uncomfortable and disturbing. The reaction is apparently due to protein material in the toxoid. By removing this and immunizing with purified toxoid, the severity of reactions is reduced. However, a small group of individuals shows sensitivity to the toxoid also, and injection of full doses may cause severe reactions. Fortunately, such individuals are readily immunized by small doses.

If individuals above the age of 10 years, who have not been previously immunized, are to receive a primary series of diphtheria toxoid, it is wise to test them for sensitivity. This is done by the Moloney test and consists of an intradermal injection of 0.1 cubic centimeter of a 1:10 dilution of fluid diphtheria toxoid. A positive result is indicated by an area of erythema at the site of injection in 24 to 48 hours. Moloney-positive individuals can be immunized safely by starting injections with 0.1 cubic centimeter of fluid toxoid subcutaneously; if no reaction occurs, the second dose of 0.5 cubic centimeter is given in a month, and the third dose of 1 cubic centimeter is given a month later. If more than a mild reaction occurs to any one dose, the subsequent dose should be the same or one half the last dose.

To determine the exact amount of antitoxin an individual has in his circulation, it is necessary to titrate the blood serum. This is a laboratory procedure and requires expert technical assistance. A much simpler, although a cruder method, is to perform a *Schick test.* Diphtheria toxin so diluted that 1/50 M. L. D. (minimum lethal dose for a guinea pig weighing 250 grams) contained in 0.1 cubic centimeter of the solution is injected intradermally in the forearm. If no antitoxin is present in the circulation, this amount of toxin will cause a local reaction at the site of inoculation. If antitoxin is present, it will neutralize the injected toxin and no reaction will occur. Reactions are usually read 3 to 4 days after injection. Since filtrates of the cultures of diphtheria bacilli contain other substances in addition to toxin, and since these substances may also cause a local reaction it is necessary to control the Schick test. This is done by injecting in the opposite arm the same material after heating to 60° C. for 15 minutes. Such heat will destroy the toxin but not the other proteins. The resulting reactions, after performing the Schick test and control are given four grades: (1) positive, (2) negative, (3) pseudoreaction, and (4) combined reaction. Descriptions of the four reactions follow.

1. At the site of toxin injection there occurs an area of redness beginning about 24 hours later and increasing for several days. At the end of 3 to 4 days there are both redness and infiltration of the skin. After about 1 week this fades, turns brown, and usually desquamates and disappears, leaving behind a pigmented area which persists for several weeks. The control arm shows no reaction. A positive reaction indicates the absence of an effective amount of diphtheria antitoxin in the circulation.

2. There is no reaction in either arm. This indicates that sufficient circulating antitoxin is present to render the individual immune to an ordinary exposure to diphtheria.

3. An area of redness appears on both arms in about 18 to 20 hours and increases for another 6 to 18 hours but does not become infiltrated; it disappears at both sites in about 3 to 4 days after the test. This reaction indicates immunity, but it indicates also sensitiveness to some proteins in the injected material.

4. This is a combination of a positive and a pseudoreaction. It consists of a positive reaction in the arm injected with toxin and a

pseudoreaction in the arm injected with the control. Its interpretation is an absence of an effective amount of diphtheria antitoxin in the circulation and a sensitiveness to proteins in the antitoxin solution.

The Schick test is a valuable tool, since it can easily be performed in the field or in a physician's office and gives a fairly good indication of the immunity of the person tested. However, it takes a certain amount of time and material to perform, requires the return of the tested individual for a reading, and means an extra visit and injection for those found to be Schick positive. The vast majority of children above the age of 1 year are usually Schick positive. In public health practice it is therefore considered uneconomical to do Schick tests. All infants are immunized during the first year. They are given a booster dose every 3 years thereafter, up to the age of 10 years. The booster dose is as simple to do as a Schick test, it eliminates the extra visit, and it does no harm even if the child is Schick negative.

Individuals above the age of 10 years who require primary immunization because of special exposure to diphtheria should be Schick tested. If negative, nothing further need be done. If positive, one should proceed as outlined above.

Passive immunizaton—Individuals who are exposed intimately to a case of diphtheria should be immunized. If they have previously received a primary series, a booster dose is all that is necessary. If they have not been previously immunized, they should receive an injection of diphtheria antitoxin. The dose is 500 units for small children and 1,000 units for older children and adults. Such immunity lasts for 3 or 4 weeks only. Children receiving such prophylactic immunization should be actively immunized with diphtheria toxoid, beginning about 1 month after the administration of the prophylactic antitoxin.

THE ENVIRONMENT

Diphtheria is rare in the tropics. Until recent years, morbidity and mortality increased as one went from the tropics to the Temperate Zones. In recent years that difference is not so great. In the United States, about 30 years ago, the mortality rates were about the same in the South as in the North, but the decline since then has been greater in the Northern states, so that mortality from this disease is now higher in the South.

Age is an important factor in morbidity as well as mortality from diphtheria. The incidence of the disease in infants under 1 year of age is low, owing to inherited immunity from the mother. It rises rapidly thereafter. The distribution of cases and deaths by age groups in New York City from 1940 to 1950 is given in the table:

Distribution of Cases and Deaths for Diphtheria in New York City, 1940–1949

Age	Number	Cases Per Cent of Total Cases	Number	Deaths Per Cent of Total Deaths
All ages	2,895	100	93	100
0 – 4	987	33	44	48
5 – 9	929	32	17	18
10 – 14	330	13	10	11
15 – 19	124	4	2	2
20 – 24	106	4	4	4
25 and over	419	14	16	17

It will be seen from the table that about 80 per cent of all cases of and deaths from diphtheria occur in children under 15 years of age. However, the youngest age group, under 5 years, is responsible for one third of all the cases but one half of all deaths. As in the other acute communicable diseases of childhood, the younger the child the greater the risk of dying. This indicates a need for the immunization of children at an early age. Although a shift in case incidence to the older age groups has occurred in recent years, it has been chiefly from the 15-24 age group to older individuals.

There is little difference in the incidence of diphtheria in the two sexes, but the disease appears to be more common in whites than in nonwhites.

In the United States a gradual decline in the incidence of diphtheria has been noted since half a century ago. In New York City the attack rate for diphtheria was 1,221 per 100,000 population under 15 years of age in 1900 and 6.4 in 1949, a decrease of 99 per cent. This decline cannot be attributed solely to the introduction of antitoxin, since its general use did not begin until 1910. Nor can it be ascribed to active immunization procedures only, since these were not employed prior to 1928. That the use of active prophylactic immunization was a factor in the decline is obvious from the chart below, which shows a sharp drop in the trend of the curve following the introduction of immunization.

History

The disease has been known since ancient times but was probably confused with other throat conditions. In 1826 the clinical aspects were clarified by Bretonneau, but the bacteriologic basis of the disease was not established until 1883–1884 when Klebs identified the diphtheria organism and Löffler indicated its etiological relationship to the clinical disease. The demonstration of an exotoxin was made in 1888 by Roux and Tersin, and its ability to stimulate antitoxin in animals was shown by von Behring in 1890–1893. Von

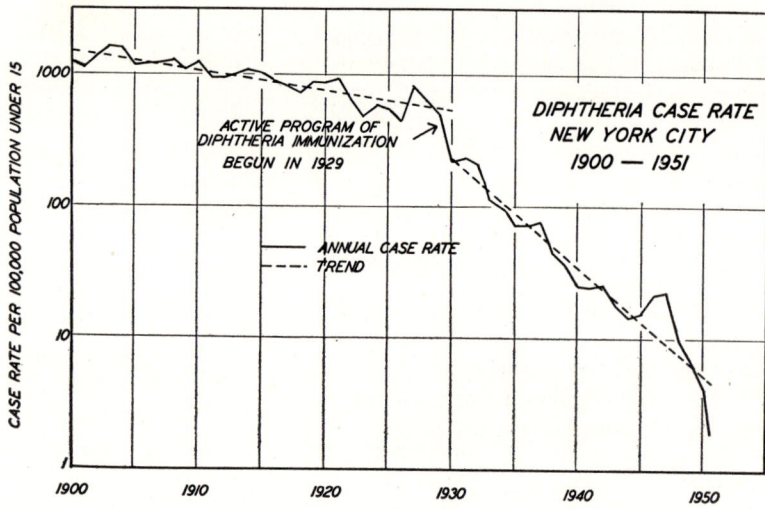

Fig. VIII. DIPHTHERIA CASE RATE IN NEW YORK CITY, 1900–1951.

Behring also showed that toxin neutralized by antitoxin could be used as an immunizing agent, and this was applied on a community scale by Park in New York, beginning in 1929. The skin test for the presence of immunity was introduced by Schick in 1913, and the development of anatoxin (toxoid) was made by Ramon in 1923.

Control

All children above the age of 6 months should be properly immunized, as indicated above, and their immunity should be kept at a high titer by booster doses, every 3 years. Cases of diphtheria should be isolated for a period of 7 days and until two sets of cultures from the nose and throat, taken not less than 24 hours apart, are negative. Contacts remaining at home should be excluded from school and from milk-handling occupations until one set of negative cultures from the nose and throat has been obtained after the case has been released from isolation. Contacts under the age of 15 who have not been previously immunized actively should be given a prophylactic dose of 500 to 1,000 units of antitoxin. Those who have been previously immunized should be given a booster dose of 0.2 cubic centi-meter of diphtheria toxoid.

Common-source outbreaks of diphtheria as a result of drinking milk contaminated by diphtheria bacilli have been reported. In practically all of them the milk responsible for the outbreak was raw. Pasteurization effectively destroys diphtheria bacilli.

Diphtheria carriers. Cases of diphtheria frequently carry the organism in their throats during convalescence. In some instances diphtheria bacilli may be recovered for several weeks or even months after recovery. However, chronic carriers, as in typhoid fever, are not known. In households with a case of diphtheria, con-tacts are frequently found to harbor the diphtheria bacillus, and they should be isolated until the organism is no longer present. With the decline in cases of diphtheria, the reservoir of carriers has also declined.

Most diphtheria carriers require no treatment. They are usually transient and cease to be carriers when contact with the case is broken. Some carriers are persistent and not too easy to clear. Sev-eral types of local applications have been used with varying results. In some, tonsillectomy has cured the carrier state. In recent years the use of penicillin given by injection and also applied locally as a spray has been reported to be of benefit in clearing up persistent carriers.

Routine cultures of children disclose a considerable number who harbor an avirulent type of diphtheria bacillus. Whether such strains contribute to the general immunity of diphtheria is not definitely known. The routine culturing for diphtheria of children admitted to hospitals, institutions, schools, or camps should be dis-couraged. Many of these cultures are morphologically positive but avirulent. The positive cases must be isolated until the virulence has been determined, and this means a considerable delay in admis-sion and a disorganization of programs. Reliance should be placed on proper immunization of all children and on culturing only those children who show suspicious clinical signs.

MEDICAL CARE PLANS

Treatment

Nonspecific treatment consists essentially of keeping the patient in bed to avoid undue exertion on the heart, which is affected by the toxin, and of proper feeding and hygienic care. Specific treat-ment consists in the early administration of diphtheria antitoxin. The toxin elaborated by the local membrane is absorbed and passes to the body cells by means of the circulation. If antitoxin is ad-ministered early, it will combine effectively with the circulating toxin and neutralize it. If given late, the toxin will already have become attached to the cells and have injured them, and the antitoxin will not have nearly the same curative effect. This is readily demonstrated in animals where the administration of antitoxin shortly after the injection of lethal doses of diphtheria toxin will save the animals, but if treatment is delayed, increasing the dose of antitoxin several hundred times will not save the animals. In humans, too, the mortality is proportional to the time when antitoxin is administered; the earlier the administration, the fewer the deaths.

If diphtheria is suspected clinically, a culture should be taken and antitoxin administered immediately, without waiting for the results of the culture. The amount needed varies with the clinical severity and the time elapsed since onset of the disease. The entire dose should be given at one time, intravenously in all but mild cases where it may be given intramuscularly. The number of units required in each case is learned by experience only. Generally, 20,000 units are given in tonsillar diphtheria, 20,000 to 40,000 units if there has been spread to the pharynx, and up to 100,000 units if there is considerable involvement. The dose administered also depends on the time elapsed between onset and treatment. With each day lost, a considerable increase in the amount of antitoxin given is necessary. The individual should first be tested for sensitivity to horse serum; if there is evidence of sensitivity, either desensitization is undertaken or a despeciated horse-serum antitoxin or a bovine antitoxin is administered.

Penicillin appears to be effective in inhibiting the growth of diphtheria bacilli and is therefore valuable as an adjuvant in treatment. It must be remembered, however, that it has no effect on the toxin and cannot be relied upon as the sole method of therapy. Nothing takes the place of diphtheria antitoxin in fixing the toxin and neutralizing its harmful effects.

The treatment of diphtheritic croup or laryngeal diphtheria requires good teamwork by doctor and nurse and careful and constant attention to details. In addition to the use of antitoxin and other drugs, it is often necessary to keep the patient in a properly constructed croup tent where he can receive steam inhalations. The trachea sometimes becomes so narrowed that suffocation is imminent unless radical measures are taken. These consist of three procedures: (1) intubation, (2) aspiration, and (3) tracheotomy.

Intubation is the procedure by which a tube is placed in the larynx with a special instrument. It was previously the method of choice, but has lost popularity on account of the danger of dislodging the tube in a coughing spell, and the irritation caused to the mucous membrane so that the throat closes up when the tube is removed.

Repeated aspiration of mucus and pieces of membrane is the method of choice in many hospitals.

Tracheotomy is the least used of the three procedures. It consists of inserting a tube into the trachea and larynx after making an incision in the neck and cutting through the rings of tracheal cartilage. None of the three procedures should be used unless indicated. However, it is unwise to wait until the child is exhausted and gasping for breath. Good clinical judgment is essential.

In laryngeal diphtheria the throat is often quite sore, and there is pain on swallowing. Patients suffering from laryngeal diphtheria should be treated in a hospital. The humidity of the room should be kept fairly high, or if that is inconvenient the patient should have steam inhalations and be kept in a croup tent. Supplies and equipment should be readily available for aspiration and for tracheotomy. The nurse should observe the patient for changes in symptoms and should keep constant watch. Any change in the child's condition, such as difficulty in respiration, change in color, rapidity of pulse, or restlessness, should be reported to the doctor immediately. If the child is unusually restless it may be necessary to administer a sedative, like phenobarbital. The diet is the same as in pharyngeal diphtheria.

Diet

The diet should be restricted to liquids and soft foods. With improvement, the diet is made more liberal.

Supportive Nursing Care

Good nursing care is of paramount importance. The room or ward should be well ventilated and the environment cheerful. The temperature in the room should be comfortable and the sleeping clothes warm but not heavy.

The application of an ice collar to the neck frequently relieves soreness and contributes to general comfort. The ice collar should be kept on for about 1 hour and then off for ½ hour to allow the skin to get back to normal. Freezing of the skin is avoided by protecting the bag with gauze or linen. When the ice collar needs refilling, it should not be taken out of the room. A basin of cracked ice and a spoon should be brought into the room and the ice collar filled. After filling, the utensils are boiled.

Mouth care is an essential part of nursing care. It should be kept clean with simple mouthwashes. When throat pain is marked, warm saline irrigations are often prescribed. To avoid resistance, the procedure should be explained to the patient in advance. The temperature of the solution should be moderate and the flow regulated so that it is not too forceful.

In nasal diphtheria, external application of a thick ointment such as zinc oxide or boric ointment to the excoriations prevents scratching and subsequent bleeding. The nursing care is the same as for pharyngeal diphtheria, except that the patient, supported by pillows or back rest, may sit up in bed.

Following recovery, the nurse should assist the family in planning the convalescent period.

In the community, home visits are made by public health nurses to all reported cases of diphtheria. The purpose of the visit is to give and to demonstrate nursing care of the patient to a member of the family. In addition, isolation procedures are explained and arrangements made for the immunization of all susceptible contacts under 15 years of age and for the adult nursing the patient.

In nursery, elementary, and secondary schools the nurse should refer students with suspicious sore throats to the family physician for diagnosis and treatment. Any outbreak of sore throats in school children should be reported to the district health officer.

The immunization status of all children in nursery and elementary grades should be checked regularly by nurses giving service in these agencies. The importance of supplementary injections for diphtheria should be emphasized by the public health nurse in all her contacts with parents, and by the nurse in the hospital pediatric clinic.

REFERENCES

1. Berman, B. B., and Spitz, S. H.: "Treatment of Diphtheria Carriers with Penicillin," *Bull. U.S. Army M. Dept.*, **87**:4, 1945.
2. Bierman, H. R., and Maxwell, R. W.: "The Present Status of the Immediate Tellurite Test for Diphtheria," *J.A.M.A.*, **117**:1255, 1941.
3. Bureau of Public Health Nursing, New York City Department of Health: *Manual of Nursing Procedures Relating to Acute Communicable Diseases*, pp. 15–17, 1949.
4. Dauer, C. C.: "Trends in Age Distribution of Diphtheria in the U.S.," *Pub. Health Rep.*, **65**:1209, 1950.
5. DiSant'Agnese, P. A.: "Simultaneous Immunization of New-born Infants against Diphtheria, Tetanus and Pertussis," *Am. J. Pub. Health*, **40**:674, 1950.
6. Frobisher, M., Jr.: "Strains of C. Diphtheriae in Various Parts of the U.S.," *Am. J. Pub. Health*, **30**:28, Suppl., 1940.
7. Goldie, W., and Maddoch, E. C. G.: "A Milk-borne Outbreak of Diphtheria," *Lancet*, **1**:285, 1943.
8. McLeod, J. W.: "The Types *Mitis, Intermedius* and *Gravis* of C. Diphtheriae," *Bact. Rev.*, **7**:1, 1943.
9. Stowman, K.: "Diphtheria Rebounds, Epidemiological Information Bulletin," *United Nations Relief & Rehabilitation Division*, **1**:157, 1945.

Chapter 14 EXANTHEM SUBITUM (ROSEOLA INFANTUM)

GENERAL DESCRIPTION

EXANTHEM subitum is an exanthematous disease of unknown origin, apparently communicable, characterized by a fever lasting a few days and a macular rash which appears after the temperature has dropped.

THE CAUSATIVE AGENT

Nothing is known of the causative agent. It has not been grown in culture, nor has the disease been transmitted to humans or animals.

THE HOST

Symptoms

The incubation period is about 2 weeks. The onset is abrupt, with fever of 103° to 104° F., or even higher, which lasts for 3 to 5 days. No other symptoms occur until the temperature has dropped to normal, when a rash appears, first on the trunk, then spreading to the head and extremities. It is macular and reddish in color, resembling the rash of German measles. It fades in 1 or 2 days, and the patient is completely well.

Diagnosis

There are no laboratory tests to aid in the diagnosis. A leukopenia is usually present. Diagnosis depends on the clinical findings which are characteristic, since in none of the other exanthems does the rash appear after the decline of the fever.

Immunity

It is believed that one attack confers immunity, but second attacks have been described.

THE ENVIRONMENT

The disease is seen almost exclusively in young children. It was first described by Zahorsky in 1910. It occurs sporadically but may also be seen in outbreaks in institutions. The highest incidence is in the spring and autumn.

MEDICAL CARE PLANS

Treatment

There is no specific treatment. The antibiotics are of no value. Recovery is the rule, no matter what treatment is used.

Diet

The fluid intake should be adequate. A soft diet is given after the temperature declines.

Supportive Nursing Care

Nursing care consists in keeping the patient comfortable, and sponge bathing during the febrile period.

Chapter 15 GERMAN MEASLES (RUBELLA)

RUBELLA is a mild exanthematous disease, presumably caused by a virus and characterized by slight fever, a macular rash, and enlargement of the posterior cervical glands.

THE CAUSATIVE AGENT

No causative agent has been isolated. The infection has been transmitted to children by inoculation of filtered nasal washings. It can also be transmitted to monkeys with filtered nasal washings or defibrinated blood of patients taken early in the course of the disease, either by nasal instillation or inoculation. It has not been grown successfully in chick embryos or tissue culture, or in ordinary laboratory culture.

THE HOST

Symptoms

The incubation period is about 18 days. The onset is usually with mild sore throat and slight fever. The rash comes out within 1 day, first on the face, and spreads rapidly to the neck, trunk, and extremities. It is in full bloom in 24 hours. It lasts 2 or 3 days and then fades. It consists of pinkish macules which are discrete but may become confluent. There are no Koplik spots, cough, or eye symptoms, as in measles. However, enlargement of the occipital and posterior cervical nodes is characteristic, the glands remaining enlarged for 1 or 2 weeks after fading of the rash. Complications are rare.

Diagnosis

No laboratory test exists to aid in diagnosis. The disease must be distinguished from measles and scarlet fever. In the former, a high fever, catarrhal symptoms, cough, and Koplik spots are distinguishing signs. In scarlet fever the throat is more inflamed, the rash more punctate, and fever is higher. In neither of the two diseases is the occurrence of enlarged cervical and occipital glands common. Leukopenia is usually present.

179

Immunity

One attack usually confers permanent immunity. There are no prophylactic immune agents available. Gamma globulin has been used experimentally in the prevention of the disease in exposed contacts, but the results have been contradictory.

THE ENVIRONMENT

The distribution of rubella is similar to that of measles. It occurs more commonly in winter and spring. Although children are more susceptible than adults, the disease is not infrequently seen in the latter. It is not nearly so contagious as measles. It may occur sporadically but frequently occurs in epidemics. The disease is transmitted by discharges from the nose and throat of patients from the beginning of illness until 2 or 3 days after the rash appears.

In 1941, Gregg called attention to the occurrence of congenital defects in infants whose mothers had German measles in the first 3 months of pregnancy. Confirmatory reports have been made by many others, especially in Australia, England, and this country. The most common defects described are cataracts, deaf-mutism, cardiac malformations, and mental retardation. Injury to the embryo by the virus must take place before the end of the third month to cause the malformations enumerated. After the third month the development of the organs has been completed, and they are not susceptible to injury any more.

Unfortunately, most of the reported statistics have started with the defective child and worked backward. Also, they have depended on the mother's memory and on vague diagnoses. On the basis of this type of data, statements have been made that from 90 to 100 per cent of infants born to mothers who have had German measles in the first or second month of pregnancy will be deformed. Only a few studies have started with cases of German measles in pregnant mothers and worked forward to find out what percentage of their children are born defective. These indicate a percentage of about 15 to 20 per cent. There is urgent need for statistics of a large series of women who have been followed during their pregnancy when they developed German measles and whose children have been examined for congenital defects. Such a series is difficult to obtain, but by pooling their resources a number of health departments or obstetrical hospitals might be able to obtain the data. All investigators agree that the risk of a defective child if the mother develops German measles beyond the third month of pregnancy is statistically and embryologically small.

Control

The patient is isolated for a period of 5 days from the beginning of the rash. Contacts are not quarantined. To avoid the chances of developing German measles, a woman in the early months of pregnancy should not be exposed to cases of the disease, particularly in her own family. If she has been so exposed, consideration should be given to the use of gamma globulin, with the knowledge that its effect in the prevention of this disease is uncertain. Since German measles is ordinarily a mild disease conferring a lasting immunity, it appears reasonable and medically sound to advise the exposure of girls to the disease so that they will not run the risk of getting it later in life during pregnancy.

MEDICAL CARE PLANS

Treatment

There is no specific therapy. The patient should be confined to bed during the acute phase of the disease. The antibiotics are of no value. Treatment is symptomatic. The disease is usually so mild that no therapy is needed.

Diet

There are no dietary restrictions.

Supportive Nursing Care

Nursing care is largely hygienic in nature. The skin should be kept clean with daily baths.

In group teaching, such as mothers' classes, the public health nurse or nurse in hospital prenatal clinics should stress avoidance of contact to cases of German measles early in pregnancy. If the pregnant woman has been so exposed, the doctor should immediately be notified so that the use of gamma globulin may be considered. Immediate notification to the department of health should be made if a pregnant woman develops German measles.

REFERENCES

1. Fox, M. J., and Bortin, M. M.: "Rubella in Pregnancy Causing Malformations in Newborn," *J.A.M.A.*, **130**:568, 1946.
2. Greenberg, M.: "Gamma Globulin in Pediatrics," *M. Clin. North America*, **31**:605, 1947.
3. Gregg, N. M.: "Congenital Cataracts following German Measles in the Mother," *Tr. Ophth. Soc. Australia*, **3**:35, 1941.
4. Hill, A. B., and Galloway, T. McL.: "Maternal Rubella and Congenital Defects," *Lancet*, **1**:299, 1949.

5. Landon, J. F.; Bass, M. H.; and Muckenfuss, R. S.: "The Efficacy of Gamma Globulin in the Prevention of German Measles," *New York Med.*, **5**:21, 1949.
6. Ober, R. E.; Horton, R. J. M.; and Feemster, R. F.: "Congenital Defects in a Year of Epidemic Rubella," *Am. J. Pub. Health*, **37**:1328, 1947.
7. Swan, C.: "Congenital Defects in Infants Following Rubella During Pregnancy," *M. J. Australia*, **1**:409, 1944.

Chapter 16 HEPATITIS, VIRAL

VIRAL hepatitis is a syndrome characterized by jaundice and other symptoms, caused by one or more viruses, which occurs sporadically and also in epidemic form. Two forms of viral hepatitis have been studied. Both have the same symptoms, but there is reason to believe that viruses causing the two are distinct or possibly variants of one virus. The mode of infection, the incubation period, the mode of spread, and certain immunological relationships are different in the two. These are discussed below. One form is infectious hepatitis, formerly spoken of as "catarrhal jaundice," and the other is serum hepatitis or homologous serum jaundice.

Infectious Hepatitis (Catarrhal Jaundice)

GENERAL DESCRIPTION

Infectious hepatitis, or epidemic jaundice, or catarrhal jaundice, is a disease of the liver which is caused by a virus and characterized by fever, nausea, vomiting, abdominal pain, and jaundice.

THE CAUSATIVE AGENT

The agent of infectious hepatitis is a virus which affects man only. Experiments have been confined to human volunteers, since the agent cannot be transmitted to animals. The virus is resistant to heat and chlorination (not destroyed at $56°$ C. for $\frac{1}{2}$ hour, and withstands chlorination 1 part per million for $\frac{1}{2}$ hour). It can be recovered from the blood and feces early in the disease and can be transmitted to humans by feeding or inoculation or by spraying the throat. The virus has been recovered from the blood of patients as early as 3 days before onset; it is not known precisely how long the virus remains in the blood of individuals ill with the disease.

THE HOST

Symptoms

The incubation period of infectious hepatitis varies from 10 to 40 days, with an average of 25. The onset may be abrupt but is often gradual, with anorexia, nausea, headache, lassitude, and abdominal pain. Fever is occasionally quite high, but usually it is low grade. These symptoms last a few days. Jaundice then supervenes and may last from 1 week to 1 or 2 months. The liver becomes enlarged and tender, and the spleen may be felt. The stools are clay-colored, and the urine shows the presence of bile. There may be itching of the skin. As the jaundice decreases, convalescence sets in, the appetite returns, the feeling of tiredness abates, and general well-being returns. This stage is usually prolonged. Recovery may not be complete for several months. Symptoms are usually more severe in adults than in children. In the former, weight loss may be considerable, and recurrence of symptoms of weakness, tiredness, and loss of appetite are not unusual. The mortality is low. A fair number of cases go through the first stage but never develop jaundice. They are usually not recognized unless they occur in the course of an epidemic and unless liver-function tests are performed.

Diagnosis

There is no specific immunologic test. Diagnosis depends on the clinical picture and evidence of liver damage as determined by liver-function tests. It should be pointed out that in epidemics of the disease, a considerable number of individuals may not have jaundice but only mild preicteric symptoms; some may have no symptoms at all, but liver-function tests will indicate damage.

In the preicteric stage the cephalin-cholesteral flocculation test is usually positive, and the bromsulfalein and phosphatase tests are abnormal. When jaundice appears there is, in addition, a high icteric index and a positive van den Bergh reaction. The urobilinogen is elevated, there is bile in the urine, and the stools are clay-colored. The white blood count is usually not elevated; on the contrary, leukopenia is not uncommon. The sedimentation rate is also not much elevated.

Immunity

An attack of infectious hepatitis appears to confer immunity. In the Army, where the disease was studied intensively, troops that had gone through an epidemic of hepatitis did not get the disease when re-exposed. Even those who had not shown signs of infection in the original epidemic had a lower incidence than fresh troops not previously exposed. Volunteers convalescing from an attack of epidemic hepatitis have been fed active virus for $\frac{1}{2}$ to $\frac{3}{4}$ year following their attack and have not come down with another attack. Furthermore, normal human gamma globulin has been administered to children exposed to epidemic hepatitis, and they have been protected by it. This would seem to indicate that the disease, possibly in subclinical form, is widely prevalent, so that immune substances are obtained when a random group of human beings is bled. The fact that the disease is epidemic and the adult population remains relatively free is added reason for believing that the attack rate in the general population is high. Second attacks are known to occur, however, in about 3 per cent of patients.

THE ENVIRONMENT

Epidemic hepatitis is a world-wide disease. In sporadic form it most commonly attacks children in the age range from 5 to 15, but it may occur in adults. Small family outbreaks and epidemics in institutions have been recognized for many years under the name of catarrhal jaundice. It has occurred in large-scale epidemics in young adults in armies as far back as the Napoleonic Wars.

The precise method of spread has not been determined. Close contact of individuals appears to play a part, but whether the virus is spread by oral discharges or by the contamination of water and food by feces has not been definitely determined. The disease is more common in the fall and winter, and this seems to argue in favor of a respiratory spread. On the other hand the virus is regularly present in the stools, the disease is more common where sanitation is poor, and outbreaks have been reported which were waterborne, milk-borne, and food-borne, so that the spread by alimentary discharges appears likely. The possibility of spread by an insect vector must also be considered, though there is little evidence for it.

Control

Since the method of spread is not known and since spread by the respiratory tract is possible, the patient should be isolated early in the disease. Contacts need not be quarantined. Discharges from the mouth and nose should be cared for as in other respiratory diseases. The stool may be emptied into a flush toilet. If this is not available, the stool should be disinfected with 5 per cent chloride of lime solution before emptying the bedpan.

In the presence of an epidemic in an institution or camp, care should be taken to maintain the purity of the water and food supply. Fecal contamination should be avoided by teaching food handlers good personal hygiene and by screening of kitchens. Contacts may be immunized with gamma globulin in a dose of 0.1 cubic centimeter per pound of body weight. Persons recovering from an attack of jaundice should not be used as blood donors for at least 1 year.

MEDICAL CARE PLANS

Treatment

There is no specific drug for the treatment of hepatitis. Of the nonspecific measures used, bed rest and adequate diet are the most important. It has been demonstrated that people who keep up their usual activity early in the disease do not fare as well as those who take to bed when symptoms first occur. It has also been shown that patients who get up early after recovery frequently have relapses.

If the prothrombin time is low and hemorrhages occur, vitamin K should be given by injection. Methionine in a dose of 5 grams a day has been recommended. Bed rest should continue until liver-function tests are normal.

Patients who have marked anorexia and those with severe nausea and vomiting may require parenteral treatment for a while. This is given in the form of 5 per cent glucose intravenously. If the vomiting is somewhat protracted, a blood or plasma transfusion may be indicated. When there is abdominal pain, a hot-water bag or an electric pad will often bring relief. If the pains are not relieved by this simple measure, atropine or a similar antispasmodic may have to be used.

Diet

A sufficient and proper diet is important in all diseases affecting the liver. The diet should be adequate in caloric and protein intake and low in fat. Vitamin preparations should be given in addition.

Supportive Nursing Care

Nursing care consists largely in keeping the patient comfortable, encouraging him to remain in bed after the acute symptoms have subsided, and maintaining adequate nutrition. The latter is not easy, since patients often have anorexia. Tepid sponge baths are given for general comfort. Placing the patient in Fowler's position may be more comfortable where abdominal cramps and distention cause distress. Since convalescence is long, the patient needs guidance and encouragement in gradual resumption of daily activities and care of self.

Serum Hepatitis (Homologous Serum Jaundice)

GENERL DESCRIPTION

Serum hepatitis is always produced by parenteral injection. It may be through the injection of blood or plasma from an infected

individual or from the use of an infected syringe or needle which
has not been properly sterilized.

The Causative Agent

The causative agent is a virus similar in its characteristics to that
of infectious hepatitis. It is resistant to heat (56° C. for 60 minutes)
and chlorination and survives for years after freezing and after
drying. Ordinary antiseptics do not destroy it. However, it may be
inactivated by ultraviolet light. This fact is taken advantage of in
the commercial preparation of plasma. The virus of serum hepatitis
can be recovered in the blood during the incubation period as well
as during active disease.

The Host

Symptoms

The symptoms of serum hepatitis are similar to those of infectious
hepatitis. The incubation period is longer than in infectious hepatitis—60 to 120 days. The disease is not spread by contact but only
by parenteral injection of infectious material. The virus does not
appear in the feces as it does in infectious hepatitis, and infection
in volunteers cannot be brought about by feeding infected serum.

Diagnosis

This is similar to the diagnosis of infectious hepatitis, page 184.

Immunity

There is no cross immunity between infectious and serum hepatitis. An individual recovering from one disease can be infected with
the other. Gamma globulin does not protect against serum hepatitis
as it does against infectious hepatitis.

The Environment

Blood and plasma are now used universally. Since individuals
with serum hepatitis carry the virus during the incubation stage,
individuals may donate infected blood. Where bloods are pooled,
as for the preparation of plasma, a large batch may become infected.
The inactivation of the virus by ultraviolet light offers one method
of protecting pooled plasma. However, cases have occurred in persons transfused with light-treated blood. The heating of albumin
(one of the fractions of plasma) at 60° C. for 10 hours also destroys
the virus without hurting the albumin. When whole blood is given,
the transfusion is taken from a single individual, so that the possibility of transfer of disease is limited. Nevertheless, all blood donors

should be questioned about a history of jaundice, and no blood should be accepted in the presence of a positive history within 1 year.

Control

Serum hepatitis may also be transferred by infected needles used for Wassermann tests, for injections of vaccines, toxoids, antibiotics, or numerous other drugs and biologicals. Since the virus is resistant to ordinary chemicals, thorough cleansing and proper sterilization of all syringes, needles, and stylettes is very important.

REFERENCES

1. Baxter, Ola M.: "Hepatitis," *Am. J. Nursing,* **46**:385, 1946.
2. Blumer, G.: "Infectious Jaundice in the United States," *J.A.M.A.,* **81**:353, 1923.
3. Capps, R. B.; Skorov, V.; and Scheifley, C. H.: "A Syringe Transmitted Epidemic of Infectious Hepatitis," *J.A.M.A.,* **136**:819, 1948.
4. Findlay, G. M., and Martin, N. H.: "Jaundice Following Yellow Fever Immunization," *Lancet,* **1**:678, 1943.
5. Havens, W. P., Jr., and Paul, J. R.: "Prevention of Infectious Hepatitis with Gamma Globulin," *J.A.M.A.,* **129**:270, 1945.
6. Letourneau, Charles U., and Fleigh, George: "Approved Hospital Techniques to Control Viral Hepatitis," *Hospitals,* **26**:97–103, 1952.
7. Murphy, W. J.; Petbie, L. M.; and Work, S. D., Jr.: "Outbreak of Infectious Hepatitis, Apparently Milk-borne," *Am. J. Pub. Health,* **36**:169, 1946.
8. Neefe, J. R., and Stokes, J., Jr.: "An Epidemic of Infectious Hepatitis Apparently Due to a Water-borne Agent," *J.A.M.A.,* **128**:1063, 1945.
9. Neefe, J. R.; Stokes, J., Jr.; and Gellis, S. S.: "Homologous Serum Hepatitis and Infectious (Epidemic) Hepatitis," *Am. J. M. Sc.,* **210**:561, 1945.
10. Paul, J. R.; Havens, W. P.; Sabin, A. B.; and Philip, C. B.: "Transmission Experiments in Serum Jaundice and Infectious Hepatitis," *J.A.M.A.,* **128**:911, 1945.

Chapter 17 HISTOPLASMOSIS

GENERAL DESCRIPTION
HISTOPLASMOSIS is an infectious disease, caused by a fungus, which usually runs a chronic course and is characterized by a variety of symptoms.

THE CAUSATIVE AGENT
The causative agent is a fungus, *Histoplasma capsulatum,* which is small and yeastlike. It grows on cultures at room temperature, like a mold. It infects the reticulo-endothelial system, causing small granulomas which may become calcified.

THE HOST

Symptoms

The incubation period is not known, since the onset is insidious. Symptoms vary and are often absent throughout. There is even no definite information as to how the organism enters the body. Most of the cases have been diagnosed postmortem. In advanced cases symptoms are those of a general cachexia, with slight fever, emaciation, anemia, and enlargement of the spleen, liver, and lymph nodes. The disease may manifest itself mainly in the lungs, resembling tuberculosis, or in the skin, resembling other granulomas. There is usually an associated leukopenia.

The importance of the disease is due chiefly to the fact that it appears to be endemic in certain parts of the country, chiefly in the Kansas City area and in the states bordering on the Mississippi River and its tributaries. Surveys conducted in these areas by means of the histoplasmin skin test have shown a large number of positive reactors. A number of these have shown calcified areas in the lungs. Since their tuberculin tests were negative, the assumption has been made that the lesions were due to histoplasmosis.

In recent years a number of cases have been diagnosed during life, and the fungus has been recovered from their sputum, blood, or stomach washings. Some of these were discovered accidentally in surveys; others were studied because they had pulmonary calcifications or symptoms resembling influenza or pneumonia.

Diagnosis

A diagnosis can be made by recovering the fungus from sputum, stomach washings, blood, bone marrow, or biopsy either by culture or by animal inoculation. Infected individuals give a positive skin test with histoplasmin, but the specificity of this has been questioned. Recently, a complement-fixation test has been used in diagnosis, but its value has not yet been definitely determined.

Immunity

Infection with *Histoplasma capsulatum* causes the development of a positive skin reaction to the filtrate of broth in which the fungus is grown. This filtrate is known as *histoplasmin*. The skin reaction is of the delayed type, resembling tuberculin. In endemic areas many individuals are found with pulmonary calcifications, negative tuberculin tests, and positive histoplasmin tests. It has been assumed by some investigators that these calcifications represent healed lesions of histoplasmosis.

THE ENVIRONMENT

The first description of the organism was made in 1906 by Darling, who found the organism at necropsy and thought it was a protozoan. Later, it was shown by others to be a fungus. It has been found in Central America, in Indonesia, and in this country. There appears to be no predilection for either sex or for any age, although the percentage of positive skin tests rises with age, as in tuberculosis. The organism has also been recovered from animals, such as dogs, cats, rats, and skunks, and has been recovered from soil. The method of transmission is not known, nor is it known how long an infected individual is communicable.

Control

Isolation is not required since the method of transmission is unknown. Discharges from lesions and articles soiled with such discharges or with sputum should be burned or properly sterilized. There are no effective control measures, since little is known about the epidemiology of the disease.

MEDICAL CARE PLANS

Treatment

There is no specific treatment. The antibiotic drugs have not proved effective. Therapy is chiefly symptomatic.

Diet

As in tuberculosis, the patient's nutrition may be below par. A diet containing essential nutrients and supplemented with vitamins is given.

Supportive Nursing Care

Plans for nursing care are dependent upon the health and social needs of the patient and family.

REFERENCES

1. Christie, A., and Peterson, J. C.: "Pulmonary Calcification in Negative Reactors to Tuberculin," *Am. J. Pub. Health*, **35**:1131, 1945.
2. Darling, S. T.: "Histoplasmosis," *Arch. Int. Med.*, **2**:107, 1908.
3. Emmons, C. W.: "The Isolation of *H. Capsulatum* from Soil," *Pub. Health Rep.*, **64**:892, 1949.
4. Emmons, C. W., and Ashburn, L. L.: "Histoplasmosis in Wild Rats," *Pub. Health Rep.*, **63**:1416, 1948.
5. Furcolow, M. L.: "Development of Calcification in Pulmonary Lesions Associated with Sensitivity to Histoplasmin," *Pub. Health Rep.*, **64**:1363, 1949.
6. ——— "Further Observations on Histoplasmosis," *Pub. Health Rep.*, **65**: 965, 1950.
7. Kingberg, W. G.: "Generalized Histoplasmosis in Infants and Children," *J. Pediat.*, **36**:728, 1950.
8. Meleney, H. E.: "Histoplasmosis: A Review," *Am. J. Trop. Med.*, **20**:603, 1940.
9. Palmer, C. E.: "Nontuberculous Pulmonary Calcification and Sensitivity to Histoplasmin," *Pub. Health Rep.*, **60**:513, 1945.

Chapter 18 INFLUENZA

GENERAL DESCRIPTION

INFLUENZA is a viral disease usually occurring in epidemic form and characterized by general symptoms of fever, chills, headache, backache, and prostration, and by mild upper respiratory symptoms.

THE CAUSATIVE AGENT

Influenza is caused by one of a number of related viruses. Two types are recognized—influenza A and influenza B. They are serologically distinct. Each of these types, however, has many strains which resemble each other but may nevertheless differ from each other serologically. Both types of virus are readily destroyed by heating and by treatment with disinfectants. They can, however, be preserved at very low temperatures. Influenza virus is able to agglutinate red blood cells, and a commonly used diagnostic test depends on this phenomenon.

The virus of influenza can be recovered from throat washings of patients from the first to the fifth day of illness, by intranasal inoculations of ferrets, mice, and hamsters, or by inoculation into the amniotic sac of chick embryos. It is not found in the blood stream or other organs. It causes inflammation of the trachea and bronchi, with necrosis and desquamation of the epithelium. The alveolar walls of the lungs may show hemorrhage and necrosis.

THE HOST

Symptoms

The incubation period is short, from 1 to 3 days. The onset is abrupt, with chills, fever, headache, backache, loss of appetite, and muscular aches and pains. Occasionally, there is nausea. Sneezing and nasal and throat irritation are often complained of, but they are mild compared to the constitutional symptoms. Cough may supervene. On examination, the striking fact is that the signs of illness are much milder than the general symptoms warrant. There is usually some injection of the nasal and pharyngeal mucosae, the face may be flushed and the skin hot. The lungs are usually clear. The duration of illness is short, most patients recovering in a few days unless complications set in. There are no characteristic differences in the symptoms of influenza A and influenza B.

Complications

Complications are not uncommon, particularly in old and debilitated persons. They are chiefly bacterial infections of the respiratory tract, such as otitis media, sinusitis, bronchitis, and pneumonia. Fortunately, they respond to antibiotic treatment.

Diagnosis

The white blood count is usually normal or may show a leukopenia. The sedimentation rate is slightly increased. Influenza virus may be recovered from throat washings in the acute stage. However, such recoveries are time-consuming and can be performed only in a laboratory equipped for the purpose. They are not of practical value in early diagnosis. Yet without recovery of the virus or the finding of an increasing titer of antibodies in the blood, a definitive diagnosis cannot be made.

A clinical diagnosis can be made with a fair degree of certainty during epidemics of influenza, particularly when recoveries of virus have been made from some cases. When influenza is not prevalent, a diagnosis is difficult. For this reason the reporting of influenza in nonepidemic years is poor indeed.

Immunity

Following an attack of influenza, immunity develops against the specific strain causing the disease. This may be demonstrated by obtaining a specimen of blood from the patient in the first few days of illness and another one 2 to 3 weeks later. The presence of antibody can be tested for by the complement-fixation reaction, by the serum neutralization test in the ferret, mouse, or chick embryo, or by the agglutination-inhibition test of Hirst. The latter method is the most commonly used because of its simplicity. It depends on the fact that influenza virus causes the agglutination of red cells, but if virus and immune serum are mixed and red cells are then added, agglutination does not result.

If an individual recovers from influenza, antibodies against the specific strain that caused the illness are present in his blood. If he suffered from influenza A, his blood serum will inhibit the agglutination of red cells when mixed with virus A but not when mixed with virus B. The reverse happens if he is recovering from influenza B. A fourfold increase in titer of antibody in the serum between the early and convalescent stages is usually considered evidence that illness was caused by the specific virus. Immunity does not last long, probably not more than 6 months.

For active immunization a vaccine made from influenza viruses A and B, grown on chick embryo and inactivated, has been used. This is injected subcutaneously in one dose of 0.5 cubic centimeter. Antibodies appear in the serum in 1 week; they reach their height in about 1 month and then decline. The immunity conferred does not last more than a few months. The vaccine has the further disadvantages that toxic reactions occur not infrequently after injection and that, since it is grown on embryonated eggs, individuals sensitive to eggs or chickens may get allergic reactions if injected with it.

From 1944 to 1946, prophylactic immunizations were given with a vaccine containing A and B virus to large groups of young adolescents. When influenza broke out in these groups the immunized individuals showed considerable protection. Commercial firms began the manufacture of the vaccine on a large scale, and the public was advised to be injected and thus immunized. In 1947, however, the previous results could not be duplicated. Investigation showed that the prevalent influenza of that year was caused by a variant of influenza A which was immunologically distinct from both A and B viruses. It was called A prime. Even when this virus was added to the vaccine it did not offer the same protection against A prime influenza as the vaccine had given against A and B influenza in the previous few years.

Further study has clearly indicated that A and B are not homogeneous types. Each is made up of a number of strains, some of which resemble the parent strain but others of which are totally different immunologically. To have an effective vaccine the least requirement is that it should contain the strains of the current epidemic. However, it is not possible to tell in advance what strains will be current in the next epidemic to come around. Practical considerations also limit the number of strains that can be put into a vaccine. Until the research workers can supply the answers to the many problems connected with development of a good vaccine, the general use of influenza vaccine is not advisable.

THE ENVIRONMENT

Both influenza A and B usually occur in epidemic form. The intervals between epidemics in the former are usually 2 or 3 years and in the latter 4 to 5 years. The attack rates are generally high in places where people are closely congested, as in schools or institutions. Outbreaks were fairly common in barracks in World War II. In rural communities, spread is slow. Recoveries are the rule, but death may occur from uncomplicated influenza. Most deaths result from complications, particularly pneumonia.

Influenza is world wide in distribution and has been known since ancient times. While it occurs most commonly in colder weather in the Temperate Zones, it has occurred even in summer months in the tropics. The greatest epidemic of the disease occurred in 1918–1919, when it was widely distributed over the globe and caused the death of large numbers of people. The viruses of influenza had not yet been discovered at the time, so that there is no way of knowing what strains were then prevalent. Certainly their virulence must have been much greater than recent ones, since mortality then was high, while the mortality in recent outbreaks of A and B influenza has not been great.

Control

The patient with influenza should be isolated during the febrile period. Contacts are not quarantined. The patient should be instructed to cover his face when sneezing or coughing and to use paper tissues for the collection of nose and throat secretions. These should be burned or flushed down the toilet.

MEDICAL CARE PLANS

Treatment

There is no specific treatment available. Bed rest is essential during the acute stage. The surrounding environment should be cheerful and pleasant, the room temperature warm, and the humidity adequate to keep the mucous membranes moist. An icecap often relieves headaches and gentle massage of the extremities and back with tepid alcohol may ease muscular aches. If there is a dry cough, steam inhalations often give relief. Reassurance that the illness is of short duration and not of serious consequence is often necessary for patients who are mentally depressed. Antipyretics are used to make the patient comfortable, and sedatives are prescribed for restlessness and insomnia. Sulfonamides or antibiotics are of no value against the virus, but they are used either prophylactically or in treatment for the bacterial complications.

Diet

A high fluid intake, including liberal amounts of citrus-fruit juices, should be given to make up for the loss caused by sweating. During the acute stage of illness, a light diet is offered. With the onset of convalescence, the diet is increased; it should contain a variety of foods, including generous amounts of protein.

Supportive Nursing Care

Routine general nursing care for the comfort of the patient is of prime importance.

During epidemics of influenza, coordinated community planning is essential to provide nursing services to all who need them. Since many patients remain at home, the public health nurse may give or demonstrate nursing care of the patient and instruct the family in isolation procedures.

REFERENCES

1. Francis, T., Jr.: "A New Type of Virus from Epidemic Influenza," *Science,* **92**:405, 1940.
2. Francis, T., Jr.; Salk, J. E.; and Quilligan, J. J., Jr.: "Experience with Vaccination against Influenza in the Spring of 1947," *Am. J. Pub. Health,* **37**:1013, 1947.
3. Hirst, G. K.: "The Agglutination of Red Cells by Allantoic Fluid of Chick Embryos Infected with Influenza Virus," *Science,* **94**:22, 1941.
4. Jordan, William S.: "Acute Upper Respiratory Infections," *Am. J. Nursing,* **50**:39, 1950.
5. Rasmussen, A. F., Jr.; Stokes, J. C.; and Smadel, J. E.: "The Army Experience with Influenza, 1946–1947, II. Laboratory Aspects," *Am. J. Hyg.,* **47**:142, 1948.
6. Salk, J. E.; Menke, W. J., Jr.; and Francis, T., Jr.: "A Clinical, Epidemiological and Immunological Evaluation of Vaccination against Epidemic Influenza," *Am. J. Hyg.,* **42**:57, 1945.
7. Sartwell, P. E., and Long, A. P.: "The Army Experience with Influenza, 1946–1947, I. Epidemiological Aspects," *Am. J. Hyg.,* **47**:135, 1948.
8. Smith, W.; Andrewes, C. H.; and Laidlow, P. P.: "Virus Obtained from Influenza Patients," *Lancet,* **2**:66, 1933.

Chapter 19 LYMPHOCYTIC CHORIOMENINGITIS

GENERAL DESCRIPTION

LYMPHOCYTIC choriomeningitis is a disease caused by a specific neurotropic virus, which manifests itself by symptoms of a respiratory infection and sometimes by signs of meningitis.

THE CAUSATIVE AGENT

The causative agent is a specific virus which is filterable. It can be preserved in 50 per cent glycerin and frozen at a temperature of $-70°$ C. It can be grown in animals, tissue culture, and chick embryos.

THE HOST

Symptoms

The commonest recognizable symptoms are meningeal. After an incubation period of a few days, there is a sudden onset with symptoms resembling grippe or influenza. Signs of meningitis may follow, and a spinal tap will show clear fluid under pressure, with increased protein, normal sugar, and a cell count of 100 to 300 lymphocytes per cubic centimeter. Symptoms persist for 2 to 3 weeks, with recovery in most cases. The disease occasionally occurs in a very mild form without meningitis, or is even clinically inapparent. Occasionally the disease may be severe and death may result; as in the following description of a small outbreak investigated by the New York City Department of Health:

A man of 31, an animal attendant in the veterinary division of a firm manufacturing biologicals, and a woman of 42, a glassware worker in the same division, became ill on the same day with fever, malaise, and a slight cough. Symptoms became worse, and each was admitted to a hospital, the man 3 days later, the woman 4 days later. Symptoms in both became more severe but were indefinite, suggesting a grippe or influenza. Both developed a rash which was macular and faded on pressure; however, in adjacent areas it was definitely petechial. The man had no meningeal signs, but the woman had a suggestion of a stiff neck, and a spinal tap was done. This, however, was negative, with 5 cells per cubic millimeter. Blood counts in both patients showed moderate leukopenia. Blood cultures were negative, and so were agglutination tests for typhoid, brucella, and typhus. They became mentally confused, lapsed into coma, and died, the man 12 days after onset, the woman 11 days after onset.

Autopsies were done in both cases. An attendant sewed up the body of the man. Six days later he became ill with fever, anorexia, and malaise. He developed symptoms similar to those of the other two patients, including evidence of hemorrhage into skin and organs. He became irrational, lapsed into coma, and died 18 days after onset.

In all three the symptoms resembled a respiratory infection. In two there were no meningeal signs, while in the third the meningeal signs were minimal and the spinal fluid was negative. Yet, the virus of lymphocytic choriomeningitis was recovered from the nervous tissue of all three.

Diagnosis

The blood shows a mild leukocytosis, with increased polynuclear count. Diagnosis is made by symptoms and signs of a mild meningitis, the spinal-fluid findings, as indicated above, and the recovery of the specific virus. This may be obtained during the febrile period from the blood, spinal fluid, urine, and nasopharyngeal secretions by injection into mice. In fatal cases the virus is found in the central nervous system and in the lungs. Many laboratory animals can be infected. Albino mice are commonly used and can be fatally infected intranasally as well as intracerebrally. However, if inoculated subcutaneously with small doses, they may be rendered immune. Serologic tests may be done with serums obtained in the acute stage and in convalescence. These consist in the finding of fourfold increases, in the later specimen, of complement-fixing or neutralizing antibodies. The former appear after about 3 weeks and the latter, after about 2 months.

Immunity

An attack of the disease confers immunity. No procedures for active or passive immunization are available.

THE ENVIRONMENT

The virus was first recovered in 1934, from a monkey, by Armstrong and Lillie, and the next year it was recovered from a human being by Rivers and Scott. It is common in mice, causing no symptoms, and passing from generation to generation. It is also found in dogs and other animals. Humans usually get it by contact with infected animals. Spread from man to man does not seem to take place. In humans it is a fairly widespread disease, most of the cases being inapparent and recognized only by the presence of antibodies in the blood. The recognized disease occurs in both sexes, more frequently in adults. It is most commonly seen in the winter and spring.

The virus is generally found in the house or field mouse and is shed in the nasal secretions, urine, and feces. It is easily transmitted to man. Although the exact method of transmission has not been demonstrated, it is believed to be through the respiratory tract, possibly in dust.

Control

This depends on measures usually taken in rodent control, trapping, poisoning, and destruction or sealing off of harborages. The patient need not be isolated, nor do the contacts have to be quarantined.

MEDICAL CARE PLANS

Treatment

No specific treatment is known. The antibiotics have no effect on this or on any other neurotropic virus. Symptomatic treatment is the same as for other forms of meningitis.

Diet

Fluids are given during the acute stage, and the diet is increased as the patient improves.

Supportive Nursing Care

Essential nursing measures are supportive and adapted to the individual needs of the patient.

REFERENCES

1. Christian, Henry A.: *The Principles and Practice of Medicine,* 16th ed., Appleton-Century-Crofts, Inc., New York, pp. 385–386, 1947.
2. Meakins, Jonathan Campbell: *The Practice of Medicine,* 5th ed., The C. V. Mosby Company, Medical Publishers, St. Louis, pp. 1401–1402, 1950.
3. Mitchell, Charles A., and Koltz, Max O.: "Lymphocytic Choriomeningitis," *Canad. Pub. Health J.,* **33**:208–213, 1942.

Chapter 20 MEASLES (RUBEOLA)

GENERAL DESCRIPTION

MEASLES is an acute exanthematous disease caused by a virus and characterized by a prodromal period of fever and catarrhal symptoms, followed by a generalized macular rash.

THE CAUSATIVE AGENT

The virus of measles is present in the blood and in nasopharyngeal washings of cases during the prodromal period and the first 2 to 3 days of the rash. It can survive at room temperature for about 1½ days and at 0° C. for several days. It has been cultivated successfully in tissue culture and in chick embryos. Egg passage virus produces a very mild disease in man and monkeys and results in immunity to measles. Measles can be transmitted to man and monkey only, none of the lower animals being susceptible to the natural disease or artificial inoculation.

THE HOST

Symptoms

The incubation period is 14 days. About 10 to 11 days after exposure, the prodromal period begins, with catarrhal symptoms, sneezing, coryza, injected eyes, cough, and fever. An enanthem appears on the inside of the cheeks from the first to the fourth day of the prodromal period. It consists of discrete, grayish spots, pin point in size, on a red base. They are seen on both sides, usually at the level of the molars, but often widely spread. They are known as "Koplik spots" and are diagnostic of measles. Fever may vary from 100° to 103° F.

By the fourth day after onset, the rash appears, first on the face, either on the forehead or behind the ears. It spreads rapidly over the face, neck, trunk, and limbs, to reach its height in 24 to 48 hours. It is a macular, red, rash beginning as small irregularly round lesions and becoming crescentic in shape. Adjacent patches may coalesce and form a large blotch. The rash fades on pressure. After reaching its height, it begins to recede and after 2 to 3 days is completely gone, leaving a brownish discoloration and fine, branny desquamation.

When the rash first appears the child is at its sickest. Fever is high, the cough is troublesome and continuous, the eyes watery and sensitive to light, the nose running, and the general appearance one of great misery—a measly appearance. After the rash has reached its full development, the temperature falls abruptly and all symptoms begin to abate. In a few days the child has fully recovered and the discolored skin is the only telltale. This, too, disappears in another few days.

Complications

The two commonest complications are otitis media and bronchopneumonia. They are caused by secondary bacterial invasion. Encephalitis is the most serious complication and does not as a rule arise until the symptoms of measles have abated. There is a secondary rise in fever, and signs of encephalitis develop. These may consist of drowsiness and stupor or of convulsions or paralyses. The neck becomes rigid, and a spinal tap shows an increase in cells and in protein. Mortality may be as high as 10 per cent. Fortunately, the complication is uncommon. Mortality from measles is low. In New York City the case fatality rate for 1950 was 0.07 of 1 per cent. For the United States the mortality rate for 1948 was 0.06 per 100,000 population.

Mortality is highest in the very young. In 1948 the age specific mortality rates for measles in the United States were 5.7 per 100,000 in infants under 1 year of age, 3.4 in children 1 to 4 years old, 1.3 in children 5 to 9 years old, and 0.4 in children 10 to 14 years of age.

Diagnosis

There are no laboratory procedures to aid in the diagnosis. A leukopenia is found, but this also occurs in a number of other diseases. The symptoms and signs are, however, so characteristic and the Koplik spots so unusual that no difficulty should be encountered after a little experience.

Immunity

An attack of measles confers a permanent immunity. There is no active immune agent available, but passive prophylactic immunization of susceptible children is possible with convalescent serum or human immune serum globulin (gamma globulin). The latter is the substance of choice since it is readily available and can be administered in small doses with no reaction. Infants under 6 months old usually possess inherited passive immunity from their mothers. This wears off during the second half of the first year. Children between the ages of 6 months and 5 years should be given a dose of 2 cubic centimeters of gamma globulin. This will completely protect the younger children and allow a modified measles in the older ones. This is desirable, since children getting a mild attack become immunized against the disease similarly to those who have regular measles. Since mortality is highest in very young infants, it is desirable to protect them completely. A dose of 2 cubic centimeters will perform the necessary function in both the very young and the somewhat older ones.

Children above the age of 5 usually go through an attack of measles without much difficulty and do not need to be protected if they are exposed and are susceptible. If, however, they are in delicate health or have recently been ill, it may be necessary to protect them. The dose for complete protection is 0.1 cubic centimeter, and for modification .02 cubic centimeter per pound of body weight. Immunization with gamma globulin confers a passive immunity and does not last more than 3 weeks. If a child is reexposed after that length of time, he should be reinjected.

THE ENVIRONMENT

Measles has been known since early times but was confused with other exanthematous diseases until Sydenham described it accurately in the seventeenth century. An excellent epidemiological investigation of the disease was made by Panum in 1846 on the Faroe Islands, and his report has become a classic in epidemiological literature. Koplik, a New York pediatrician, first pointed out the diagnostic importance of the enanthem which appears on the inside of the cheeks before the rash, and the spots are now known by his name. Measles was transmitted to humans with the blood of measles patients by Hektoen in 1905, and was produced in monkeys by Goldberger and Anderson 5 years later. Convalescent serum as a passive prophylactic agent was first used in 1918, and gamma globulin was introduced in 1944.

The disease occurs all over the world. It is extremely infectious, particularly during the prodromal stage, but the infectivity rapidly disappears after the rash comes out. Transmission is usually direct, through respiratory discharges from person to person. There is ample evidence to indicate that it may also be air-borne, and that it may also be spread by articles freshly soiled with the discharges from the upper respiratory tract. In New York City, children with measles are isolated until 5 days after the appearance of the rash. Contacts are not quarantined. Experience has shown that the quarantine of contacts does not lessen the spread of the disease.

In 1941, when contacts were still prohibited from attending school, New York experienced the worst epidemic it had ever had, with about 80,000 reported cases. Quarantine was abolished that year, and the number of cases reported annually varies little from the number reported previously.

Measles occurs cyclically every 2 or 3 years. High measles years usually alternate with low measles years. Occasionally, a high year will be followed by 2 low years. In New York City the even years are usually high measles years and the odd years low ones. In other communities, the cycle may vary. Several explanations, none completely satisfactory, have been offered for this periodicity. The most common explanation is that all susceptibles are exhausted during epidemic years. About 2 years are required for a new crop of susceptibles to arise.

The disease usually confers a solid immunity. Because of its high contagiousness, most adults have had the disease in childhood and carry antibodies against the disease in their blood. When blood is obtained from large pools, it is sure to contain a considerable concentration of antibodies. When the blood is fractionated and gamma globulin obtained, the immune bodies are concentrated about twenty-five times as much as in the serum. This is why gamma globulin is so effective in the prophylaxis of measles.

In urban areas measles occurs almost exclusively in young children. In rural areas where contact is not so close, children may escape the disease and develop it later in life when they come in contact with a case. Sex and race appear to play no part in the prevalence of the disease. In most communities measles occurs in the winter and spring, with the peak incidence in April or May or even in June.

Control

A separate room or ward or isolation unit should be maintained in hospitals admitting patients with measles, because the disease is highly communicable. In the home a patient should be isolated. Susceptible children in good health should be injected with gamma globulin and then permitted to come in contact with the sick child. They will develop a mild case of measles and become permanently immune.

If a case of measles occurs in the general ward of a children's hospital, it should be properly isolated. All susceptible contacts on the ward should be injected with a protective dose of gamma globulin. The ward may be kept open to admissions. Should a secondary case occur, all susceptible contacts who have not been immunized within the past 3 weeks should receive a protective dose of gamma globulin.

MEDICAL CARE PLANS

Treatment

There is no specific treatment for the disease. Rest in bed is necessary until after the subsidence of fever and after the cough has abated. The room should be well ventilated and the temperature comfortable. The clothing should be the usual type worn in bed. The eyes should be shielded from bright light. In a sunny room this can usually be arranged by having the patient face away from the window. There is a superstition among many people that a patient with measles should be kept very warm and that the room must be dark. Neither of these beliefs has any validity in medical experience.

Some physicians like to use antibiotics to prevent the complications of measles. A disturbing symptom is the cough, which may be severe and persistent. It is usually necessary to prescribe a sedative like codeine to control it.

Diet

The diet is chiefly liquid during the period of high fever. As the fever subsides, other foods are added until there is a return to a normal diet.

Supportive Nursing Care

Skilled nursing care is important. The skin needs special care and the use of soap in bathing the patient is occasionally irritating. Sometimes the addition of cornstarch, oatmeal, or soda bicarbonate to the bath water produces a soothing effect. Tepid sponge baths may be given if the body temperature is high. Alcohol may be added to the water for its cooling effect.

Oral and nasal hygiene need special emphasis. When thick mucus is present, mechanical suction, applied gently, aids in removing it and may prevent extension of the infection to the middle ear.

Many families in a community regard measles lightly and do not call a physician when a child is ill unless complications arise. Education of parents is important in control of measles. In some communities public health nurses make home visits to families where children under 3 years of age are reported ill with measles and no doctor is in attendance. The instructions to the family include the importance of medical care, isolation, prevention or modification of measles in familial contacts, and demonstration of nursing care procedures.

All nurses should be aware of the psychological factors in measles. Children who suddenly erupt with measles develop anxieties about the cosmetic effect of the rash and occasionally have fears because of the sudden isolation and withdrawal of playmates and siblings. The temporary nature of the condition should be explained and reassurance given to dispel their fears.

In nursery and elementary schools the nurse should enlist the aid of teachers in the control of the disease, particularly during epidemic periods. She should provide them with pertinent information about early symptoms and signs. All suspicious cases should be referred to the school nurse and isolated until seen by a doctor.

REFERENCES

1. Greenberg, M.: "Measles," in *Conn's Current Therapy*, W. B. Saunders Company, Philadelphia, 1951.
2. Greenberg, M.; Frant, S.; and Rutstein, D. D.: "Gamma Globulin and Placental Globulin," *J.A.M.A.*, **126**:944, 1944.
3. Karelitz, S.: "Does Modified Measles Result in Lasting Immunity?" *J. Pediat.*, **36**:697, 1950.
4. Ordman, C. W.; Jennings, C. G.; and Janeway, C. A.: "The Use of Concentrated Normal Human Serum Gamma Globulin (Human Immune Serum Globulin) in the Prevention and Attenuation of Measles," *J. Clin. Investigation*, **23**:541, 1944.
5. Stokes, J., Jr.; Maris, E. P.; and Gellis, S. S.: "The Use of Concentrated Normal Human Serum Gamma Globulin (Human Immune Serum Globulin) in the Prophylaxis and Treatment of Measles," *J. Clin. Investigation*, **23**:531, 1944.
6. Towsley, H. A.: "Measles," *Am. J. Nursing*, **47**:278, 1947.

Chapter 21 MENINGOCOCCUS MENINGITIS (EPIDEMIC CEREBROSPINAL MENINGITIS)

GENERAL DESCRIPTION

MENINGOCOCCUS meningitis is an acute infectious disease caused by the meningococcus and characterized by fever, the occurrence of a petechial rash, a rigid neck, and the presence of an increased number of cells and of meningococci in the spinal fluid.

THE CAUSATIVE AGENT

The causative agent is the meningococcus, known technically as *Neisseria intracellularis*. It is a gram-negative coccus, somewhat kidney-shaped, occurring in pairs with the indented sides adjacent. It grows best on mediums to which animal proteins have been added. It is readily destroyed by heat, the common antiseptics, and drying, and is very sensitive to sulfadiazine and the antibiotics. It occurs in nature in man only.

An attempt has been made to classify meningococci by types. The original classification had four types, but more recent classification divides them into two general types or groups called Group I and Group II. The typing of meningococci is not of much value since specific antiserums are no longer used.

THE HOST

Symptoms

The incubation period of meningococcus meningitis is from 3 to 10 days. Although the term "meningococcus meningitis" is commonly used, it would be more correct to refer to the disease as "meningococcal infection," since meningitis is only one of its manifestations. The meningococcus enters the body by the nasopharynx. It sets up a localized infection there. However, this is so mild that no attention is paid to it. On questioning, however, many patients with manifest symptoms of meningococcus infection state that they had a mild sore throat or nasal discharge at the beginning of their illness.

The next stage is usually that of sepsis, which manifests itself by fever, chills, a rapid pulse, irritability or drowsiness, and the appear-

206

ance of a petechial rash over the body. The rash is discrete and consists of pin-point- to pinhead-sized lesions which are flat and which do not disappear on pressure. Occasionally, in addition to the petechiae, there are larger hemorrhagic areas in the skin. This is the stage in which meningococci are present in the blood stream, and the petechiae and hemorrhagic areas represent the result of thrombi in the capillaries. Since meningococci are present in the blood stream, this stage is spoken of as one of *meningococcemia.*

Occasionally, the stage of sepsis is extremely severe and fulminating. The symptoms, as indicated, come on very abruptly, shock rapidly supervenes, stupor and coma develop, and the patient may die in a few hours or in 1 or 2 days. At autopsy it is common to find hemorrhage into the adrenal glands. This type of fulminating infection is known as the *Waterhouse-Friderichsen syndrome.*

In some cases the stage of sepsis merges into the stage of meningitis. In others the stage of sepsis is so mild as to be overlooked, and the illness appears to begin with meningitis. The onset is acute, with fever, severe headache, vomiting, and pain in the back of the neck. As a rule, a petechial rash is already present on the skin. Examination shows a marked cervical rigidity, so that it is impossible to approximate the chin to the chest. Abnormal neurologic signs can usually be elicited. Of these, the more important ones are the Kernig and the Brudzinski. The former is an inability to straighten the leg to a right angle when the thigh is flexed on the abdomen; the latter is manifested by a flexion of the knees and hips when an attempt is made suddenly to flex the head on the chest.

The severity of the symptoms of meningitis varies. The patient is always quite ill, but in some cases he is alert, restless, or irritable, and complains of discomfort and headache. In other cases he is drowsy, stuporous, or even in coma. There may be involvement of the cranical nerves resulting in deafness or strabismus.

Complications of various kinds may follow infection with the meningococcus. These are due to the localization of the bacteria in certain tissues or organs. Among the commoner ones are ophthalmitis, arthritis, pericarditis, and pneumonia. These complications are less common since the use of sulfadiazine and the antibiotics.

Diagnosis

The diagnosis can be confirmed by recovery of the meningococcus from the blood or spinal fluid. In the early stage of meningococcal infection, positive blood culture can be obtained in more than half the cases. When meningeal signs supervene, a lumbar puncture should be performed. This will show cloudy fluid under pressure, with a high cell count, mostly polymorphynuclears, increased pro-

tein, and decreased sugar content. Pandy's test for globulin is positive. After sedimentation, a stained smear will show gram-negative
diplococci. Culture of the fluid will yield meningococci. Nasopharyngeal cultures are usually positive for meningococci early in
the disease, and smears made from petechial lesions are also occasionally positive.

The blood count shows an increased number of white cells with
a predominance of polymorphonuclear leukocytes.

Immunity

The degree of immunity conferred by an attack of meningitis is
not known, since there is no practical method of testing for it.
Second attacks are rare, but this may be due to the statistical im-
probability that the disease will hit the same individual twice, since
the incidence is low. There are no available methods for active
or passive immunity.

THE ENVIRONMENT

Although meningitis was probably recognized in early times, a
differentiation of meningococcus meningitis from other meningitides
was not made until the discovery of the organism by Weichselbaum,
in 1887. The disease is spread by discharges from the nose and
throat of patients or carriers, by respiratory contact, or by articles
contaminated with respiratory secretions. The portal of entry is
the upper respiratory tract. It occurs in all climates and at all
seasons of the year, but it is more prevalent in the winter and
spring.

Meningococcus meningitis occurs both endemically and epidemically. Epidemics frequently occur in wartime, in both the civil
and the military population. In the latter it is more common among
new recruits. Occurrence of epidemics is probably related to sudden
and intimate association of large numbers of individuals, shifts in
population, and overcrowding. Epidemics usually spread over a
period of several years. In the United States epidemics occurred in
1917–1918, 1929–1930, 1935–1937, and 1942–1944, with reported
case rates per 100,000 of 7.5 in 1918, 9.6 in 1929, 5.5 in 1936, and 14.1
in 1943.

Males are more commonly attacked than females, the ratio being
about 2 to 1. Although all ages are susceptible, infants and young
children have a higher attack rate and a higher case fatality than
older children and young adults. There is no influence of color on
incidence or mortality.

The introduction of the sulfonamides and penicillin has caused a marked decrease in mortality from meningococcus meningitis, as can be seen from the table below:

Mortality from Meningococcus Meningitis, New York City

PERIOD	DEATH RATE PER 100,000 POPULATION
Presulfonamide (1919–1933)	2.85
Sulfonamide (1934–1944)	1.50
Sulfonamide and penicillin (1945–1949)	0.63

The reservoir of infection in meningococcus infections is the case and the carrier. How much of a part each plays is difficult to determine. Case-to-case spread is usually not observed. In surveys during nonepidemic periods, carrier rates varying from 5 to 50 per cent have been found among noncontacts by different investigators. During epidemic periods, carrier rates as high as 90 per cent have been obtained. Furthermore, the organism carried in the nasopharynx is usually of the specific strain found in cases. The organism is not carried for long periods of time. It may remain in the nasopharynx for several weeks or months and disappear and may then again be found on culture some time later.

It is obvious that subclinical infection is very widespread. The incidence of the disease is low. Even in epidemic periods it is rarely more than 10 per 100,000 population. This, and the fact that the disease shows a predilection for young children, would indicate that there is widespread immunity in the population.

Control

The patient should be isolated until clinical recovery, by which time the meningococci will have disappeared from his nasopharynx. Contacts need not be quarantined. It is obvious that with a high carrier rate in the population there is no point in quarantining a few carriers and allowing others at large. The administration of sulfadiazine to carriers clears up their carrier state in 24 to 48 hours. It is therefore advisable to administer sulfadiazine to contacts for 2 or 3 days.

MEDICAL CARE PLANS

Treatment

The introduction of sulfadiazine has changed the outlook in patients with meningococcus meningitis. The organism is highly susceptible to the drug. It is not unusual to see a child admitted with the signs of meningitis, in stupor or even in coma, sit up in bed and play after treatment with sulfadiazine for 24 to 48 hours. This drug is the drug of choice, although the meningococcus is also sensitive to penicillin, Aureomycin, chloramphenicol, and Terramycin. Symptomatic therapy is the same as for other types of meningitis.

Diet

Fluids in liberal amounts are given during fever. A soft diet is served as soon as the fever subsides.

Supportive Nursing Care

The plans for nursing care are adapted to the individual needs of the patient. Tepid sponge baths may be given for high elevations in body temperature.

Routine home visits by public health nurses are not usually made to cases of meningococcus meningitis. If the physician requests nursing service for a patient at home, the public health nurse may either give or demonstrate nursing care to a member of the family. The contacts should be referred to the doctor for the prophylactic administraton of sulfadiazine.

Chapter 22 MONONUCLEOSIS, INFECTIOUS (GLANDULAR FEVER)

General Description

INFECTIOUS mononucleosis is an acute infectious disease of unknown origin which is characterized by a fever, sore throat, enlarged glands and spleen, the finding of a pathognomonic blood picture, and the presence of a heterophile antibody in the blood.

The Causative Agent

The causative agent is believed to be a virus but has not been recovered. Experimental work, using monkeys and human volunteers, is inconclusive.

The Host

Symptoms

The incubation period is 4 to 14 days. The onset is usually acute but may be insidious, with general malaise, lack of appetite, and irritability. Fever occurs in all cases and may be quite high, and is usually accompanied by chills and sweats. A sore throat is almost always present; it may be mild or it may be so severe as to simulate diphtheria or streptococcus sore throat. The lymph glands, particularly the cervicals, become enlarged and tender, and the spleen also becomes enlarged. Occasionally, a rash is seen on the body. Jaundice is also sometimes present. The acute symptoms subside in 1 week to 1 month. Usually, the enlarged glands persist for some time after the fever has abated.

Sometimes there occurs involvement of the central nervous system at about the second week, with headache, cervical rigidity, and other symptoms of encephalitis, including an increased number of cells in the spinal fluid, mostly lymphocytes, and an increase in the concentration of protein. The prognosis in all cases of infectious mononucleosis is good.

Diagnosis

The clinical picture is often quite characteristic. Laboratory confirmation consists of the blood count and the presence of heterophile antibody in the serum. The blood count usually shows a leukocytosis, which may be as high as 100,000 white cells, although early in the disease there may be a leukopenia. There is a tremendous increase in lymphocytes and usually the finding of a characteristically abnormal cell.

Tests to establish the presence of heterophile antibody are made by mixing a dilution of the patient's serum with sheep red cells; these become agglutinated (Paul-Bunnell test). Normal human serum also agglutinates red cells of sheep but usually at a low titer of the serum. After injection of horse serum, the agglutination may occur at a high titer. However, the heterophile antibodies in normal human serum and after injection of horse serum are adsorbed by guinea-pig kidney. The test should, therefore, be performed with sheep red cells and dilutions of human serum from the patient both before and after adsorption with guinea-pig kidney. A positive test after adsorption, in a dilution of 1:80 or higher, occurs in more than half the cases.

Immunity

Although relapses may occur in the course of the disease, second attacks are rare. There are no known procedures for active or passive immunization.

THE ENVIRONMENT

The disease has a wide distribution and occurs in all climates and seasons. Since it frequently occurs in a mild form, and since laboratory confirmation is usually necessary, it may be overlooked. It affects people of all ages but is most common in children and young adults. It occurs in whites and nonwhites and in both sexes. Since it is not a reportable disease in most states or countries, its extent is not known. It may occur sporadically but occasionally breaks out in epidemics, particularly in institutions for children. The exact method of transmission is not known but is believed to be by way of the respiratory tract through droplet infection.

Control

The patient should be kept in bed until the subsidence of fever, and the discharges from the mouth and nose should be properly disposed of. Contacts need not be quarantined.

MEDICAL CARE PLANS

Treatment

No specific treatment is available. The antibiotics have no effect on the disease, although penicillin is frequently used to prevent secondary infection of the throat. The nonspecific treatment is similar to that used for any acute illness. Alcohol sponges and aspirin are given for high fever. Sedatives are used to make the patient comfortable. An ice collar may be applied to the neck.

Diet

The appetite is very poor, and the dietary needs of the patient need special consideration. An increased fluid intake, including liberal amounts of citrus-fruit juices and protein liquids, is given when fever is present. The diet should consist of carefully selected foods which are palatable to the patient and served attractively to coax and stimulate the appetite.

Supportive Nursing Care

The measures in nursing care are essentially palliative. Recovery from infectious mononucleosis is slow, and there is general debilitation. The patient feels very fatigued and is unable to carry out any activity for a reasonable period. He frequently develops anxieties and fears regarding return to work. The nurse should recognize these factors and give guidance and support in gradual resumption of work and social activities.

REFERENCES

1. Bolton, William.: "Rival of the Common Cold," *Hygeia*, **28**:52, 1950.
2. Julianelle, L. A.; Bierbaum, U. S.; and Moore, C. V.: "Infectious Mononucleosis," *Ann. Int. Med.*, **20**:281, 1944.
3. Paul, J. R., and Bunnell, W. W.: "Presence of Heterophile Antibodies in Infectious Mononucleosis," *Am. J. M. Sc.*, **183**:90, 1932.
4. Press, J. H.; Schlevin, E. L.; and Rosen, A. P.: "Infectious Mononucleosis," *Ann. Int. Med.*, **22**:546, 1945.
5. Reed, J., and Helwig, F.: "Infectious Mononucleosis," *Arch. Int. Med.*, **75**:376, 1945.

Chapter 23 MUMPS
(EPIDEMIC PAROTITIS)

GENERAL DESCRIPTION

MUMPS is an acute infectious disease caused by a virus and characterized by enlargement of one or more of the salivary glands, most commonly the parotid.

THE CAUSATIVE AGENT

The causative agent is a virus which may be grown in chick embryo and which is filterable. It is destroyed by heat but can be preserved at a temperature of −70° C. and is fairly stable at a temperature of 40° C. At room temperature, its infectivity is destroyed in about 4 days. It is also destroyed by ultraviolet radiation and by Formalin. The virus causes agglutination of the red cells of chickens and humans. The virus is found in involved glands and in the saliva, blood, and cerebrospinal fluid. The only other animal besides man that can be infected by the mumps virus is the monkey.

THE HOST

Symptoms

The incubation period is 18 days. The onset is acute, with fever, malaise, and pain or tenseness under the ear, followed in 24 to 48 hours by swelling of one or both parotid glands. These remain enlarged for about 1 week or 10 days. Sometimes one parotid enlarges and the other does not swell until a few days later, or remains normal. Frequently, the submaxillary and sublingual glands also enlarge, and occasionally they become enlarged while the parotids remain normal. At the height of enlargement the glands are firm and tender, and the skin over them is tense and slightly reddened. In about 20 per cent of the cases orchitis or ovaritis occurs. This complication is more common at puberty and in adults than in children. It usually occurs in the second or third week of illness and is ushered in by high fever and pain in the affected gland. Rarer complications are pancreatitis and encephalitis. Sterility is rare following orchitis, and recovery from encephalitis is the rule.

Mumps sometimes occurs without swelling of the salivary glands. It may manifest itself clinically by the occurrence of orchitis or pancreatitis or by symptoms of encephalitis. Encephalitis is manifest by cervical rigidity and by the finding of an increased number of cells, usually lymphocytes, in the spinal fluid, and an increase in globulin. Occasionally, no clinical symptoms appear. Diagnosis can then be made only by serological methods. Similarly, in cases where other organs are involved and there is no swelling of the salivary glands, the diagnosis must be confirmed by serological methods.

Diagnosis

In the presence of an epidemic the diagnosis is readily made by the symptoms. Sporadic cases are not so easy to diagnose, particularly if only one parotid is enlarged, since other agents may cause enlargement of this gland. The most common conditions which may resemble mumps are symptomatic and purulent parotitis. The former is a nonspecific enlargement of the parotid gland which occasionally occurs following an operation. It is not infectious and it usually subsides without treatment. Purulent parotitis is an infection with a pus-producing organism. The gland is more swollen than in mumps and more tender, and pus can usually be expressed from Stensen's duct in the mouth. The most common condition which is confused with mumps is cervical adenitis. It should not be difficult for a physician to distinguish between the two by palpation. The parotid extends in front of the ear, while the cervical glands lie under the jaw. The error is most commonly made when the parotid is not enlarged and the swelling is limited to the submaxillary or sublingual glands.

The blood count is within normal limits, although a relative lymphocytosis is usually found. The clinical diagnosis can be confirmed by the neutralization, complement-fixation, or hemagglutination-inhibition tests. The latter test is performed as in influenza. If immune serum is mixed with mumps virus, it prevents the latter from agglutinating red cells. For serological diagnosis a specimen of blood should be obtained early in the disease and in convalescence. A fourfold or more increase in titer of the antibody is considered evidence that the suspected illness was mumps.

When mumps virus is grown in chick embryos, two types of antigen are obtained. One is a soluble antigen (S) which is obtained from the amniotic fluid, and the other is a fixed antigen (V), obtained from the membrane. The complement-fixation test can be performed with the patient's serum for each of these antigens, but the test with the former is positive earlier than with the latter. This fact is made use of in epidemiological investigations of the disease.

A skin test has been perfected for testing previous infection with mumps. It consists of the intradermal injection of the virus in the forearm. A positive reaction consisting of redness and induration appears in immune individuals 48 to 72 hours later. The test is positive only in recovered cases and should not be used for diagnosis.

Immunity

An attack of mumps confers a permanent immunity. Second attacks are rare. The development of antibodies in the patient's serum has been discussed under diagnosis. The development of a vaccine made from inactivated or attenuated virus for active immunization is in the experimental stage. Attempts to confer passive immunity with gamma globulin or convalescent serum have not been successful. There is some evidence that gamma globulin obtained from convalescent serum may prevent orchitis when used in large amounts, but such use is not practical.

THE ENVIRONMENT

Mumps has been recognized as a clinical entity since Hippocrates. The causative agent was proved to be a virus in 1934. The disease is world wide in distribution and occurs epidemically and sporadically, chiefly in the winter and spring. It affects all races and both sexes equally. It is more common in children but is not unusual in adults, in whom orchitis and ovaritis are more common than in children. It frequently occurs in inapparent form, as judged by positive antibody response in surveys of normal adults without a history of the disease, and in normal children in a community where the disease is epidemic. It is transmitted from person to person by droplet infection and may be transmitted by linen freshly soiled by saliva. Patients with mumps are infectious from about 2 days before onset until the swelling of the glands has subsided. The disease is not carried by an intermediary unless he has an inapparent infection.

Control

This consists of isolating individuals with the disease until swelling of salivary glands has completely subsided. Contacts need not be quarantined.

MEDICAL CARE PLANS

Treatment

There is no specific treatment for mumps. Antibiotics are of no value. If there is pain, mild analgesics are used, and if fever is high, antipyretics are of value. If orchitis develops, the patient should be kept strictly in bed and the scrotum adequately supported.

Diet

Food may be given freely. The patient may select those foods which do not cause him discomfort in chewing.

Supportive Nursing Care

The comfort of the patient is the primary concern of the nurse. If there is no fever, he may be permitted to be up and about but should be kept away from susceptible persons until recovery.

If orchitis develops, there may be considerable pain of the testicle. Proper support of the scrotum with a small pillow between the thighs and the application of an ice bag frequently give relief. The ice bag should not be left on continuously. It should be kept on for about 1 hour and removed for about $\frac{1}{2}$ hour. If the pain and discomfort are severe, codeine will probably have to be prescribed.

Routine home visits by the public health nurse are not usually made for mumps. Instruction in nursing care for ill children should, however, be given if mumps is found in a family during the course of home visiting. In school situations the nurse recommends exclusion of children with suspicious symptoms and refers them for medical diagnosis and treatment. If an outbreak of mumps occurs in a classroom, it should be promptly reported to the district health officer.

REFERENCES

1. Enders, J. F., and Cohen, S.: "Detection of Antibody by Complement Fixation in Sera of Man and Monkey Convalescent from Mumps," *Proc. Soc. Exper. Biol. & Med.*, **50**:180, 1942.
2. Gellis, S. S.; McGuiness, A. C.; and Peters, M.: "Study on Prevention of Mumps Orchitis by Gamma Globulin," *Am. J. M. Sc.*, **210**:661, 1945.
3. Habel, K.: "Cultivation of Mumps Virus in the Developing Chick Embryo and Its Application to Studies of Immunity to Mumps in Man," *Pub. Health Rep.*, **60**:201, 1945.
4. Henle, G.; Harris, S.; and Henle, W.: "The Reactivity of Various Human Sera with Mumps Complement Fixation Antigens," *J. Exper. Med.*, **88**:133, 1948.
5. Montgomery, J. C.: "Mumps Meningoencephalitis," *Am. J. Dis. Child.*, **48**:1279, 1934.
6. Rambar, A. C.: "Mumps," in *Recent Advances in Nursing*, American Journal of Nursing, New York, p. 28, 1948.

Chapter 24 PNEUMONIA

PNEUMONIA is an infectious disease of the lung caused by a variety of pathogenic organisms and characterized by the exudation of cells and fluid into the alveoli, resulting in a consolidation.

Pneumonia may be classified on the basis of clinical findings, or, in other words, on an anatomic basis, into lobar and bronchopneumonia. In the former, the consolidation involves all or a large part of the lobe or even more than one lobe. In bronchopneumonia the inflammation is chiefly in the terminal bronchioles and only the adjacent air vesicles are affected; the consolidation is, therefore, patchy. About 95 per cent of all cases of lobar pneumonia are caused by the pneumococcus; the rest are caused chiefly by the streptococcus, staphylococcus, *Klebsiella pneumoniae,* and influenza bacillus. Bronchopneumonia usually involves both lungs, with a patchy distribution, chiefly at the bases. A little more than half of all cases of bronchopneumonia are caused by the pneumococcus, the balance being caused by the organisms indicated above.

Pneumonia may also be classified according to the organism causing the disease. On this basis the most common type is pneumococcal pneumonia, which is responsible for most cases of lobar pneumonia and for more than half of bronchopneumonia. Next in importance are streptococcus pneumonia, which makes up about 2 or 3 per cent of the total, *Klebsiella pneumoniae* (Friedländer's bacillus) pneumonia, and staphylococcus pneumonia. Other microorganisms frequently causing inflammation and consolidation of the lungs, such as the tubercle bacillus, the bacillus of tularemia, and the fungus causing coccidioidomycosis, are discussed under their respective headings.

In recent years a form of pneumonia in which no specific pathogenic bacteria have been found either in the sputum or in the blood stream has been reported. In some of these a specific virus like psittacosis or Q fever has been found. In others, no virus has been recovered, but the disease suggests a virus as the cause. The term "primary atypical pneumonia" is one commonly used for this type. The following discussion will take up the bacterial pneumonias and primary atypical pneumonia, presumably of virus origin.

Pneumococcus Pneumonia

THE CAUSATIVE AGENT

The pneumococcus is responsible for most cases of lobar pneumonia and about half the cases of bronchopneumonia. It is a gram-positive, lancet-shaped organism usually occurring in pairs and possessing a capsule. It is nonmotile and nonsporeforming. It grows readily on laboratory mediums to which blood or serum has been added. It is dissolved by bile. The pneumococcus is readily destroyed by heat and by the usual antiseptics.

Pneumococci are made up of a number of strains. About seventy-five different types have been isolated, and they are immunologically distinct. Types I, II, and III are the commonest found, Type I accounting for about one fourth of all cases of pneumonia, and the first eight types responsible for about four fifths of all cases. The differentiation is made on the basis of antigens present in the capsule of the pneumococcus. An antiserum can be obtained against any type by injecting the specific type of organism into a rabbit. The resulting antiserum will protect an animal against that type of pneumococcus but not against another type. To determine to which type a pneumococcus belongs, a loopful of emulsified sputum is added to a loopful of each of the specific antipneumococcal serums, and a loopful of methylene blue dye is added for coloring purposes. Examination is then made under the microscope. In the preparation containing the pneumococcus and its homologous antiserum, the capsule will have a swollen appearance and will be sharply marked off from the surrounding medium. This is known as the Neufeld or quellung phenomenon. Although pneumococci can also be typed by the agglutination and precipitin tests with homologous antiserums, the Neufeld phenomenon is much simpler.

THE HOST

Symptoms

The incubation period is 24 to 48 hours. The onset is sudden, with a chill and fever. In children a chill is uncommon, but a convulsion may occur. The temperature rises to 103° F., the cheeks become flushed, and the respirations rapid. Cough is common and often annoying, and the expectoration has a reddish or rusty color. Pain in the chest is common, particularly on deep breathing. Cyanosis is frequently seen. The symptoms continue for a period of 5 to 10 days, and then there is an abrupt crisis with a rapid drop of fever and subsidence of symptoms, leaving the patient rather washed out. The patient may die from sepsis or some complication either during the course of the acute illness or some time later.

At the height of illness a patient presents a characteristic picture which enables physicians to make a presumptive diagnosis before an examination has been made. The patient looks ill, with flushed cheeks and an alert, anxious expression. He breathes rapidly with short, rapid gasps and obvious pain. His lips are somewhat bluish, and he has a short, frequent cough which distresses him. He is wide awake to all that goes on around him, makes frequent demands, is irritable, and quite unhappy.

In bronchopneumonia the clinical picture is not so clear-cut as in lobar pneumonia. The onset may be gradual and may be preceded by malaise and upper respiratory symptoms. There may be no chill at onset, and the fever may be remittent rather than continuous. There may be no crisis with a sharp drop in temperature but rather a gradual descent or lysis. The sputum in bronchopneumonia does not have the characteristic rusty appearance that it has in lobar pneumonia.

The picture painted above was much more common prior to the introduction of the antibiotics. These have reduced the seriousness of the disease as well as of the clinical manifestations. Nevertheless, in 1948 there were still more than 18,000 deaths from lobar pneumonia in the United States.

Complications

There are many complications in pneumonia. Acute fibrinous pleurisy or dry pleurisy occurs very commonly and is usually responsible for the cough and pain in the chest. In pleurisy with effusion, or wet pleurisy, there is an accumulation of fluid between the lungs and the chest wall; if it is considerable in amount, it may cause respiratory embarrassment and have to be withdrawn. The fluid that accumulates may become purulent. This is known as empyema; it is a serious complication. The pus is often very thick and cannot be effectively aspirated, so that resection of a rib may become necessary to allow for adequate drainage. Other complications that occasionally occur are pericarditis, peritonitis, thrombosis, and meningitis.

Diagnosis

The diagnosis of a typical case of lobar pneumonia is not too difficult from the symptoms and physical signs. The latter consist of relative lack of mobility of the affected side of the chest, dullness over the consolidated area, bronchial breathing, and crackling rales. Both signs and symptoms vary in cases that are not typical, and skill on the part of a physician is required to diagnose atypical cases. The

X ray is of considerable help, since the consolidated area throws a shadow on the plate.

In bronchopneumonia there are rales and scattered areas of dullness over involved parts of one or both lungs. Changes in breath or voice sounds are sometimes difficult to elicit. If several areas of bronchopneumonia are adjacent to each other, the signs will be similar to those in lobar pneumonia. The blood count shows a leukocytosis with a relative increase in polymorphonuclear cells. Blood culture is positive early in the disease in about a third of all cases. Typing of the pneumococci from the sputum has been discussed above. If the sputum does not contain many pneumococci, it is often advisable to inject a small amount, after washing in salt solution, into the peritoneum of a mouse. In a few hours a drop of peritoneal exudate is withdrawn by means of a sterile syringe or pipette. Sufficient organisms will usually be present for typing.

Immunity

An attack of pneumonia confers very little immunity against other attacks. Whether this lack of immunity is chiefly against other types or also involves the homologous type is not quite clear. Certainly individuals may have several attacks of lobar pneumonia, the majority of which are caused by Type I pneumococcus. Apparently, whatever immunity is conferred is short-lasting.

Attempts to vaccinate against pneumonia are still in the experimental stage. A vaccine has been prepared and used with a certain amount of success in active immunization. However, it immunizes only against the strains of pneumococci present in the vaccine, and these are limited. The amount of and length of time for which protection is afforded have not been definitely determined.

THE ENVIRONMENT

Pneumonia occurs in all climates and in all seasons. In the Temperate Zones it is a cold-weather disease, the highest incidence occurring from December to March. Males are more commonly affected than females in all age groups. Infants and old people have a much higher death rate than children and young adults. In older people pneumonia is frequently the terminal condition in chronic illnesses or serious accidents. Pneumonia occurs more frequently in Negroes than in whites.

There are no chronic carriers as there are in typhoid fever. Most normal people carry the pneumococcus in the upper respiratory passages for varying periods of time. However, only a small percentage of individuals not in contact with a case of pneumonia carry Types I or II pneumococci, which cause most of the pneumonias.

Contacts to cases carry the homologous organism in a fair percentage, the closer the contact the greater their percentage. In a household with a case of pneumonia, a quarter of the contacts may carry the same type of pneumococcus. The secondary attack rate is thirty to forty times greater in such a household than in the general population.

Certain occupations are a greater hazard for the development of pneumonia than others. They include occupations in which there are marked changes in temperature or exposure to dust, such as in foundry workers, stevedores, and miners. The disease is more common in those in the low economic scale than in those who are financially better off. This is probably related to nutrition, housing, crowding, rest, and other factors.

The death rate from pneumonia has been gradually decreasing in the United States from 140 per 100,000 population in 1920 to about 30 in 1948. The disease is still one of the chief causes of death, in spite of the excellent response to antibiotics. One must remember, however, that many of these deaths are terminal, in the course of some other disease, usually chronic. If one omitted these one would find that a very marked reduction in mortality has occurred since the introduction of the antibiotics.

Control

Pneumonia is undoubtedly communicable, but other factors than the mere presence of the pneumococcus in the throat of an individual determine whether the person will become ill or not. Patients are therefore permitted to remain on general wards. However, it is wise not to allow patients with chronic or debilitating illness or very old people in the same room with a pneumonia patient. Crowding of people in hospitals, institutions, or barracks should be avoided. No other measures can be recommended until more is known of the disease.

MEDICAL CARE PLANS

Treatment

The treatment of patients with pneumonia involves symptomatic relief, use of oxygen, specific therapy, nutrition, and supportive nursing care. Good nursing is extremely important and is intimately involved in all aspects of treatment.

Symptomatic relief—Chest pain and cough are common complaints and should be treated with codeine. Local application of heat is often soothing for the pain. In severe cases restlessness is common, and occasionally delirium occurs. Phenobarbital may be used to advantage. Distention is, at times, a very troublesome symptom. An enema frequently relieves this. If the distention persists, the insertion of a soft rectal tube combined with the external application of stupes may help. Neostigmine, 1:2,000 solution, injected subcutaneously in a dose of 1 cubic centimeter should be given at the same time.

Oxygen—In recent years oxygen therapy has been used more and more in the treatment of pneumonia. It is of great value in combating anoxemia. Clinically, the most important symptom of anoxemia is cynanosis, and it is for this symptom that the treatment is mainly used. However, patients with dyspnea or rapid respirations or rapid pulse are also benefited by oxygen and should be given the advantages of its use. The oxygen tent is the best method of administration of the gas. A flow of 8 to 12 liters per minute gives an oxygen concentration of from 40 to 60 per cent. If a tent is not available, a nasal catheter may be used, with oxygen flowing at the rate of about 6 liters a minute. Nasal catheters are irritating to some individuals and must be removed and cleaned every few hours. Still another method of administration is by means of the gas mask. This also is often irritating to the patient.

When oxygen is used, safeguards to protect the patient against injury are very important. The nurse should make sure that no flame is used in the same room. The tent must be checked constantly to see that the sides are properly tucked in and that there is no leak. If the patient is quite cyanotic he must be fed while in the tent. The general care of the patient requires much time and a great deal of gentleness and deftness.

Specific treatment—Specific treatment began with the use of antipneumococcic serum. With the introduction of the sulfonamides and the antibiotics the results have been so good that serum has been discarded. Penicillin is effective and can be given in two or three doses a day, intramuscularly. Aureomycin, chloramphenicol, and Terramycin are also effective and can be given by mouth.

Pneumonia caused by the streptococcus and staphylococcus is treated similarly to pneumococcus pneumonia. Pneumonia caused by *Hemophilus influenzae* or by *Klebsiella pneumoniae* (Friedländer bacillus) is treated with streptomycin instead of penicillin.

Diet

Patients with pneumonia are not keen about food. Since the illness is of short duration, no great efforts need be made to keep up their caloric requirements. Fluids, however, are necessary to make up for natural loss. Liquids of all kinds may be given. A pitcher of water should be close at hand. Since the patient is often too weak to help himself, he should be spared the effort of helping himself. If complications ensue and recovery is delayed, a high-calory diet with vitamin supplements should be offered. Small meals, at fairly frequent intervals, are better tolerated than three large meals a day.

Supportive Nursing Care

Rest in bed is essential until convalescence is well established. Restriction of visitors aids in keeping the patient quiet, physically and mentally. The use of a light, cheerful room or ward should be stressed, since pneumonic patients are alert and apprehensive, and quite aware of their environment. Bedcovers should be warm and light in weight. The patient may lie flat or be raised on pillows or a bed rest, depending on which he finds most comfortable. Tepid sponge baths should be given for general comfort. Alcohol rubs have a cooling effect and aid in keeping the skin in good condition. If constipation is present, soapsuds enemas should be used.

The position of the patient should be changed frequently to avoid the possibility of bedsores. The bony prominences should be protected from pressure and relieved by pillows, rubber rings, or cotton doughnuts. If there is extreme restlessness or delirium, sideboards may be needed to prevent injury and falling out of bed.

During convalescence the patient is easily fatigued and needs constant reassurance to prepare him for return to his occupational tasks.

Sputum and other respiratory discharges are received in paper tissues which should be placed in a bag pinned to the side of the bed. If a specimen of sputum is needed for the laboratory or is desired for inspection by the physician, it may be expectorated into a receptacle, properly labeled, and sent to the laboratory at once.

The public health nurse is frequently called to give nursing care to patients with pneumonia or to supervise care given by a member of the family.

Primary Atypical Pneumonia

General Description

Primary atypical pneumonia is an acute infectious disease of unknown etiology but believed to be viral in nature, in which there are fever, a variety of general symptoms, and bronchopneumonic consolidation of the lungs.

The Causative Agent

No causative agent of the disease has been found. Bacterial agents do not seem to play a part in its causation, nor has any specific virus been implicated. The disease has been transmitted in human volunteers by filtered pharyngeal secretions, but no successful infection has been caused in animals or in chick embryos.

The Host

Symptoms

The incubation period is 7 to 14 days. The onset is insidious, with lassitude, a feeling of tiredness, and lack of desire for food. Symptoms of an upper respiratory infection may be present. There is usually some fever, frequently low grade but sometimes high, slow pulse, headache, and a cough with mucoid sputum. The respirations are normal and there is no cyanosis. Often, the symptoms are so mild that there is no suspicion of the presence of pneumonia.

The examination of the chest is also not very striking. Sometimes, no abnormal signs are found. Occasionally, patches of slight dullness and rales are found. The diagnosis is frequently made by the X ray, which shows pneumonic consolidation, usually more extensive than suspected by symptoms and signs. The patches are not well defined and may occur in any part of the lungs, although they are more commonly seen in the lower lobes.

The duration of the disease varies from 1 to several weeks.

Diagnosis

In addition to the symptoms and signs and the X ray findings, there must be certain laboratory findings present and others absent to justify a diagnosis. The blood count is usually normal, and the sedimentation rate is increased. Blood culture is sterile, and culture of sputum does not show a predominant pneumococcus. The virus of influenza, Q fever, psittacosis, or lymphocytic choreomeningitis, any of which may cause a similar lung picture, is not recovered in the sputum, nor do antibodies to any of them appear in the patient's serum.

In more than half the patients there are present cold agglutinins. These are antibodies in the patient's blood which have the property of agglutinating red blood cells at low temperatures but not at body temperature. They appear in the serum in the second week of illness and increase in titer up to the fourth week. Another positive finding is the presence of agglutinins to the MG streptococcus. It is not clear why these two agglutinins are present in cases of primary atypical pneumonia, but the fact is that they are.

It is obvious that the diagnosis of primary atypical pneumonia is beset by many difficulties. No etiologic agent is known, the clinical picture may simulate a number of other diseases, and no specific diagnostic feature is present. The diagnosis is made largely by exclusion and cannot be made unless there has been adequate laboratory study in addition to the clinical and X ray examinations. One should be cautious in accepting statements of effectiveness of drugs in primary atypical pneumonia, since the disease is so difficult to identify.

Immunity

Very little is known about immunity to the disease. There are no effective procedures for active or passive immunization.

THE ENVIRONMENT

The disease has been recognized only in recent years. It is not possible to state whether it existed before but was not recognized. The general incidence is not known. It appears to attack all ages and both sexes and is found in nonwhites as well as in whites. It is more common in cold weather. Transmission appears to be by way of the respiratory tract, from person to person. Little is known about carriers, since the etiologic agent has not been recovered. It is apparently transmitted more frequently under conditions of close aggregation of populations, as in army barracks.

Control

This is similar to that described under Pneumococcus Pneumonia, page 222.

MEDICAL CARE PLANS

Treatment

No specific treatment is available. Claims have been made for some antibiotics. These should be accepted with caution, in view of the uncertainty of diagnosis. The disease is usually mild, and recovery is the rule.

Diet

Fluids are given in liberal amounts during fever, and a light diet as soon as the fever subsides.

Supportive Nursing Care

Nursing care is similar to that described under Pneumococcus Pneumonia, page 224, except that oxygen, the antibiotics, and the nonspecific drugs are not frequently employed.

REFERENCES

1. Commission on Acute Respiratory Diseases: "Primary Atypical Pneumonia," *Am. J. Pub. Health*, **34**:347, 1944.
2. Conference on Therapy: "Treatment of Pneumonia," *Am. J. Med.*, **4**:423, 1948.
3. Curnen, E. C.; Mirick, G. S.; Ziegler, J. E., Jr.; Thomas, L.; and Horsfall, F. L., Jr.: "Studies on Primary Atypical Pneumonia," *J. Clin. Investigation*, **24**:209, 1945.
4. Finland, M.: "Recent Advances in the Epidemiology of Pneumococcal Infections," *Medicine*, **21**:307, 1942.
5. Heffron, R.: *Pneumonia*, Commonwealth Fund, Harvard University Press, Cambridge, Mass., 1939.
6. Hodges, R. G., and MacLeod, C. M.: "Epidemic of Pneumococcal Pneumonia; Description of Epidemic," *Am. J. Hyg.*, **44**:183, 1941.
7. Kneeland, Y., Jr.; Rose, H. M.; and Gibson, C. D.: "Aureomycin in the Treatment of Primary Atypical Pneumonia," *Am. J. Med.*, **6**:41, 1949.
8. Reimann, H. A.: "Viral Pneumonias," *Bull. New York Acad. Med.*, **19**:177, 1943.
9. Smillie, W. H.: "Epidemiology of Lobar Pneumonia," *J.A.M.A.*, **101**:1281, 1933.

Chapter 25 POLIOMYELITIS

GENERAL DESCRIPTION

POLIOMYELITIS is an acute infectious disease of viral origin, characterized by fever and meningeal symptoms, and by paralysis in about half the cases.

THE CAUSATIVE AGENT

The causative agent is a very small virus, which is quite stable and not destroyed by the usual antiseptics. It may be preserved at a temperature of −70° C. but is readily destroyed by heat. It is inactivated by free chlorine in 10 minutes in a concentration of 0.2 parts per million.

The virus of poliomyelitis is found in nature in man only. It may, however, be transmitted to other animals. There are a number of strains which can be separated into three types, Brunhilde (Type 1), Lansing (Type 2), and Leon (Type 3). Two of them, Types 1 and 3, have been transmitted to monkeys only. The Lansing strain has been adapted to mice also. The three types are immunologically distinct, and all the present known strains can be placed in one of them. That other types may be discovered is quite possible or even probable. The virus has also been cultivated in tissue culture.

The virus is rarely found in other than nervous tissues, in the blood stream and in lymph glands. It is, however, found regularly in the pharynx, gastro-intestinal tract, and in the cerebrospinal nervous system. It has also been recovered from the blood of orally infected monkeys and chimpanzees during the incubation period. It is only in the nervous system that the virus causes recognizable lesions sufficient to show clinical symptoms. These consist of destruction of neurons, chiefly in the motor areas of the brain and cord. In this respect the lesions of poliomyelitis differ from those in the various types of encephalitis, which are distributed generally throughout the brain.

The Host

Symptoms

The incubation period is usually 7 to 14 days but may vary from 3 to 35 days. Onset is acute with fever, headache, vomiting, and general discomfort. The patient usually is irritable and hypersensitive. Within a day or two the general symptoms increase in severity and there are, in addition, localizing symptoms and signs. The patient complains of pain in the back and in the muscles. If he is now examined there are found stiffness of the neck, as manifested by an inability to approximate the chin to the thorax; Kernig's sign, or pain and resistance to extension of the knee when the thigh is flexed; and Brudzinski's sign, which is a flexion of the thighs and knees when an attempt is made to flex the neck. The deep reflexes are normal or exaggerated. Paresthesia of the skin is not uncommon. A spinal tap done at this stage will yield a clear fluid under pressure, with increased cells, chiefly of the mononuclear leukocytes, increased concentration of protein, normal sugar concentration, and no bacterial growth on culture.

Paralysis occurs in more than half the cases and comes on within 24 hours to a few days after onset. It is flaccid in type, and the tendon reflexes of the affected muscles become diminished or disappear. The legs alone are most commonly paralyzed, and the legs and other muscles make up the vast majority of paralyses. Paralysis may, however, occur in the arms alone, where it usually affects the shoulder or the hand muscles, or in parts of the trunk or head. The paralysis reaches its height within a few days and after that ceases to progress. Regression of the paralytic state may continue for as long as a year. About 50 per cent of all paralytic cases recover completely; another 25 per cent retain some paralysis but are able to function well; about 15 per cent remain seriously paralyzed; and about 10 per cent die of the disease. These percentages are not absolute and may vary in different epidemics and in different years, but they are a rough guide to prognosis.

Occasionally, the general symptoms which occur at onset persist for a few days and then subside without the occurrence of localizing signs. After a few days of apparent recovery there is a recurrence of illness which continues with the development of definite symptoms and signs of poliomyelitis. This type of the disease is sometimes referred to as the "dromedary type," from analogy to the dromedary camel, which was mistakenly believed to have two humps.

The illness may not proceed beyond the first, or general stage. The temperature and other symptoms may subside without the development of pain and stiffness of the muscles and cervical rigidity, and the patient may go on to complete recovery. One speaks of this type as the "abortive" type. Actually, the diagnosis is made by inference. One cannot be sure that the illness is poliomyelitis. One assumes that it is because no other diagnosis has been made, because the illness occurs during an outbreak of poliomyelitis, or because it has occurred in contacts to cases of poliomyelitis. The fact that a large percentage of individuals who have never had symptoms and signs of manifest poliomyelitis develop antibodies to the disease leads one to suspect that many mild illnesses are really abortive types of the disease.

Generally, the acute illness does not last more than a week. Fever often subsides after 3 or 4 days. Convalescence depends on whether there has or has not been paralysis and on the extent and location of the involved muscles.

Clinically, the disease is often divided into the (1) abortive, (2) nonparalytic, and (3) paralytic forms. The last category is further subdivided into the (a) spinal, (b) bulbar, (c) bulbospinal, and (d) encephalitic forms, the last three occasionally being lumped together as bulbar forms. Since the abortive form cannot be diagnosed clinically, it should not be included in a clinical classification of the disease except to indicate its probable occurrence. The nonparalytic form is one in which there are neurologic symptoms as indicated by cervical rigidity, Kernig's sign, and Brudzinski's sign, and an abnormal spinal fluid, as manifested by a high cell count and an increased concentration of protein but in which no muscular paralysis occurs. The paralytic form is one in which paralysis follows.

Paralysis may be confined to the muscles of the trunk and extremities; it is then called "spinal." On the other hand, it may be limited to the muscles supplied by the cranial nerves or to the vital centers in the medulla, when it is known as the "bulbar" form. When both cranial and spinal nerves are involved, the disease is spoken of as "bulbospinal." There are some cases of poliomyelitis in which the manifestations are chiefly cerebral, such as drowsiness, irritability, stupor, or even coma. Since these symptoms are indistinguishable from those of encephalitis, this form of the disease is sometimes referred to as "encephalitic."

Diagnosis

The clinical diagnosis is not difficult in paralytic cases. In nonparalytic cases the diagnosis is made on the basis of an acute onset with fever, the presence of cervical rigidity, and positive spinal-fluid findings. These consist of clear fluid, an increase in the number of cells, an increase in the nonprotein nitrogen content, a positive test for sugar, and absence of organisms on smear and culture. The number of cells may vary from ten to several hundred. Early in the disease they may be predominantly polymorphonuclears, but later they are chiefly lymphocytes. The blood count is of little value in diagnosis; it is usually normal, with a slight increase in polymorphonuclear leukocytes. The abortive type of poliomyelitis cannot be diagnosed clinically.

The serologic laboratory offers little help in the diagnosis of this disease. Paired serums obtained from the patient early in the disease and during convalescence can be used in the neutralization test. However, the test is difficult to perform and requires the use of monkeys, which are expensive and hard to obtain, so that it is not of practical value.

Immunity

One attack of the disease seems to confer a permanent immunity. Second attacks of poliomyelitis have been reported, but they are extremely rare. That immunity is developed to homologous strains as a result of infection appears to be true even in monkeys in the laboratory. Whether the immunity extends to heterologous strains is not so clear. Since the incidence of clinical poliomyelitis is low, it may be that a second attack with a heterologous strain occurs rarely, because, statistically, the chances of an individual being infected a second time are small. It may be, on the other hand, that immunity, partial or complete, extends to heterologous strains. Immune bodies to one type of poliomyelitis appear to be quite prevalent. Beginning in childhood and continuing to adulthood, there is an increasing percentage of individuals whose serums contain neutralizing antibodies for the Lansing type of virus.

THE ENVIRONMENT

History

Poliomyelitis has probably existed for a long time, but it was not recognized until fairly modern times. It was first described as an entity by Heine in 1840, and a description of an epidemic was first written by Medin in 1891. The disease is, therefore, sometimes spoken of as Heine-Medin disease. Its epidemic nature was demonstrated in the laboratory by Landsteiner in 1909, when he caused paralysis in a monkey by the injection of an emulsion of spinal cord from a fatal human case.

Poliomyelitis occurs in all countries and in all types of climate. In the Temperate Zone it is a warm-weather disease, beginning in June and reaching a peak in August or September, after which the incidence declines. Epidemics have been described, however, among Eskimos in the middle of winter. In more primitive countries poliomyelitis is an endemic disease occurring the year round and affecting chiefly children under 5 years of age who make up from 80 to 90 per cent of the cases. As a result, the adult population is largely immune, much the same as is the case in measles in this country. As one progresses from the more primitive to the more advanced countries, the disease tends to become less endemic and more epidemic in type. Furthermore, as will be noted in the chart, since 30 years ago there has been a shift in incidence to the older age groups.

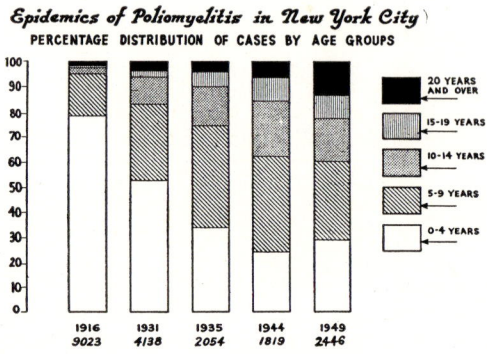

Fig. IX. EPIDEMICS OF POLIOMYELITIS IN NEW YORK CITY. PERCENTAGE DISTRIBUTION OF CASES BY AGE GROUPS.

This shift has occurred in the Northern states of this country to a greater extent than in the Southern states. In 1916, 80 per cent of the cases in New York City were in the 0–4 age group, but in 1949 the percentage of cases in this group was only 29, less than in the 5–9 age group. In spite of the shift, poliomyelitis in this country is still mainly a disease of children, since 80 per cent of reported cases are in those under 15 years of age. In rural districts, where opportunities for contact are not so great as in urban communities, epidemics of poliomyelitis are apt to involve a higher percentage of the older age groups than in the cities. This is also true of a disease like measles.

That many individuals have poliomyelitis in subclinical form is indicated by the fact that virus can be recovered from them and that they do not become ill in spite of repeated and intimate exposure. It is difficult to determine the number in this group. Various estimates have been made, a common one being that there are 100 inapparent cases to every diagnosed case.

Poliomyelitis is a much dreaded disease, largely because of the resultant crippling. Yet its incidence is not higher than 1 to 10 per 100,000 persons per year. In epidemic years the rate may be 25 or more per 100,000 persons in Southern communities, and 35 or more per 100,000 persons in Northern communities. The rates vary for the different age groups, being highest in the 5–9 age group and next highest in the 0–4 age group. Infants under 1 year of age make up only a small percentage of the total. The percentage distribution of cases by age group is given in the following table.

Percentage Distribution of Cases of Poliomyelitis by Age, New York City, 1949

Age	Cases	Per Cent of Total Cases	Age Specific Rate per 100,000
Total	2,446	100.0	29.7
0– 1	67	2.0	43.8
0– 4	718	29.3	99.0
5– 9	784	32.1	136.3
10–14	415	17.0	75.5
15–19	202	8.3	41.1
20 and over	327	13.4	5.6

Males are more frequently attacked than females. Negroes appear to have a lower attack rate than do white people. In New York City, in 1949, 6 per cent of the reportable cases were among Negroes.

Deaths from poliomyelitis vary but average about 5 to 7 per cent. Practically none occur in the nonparalytic cases. Most of the deaths occur in the bulbar types, although these are responsible for only about 15 per cent of the total cases. Mortality is higher in the older age groups than in the younger.

The method of transmission of poliomyelitis has not been definitely determined. It is known that human beings are the only animals who carry the virus in nature. This has been recovered from the pharynx of cases of poliomyelitis in the first few days of illness and from the feces for as long as 1 month or more after onset of illness. It has also been recovered from the pharynx and the intestinal contents of normal carriers, the recovery of virus being greatest from those in immediate and close contact and less and less as the distance from the cases increased. In epidemic periods virus has been recovered from sewage and from houseflies which had access to human feces. How the virus is transmitted from these sources to new cases is not clear.

It does not appear that water plays a part as a common source because epidemics cut across water sources, spread concentrically rather than along a line of supply, hit rural communities with many small sources of water as well as large communities with only one large supply, and show no correspondence between attack rates and the amount of water drunk. Furthermore, no authentic water-borne outbreak has been recorded. Milk has been implicated in several reports, but the evidence in all of them is suggestive rather than convincing. Milk is certainly not the common vehicle of spread. The virus of poliomyelitis is destroyed during pasteurization, yet epidemics do not have a different pattern in communities where milk is pasteurized than in those where it is sold raw. Epidemics ought not to occur in communities where only pasteurized milk is permitted to be sold by law, yet they do occur as frequently in such places as in other areas.

Flies can carry the virus of poliomyelitis when their bodies become contaminated as a result of lighting on infected fecal material, and it is theoretically possible that such infected insects might contaminate food, which, in turn, would infect humans. It seems extremely improbable that this occurs, however. Although the height of epidemic periods is usually in the summer, when flies are abundant, the epidemics do not die out until the winter. Furthermore, epidemics have occurred in the frozen North as well as in warmer climates. Also, epidemics occur in urban communities with modern plumbing facilities where flies do not have access to feces as well as in rural communities where the sanitation is more primitive. In epidemics, no selection has been noted in homes in which there is free access to flies over those which are well screened and in which flies are rarely seen. The conclusion must be reached that if flies play any part in transmission, it is such a minor one as to be negligible.

Poliomyelitis virus has been repeatedly recovered from sewage during epidemic periods. It probably is due to the suspension of infected fecal material and indicates the abundance of virus in such fecal material. Yet sewage appears to play no part in transmission. It could do so only by infecting water supplies. The reasons why water supplies do not appear to act as a vehicle of transmission have already been given. Furthermore, adequate treatment of sewage and of water destroys the virus, but epidemics of poliomyelitis occur in communities where both the water and the sewage are adequately treated as well as in communities where they are not.

Bathing at beaches has not been implicated by investigators as a method of transmission. Yet there is a popular belief that it may contribute to the spread. This appears to be fallacious for a number of reasons. Epidemics of poliomyelitis in the Temperate Zone usually begin in June, when very few people go to the beaches, and continue into the fall and winter. They have occurred in landlocked communities and in the cold, far North where bathing could not have been a factor in spread. They are not more abundant in coastal regions than inland. Finally, no epidemic has been reported where bathing might have been the method of transmission.

The only factor that appears to be present in all outbreaks of poliomyelitis is intimacy of contact. Again and again it has been demonstrated that the closer the contact to cases of poliomyelitis the greater the chance of acquiring the disease. Intimacy of contact is greatest in the home, and the secondary attack rate in the home should be greater than elsewhere. Actually, it is. In the 1949 outbreak in New York City, there were 83 instances in which poliomyelitis attacked more than one individual in a home. Excluding instances in which the secondary case occurred within 5 days of the primary one, on the assumption that it was really a primary case exposed to the same person, there remained 37 secondary cases. The total number of individuals exposed in these households was 8,256, giving an attack rate of 450 per 100,000 persons exposed. This compared to an attack rate of 30 per 100,000 in the city as a whole. The attack rate for household contacts was fifteen times as great as in the community. The epidemiologic features of the disease appear to indicate a respiratory rather than any other type of spread. It is possible, of course, that several methods of spread play a part in the general transmission, but the indications are that if such is the case the respiratory method is probably the most important one.

Experimentally, monkeys that are chilled or exhausted as a result of exercise are more apt to develop a serious form of paralytic poliomyelitis than do the controls. In humans it has been shown that children who have been exhausted by exercise during the preparalytic stage of poliomyelitis are more apt to develop paralysis than those who have had adequate rest during that period. Apparently, this does not extend back to the preinvasion period. Children who are very active are not more susceptible to poliomyelitis than those who are not, but if they are active when they first become ill, their chances of developing paralysis are greater than if they stay in bed. This points to a control measure. During an epidemic of poliomyelitis, children should be permitted normal activity, but if they develop an acute illness, no matter how slight, they should be put to bed, so that if it turns out to be poliomyelitis, they will have had the advantage of bed rest.

A number of authors have pointed out the relationship between tonsillectomy and other operations in the head region and the development of bulbar poliomyelitis. An increased incidence of bulbar poliomyelitis appears to occur in individuals who have had a recent operation in the head or neck region. It is, therefore, a wise precaution to defer tonsillectomies, removal of teeth, operations on the sinuses, plastic operations on the nose, and similar elective operations to those months during which the incidence of poliomyelitis is not above expectancy and which are not apt to be followed by months of high incidence. The first 3 months of the year are the safest from the point of view of poliomyelitis.

Reports from Great Britain first called attention to a possible relationship between immunization and poliomyelitis. The data indicate that the incidence of paralysis in the limb injected with pertussis vaccine, diphtheria toxoid, or a combination of the two is greater than would be expected by chance. There is also evidence that cases of poliomyelitis show a higher incidence of recent immunization than do control cases. The British figures do not give the incidence of poliomyelitis among immunized and nonimmunized children. Such data would be extremely helpful in deciding whether recent previous immunization is or is not a risk to the development of poliomyelitis. They are, unfortunately, difficult to obtain.

Several studies of this problem have been made in this country. These seem, in general, to confirm the British studies. However, it should be pointed out that the correlations obtained by all workers are chiefly in children above the age of 1 year, in whom the incidence of poliomyelitis is high. In the United States most immunizations are performed in the first year of life. The incidence of poliomyelitis in this age group is only about 2 to 3 per cent of the total. The risk in this age group, if it exists, must be very small. Further studies are needed to clarify the relationship. Stress should be laid on the fact that the occurrence of poliomyelitis is not at all influenced by injections of immunizing substances or other materials given more than 1 month before onset of illness. If immunization programs are modified, they should be discontinued only during the period when the incidence of poliomyelitis is high.

Many people appear to be worried about sending their children to summer camps. There is evidence that the incidence of poliomyelitis in camps is no greater than in the surrounding communities. Epidemics occasionally occur in camps but to no greater extent than in other communities. If a single case occurs in a camp and no others occur in a period of a few days, the chances are that there will be no outbreak. If, however, several cases occur together or soon after each other, the probabilities are that there is a heavy seeding of virus, and an outbreak of poliomyelitis becomes probable. If only a sporadic case or two occurs in a camp, there is no good reason for closing it. The cases should be isolated and the camp permitted to continue its usual activity. One should remember that removing children from the camp does not help them. They have already been exposed, and if they have been infected, removal to another location will not decrease their chances of becoming ill.

A question that is always brought up in epidemic years is whether schools should reopen on time in September. The evidence is all in favor of opening the schools. The incidence of poliomyelitis does not increase in school children after the schools are opened, nor is there a decrease in incidence beyond expectancy if the schools are kept closed. In the 1949 epidemic in New York City, about 50 per cent of all cases occurred in the school-age groups before the opening of schools, and about 47 per cent after the opening.

There is evidence to indicate that women who are pregnant are more susceptible to poliomyelitis than those in the same age group who are not pregnant. It is, therefore, a wise rule for pregnant women not to expose themselves to cases of poliomyelitis. Children born of women who have poliomyelitis during their pregnancy are, however, normal.

Coxsackie Virus

In 1948 Dalldorf reported the recovery of a virus from the stools of two cases of nonparalytic poliomyelitis in Coxsackie, N. Y. This virus differed from that of classic poliomyelitis in its inability to infect monkeys or adult mice but its predilection for suckling mice, 6 to 8 days old. The virus could be readily passed in other mice and produced lesions in the muscles, which showed evidence of degeneration, but not in the central nervous system. In this respect, too, it differed from the virus of classical poliomyelitis, which causes degeneration of the neurons of the central nervous system but does not affect muscles. The Coxsackie virus can be recovered from stools, from pharyngeal washings, from contaminated flies, and from sewage. It can also be recovered in great abundance from the affected muscles of injected suckling mice.

Since the original announcement, numerous workers have recovered the virus from humans in various parts of the country. It has been recovered from persons diagnosed as paralytic and as nonparalytic poliomyelitis, from contacts to such cases, and from normal individuals. It has also been recovered from people suffering from a variety of illnesses, such as summer colds, herpangina, and epidemic pleurodynia. It has also been recovered from cases of poliomyelitis from whom the virus of classic poliomyelitis was also recovered. It is not known what the relationship of the Coxsackie virus to poliomyelitis is. A great deal of investigation is going on in an attempt to clarify the relationship. From the available evidence it does not appear to be causal.

Control

Cases of poliomyelitis should be isolated until the febrile period is over. Discharges from the nose and throat are infectious early in the disease and should, therefore, be received in tissues, placed in a paper bag, and burned. Fecal discharges are infectious for a long period. The bedpan should, therefore, not be used by other persons until it has been sterilized. Contacts to cases need not be quarantined. The virus is believed to be present in apparently normal individuals in large numbers. It has been estimated that for every case there are 100 normal persons harboring the virus. Since there is no practical method of identifying them, it appears unreasonable to quarantine the household contacts only. Children may be permitted to attend camps during years of high incidence, and schools may be opened on time.

Children developing an acute illness during an epidemic period should be put to bed immediately and kept there until a definite determination has been made of the nature of the illness. Tonsillectomies and other elective operations in the nose, mouth, and throat should be deferred. Immunizations and other elective injections might best be deferred also, particularly in children above the age of 1 year. Bathing at beaches and pools may be permitted, but unnecessary crowding of children should be discouraged in all places.

MEDICAL CARE PLANS

Treatment

There is no specific treatment for poliomyelitis. The antibiotics are of no value. Gamma globulin is of benefit for passive immunization. No prophylactic measures are available for active immunization.

Symptomatic treatment includes bed rest early in the disease, since there is evidence that activity at this stage increases the chances of paralysis. The use of hot packs has been emphasized in recent years by Sister Kenny, who has ascribed miraculous cures to it. That it gives relief to the pain of muscle spasm seems to be generally accepted; that it influences the course of poliomyelitis is doubtful. In the application of moist packs, care should be taken to prevent burns, chilling, and exhaustion. The packs are made of light, woolen material and are cut large enough to cover the affected part. They are soaked in hot water, wrung dry, and applied quickly over rather than around the affected area.

The greatest risk to life is in the bulbar types of poliomyelitis which account for almost all deaths from the disease. In the spinal

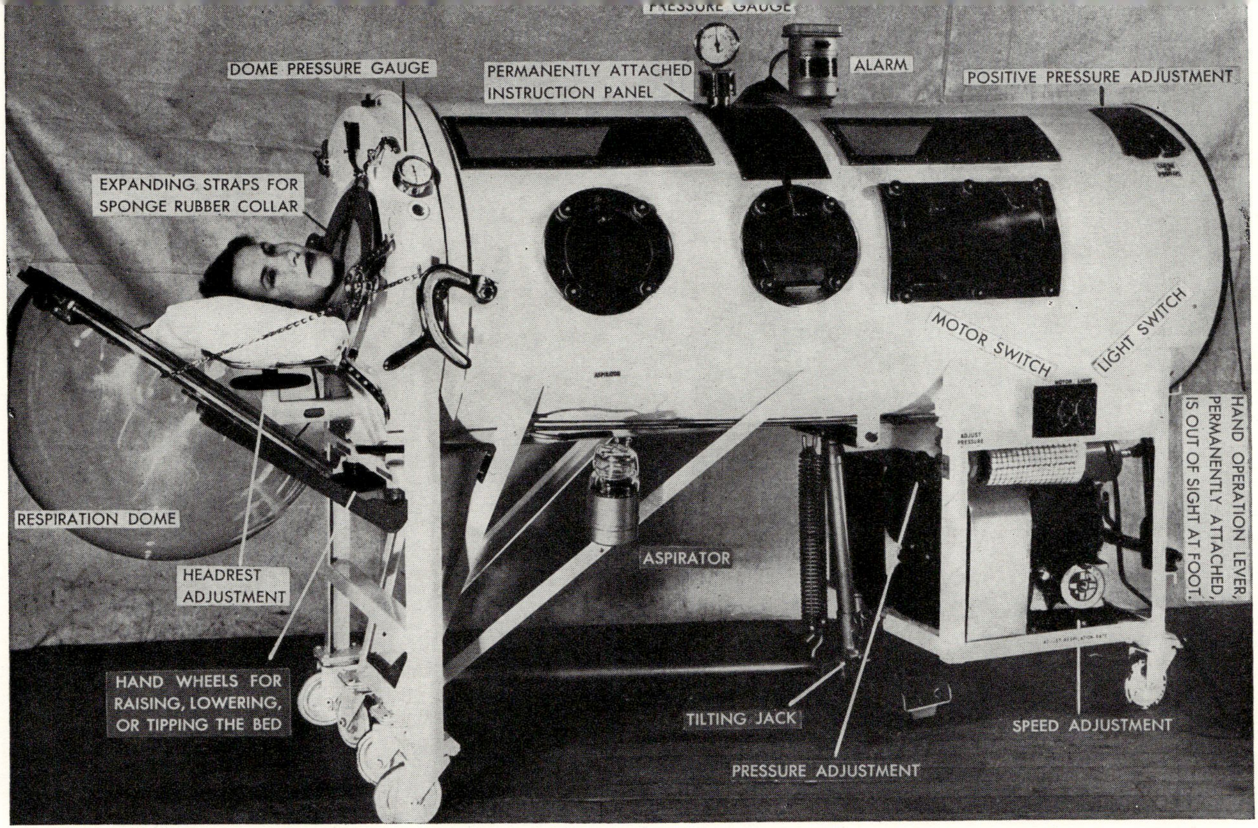

PRESSURE GAUGE

POSITIVE PRESSURE ADJUSTMENT

HAND OPERATION LEVER,
PERMANENTLY ATTACHED,
IS OUT OF SIGHT AT FOOT.

LIGHT SWITCH

MOTOR SWITCH

SPEED ADJUSTMENT

ALARM

PERMANENTLY ATTACHED
INSTRUCTION PANEL

TILTING JACK

PRESSURE ADJUSTMENT

ASPIRATOR

DOME PRESSURE GAUGE

EXPANDING STRAPS FOR
SPONGE RUBBER COLLAR

RESPIRATION DOME

HEADREST
ADJUSTMENT

HAND WHEELS FOR
RAISING, LOWERING,
OR TIPPING THE BED

Fig. X. RESPIRATOR USED IN BULBAR POLIOMYELITIS.

(Courtesy of J. H. Emerson Company, Cambridge, Mass.)
(Photograph by David Wing Nilsson)

types, paralysis of the intercostals or the diaphragm offers the greatest hazard. Patients with respiratory paralysis, resulting either from
involvement of the center in the medulla or from paralysis of the
intercostal muscles or the diaphragm, usually have to be placed in
a respirator. They require continuous and expert nursing care, not
only to keep up their nutrition but also to keep the respiratory passages free from accumulating mucus. In recent years the use of
tracheotomy in addition to the respirator in cases of respiratory
paralysis has been advocated by some physicians.

The psychic factor in recovery from poliomyelitis has been stressed
in recent years by a number of physicians. Both nurses and doctors
with an intelligent and sympathetic approach have an opportunity
to allay the fears, frustration, and shame that assail many children
who realize that they will remain permanently crippled. Those that
have become accustomed to a respirator or a tracheotomy tube are
the most difficult to treat. Their dependence on these aids is often
so great that even when they can go without them, the realization
that they are without a prop sends them into a panic. A great deal
of intelligent handling by a nurse is often needed at this stage. The
use of a rocking bed may be of value in weaning patients from their
dependency on a respirator.

Diet

During fever, fluids are given in generous quantities, and soft
foods are added as the patient improves. A full diet is given as soon
as the patient is able to take more food. Supplements of vitamins C
and D are given to aid in muscle restoration.

Supportive Nursing Care

Specific procedures include fundamentals of good general nursing
with adaptations to the specific needs of the patient and to the
nature and progress of the disease. Such factors as a cheerful environment, protection from draughts, unnecessary noise, and tender lov-
ing care are basic in making the patient comfortable. Since patients
require frequent changes in position, gentleness and skill in turning
or moving affected parts is very important. Proper support of limbs
and teamwork by assistants are essential. In bathing the patient,
warm hands and gentle movements should be used, and the body
should be dried by patting with a towel.

Keeping the patient in good body alignment has special significance in poliomyelitis because there is muscle imbalance and
there are greater hazards of deformity.

A firm hair mattress and a footboard of sufficient height should
be provided. The footboard should be held in place by 4-inch blocks

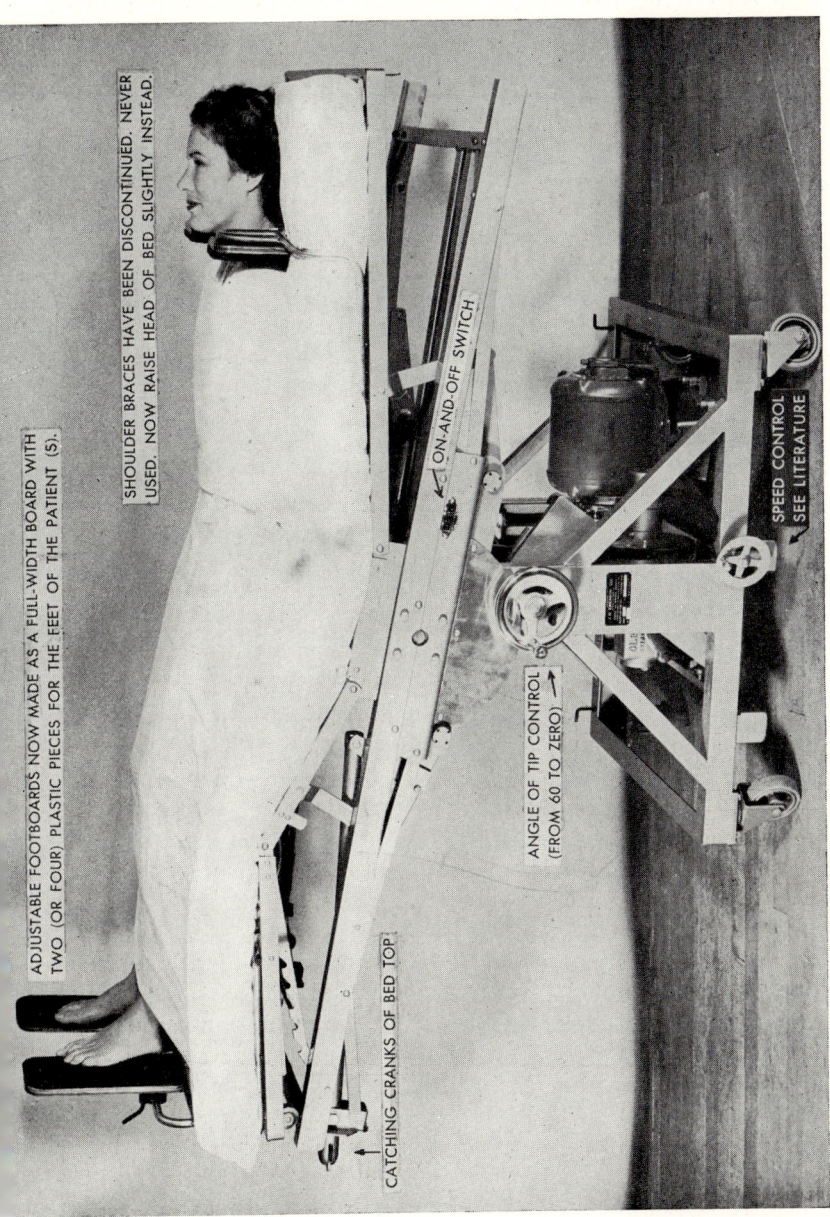

ADJUSTABLE FOOTBOARDS NOW MADE AS A FULL-WIDTH BOARD WITH TWO (OR FOUR) PLASTIC PIECES FOR THE FEET OF THE PATIENT (S).

SHOULDER BRACES HAVE BEEN DISCONTINUED. NEVER USED. NOW RAISE HEAD OF BED SLIGHTLY INSTEAD.

ON-AND-OFF SWITCH

CATCHING CRANKS OF BED TOP

ANGLE OF TIP CONTROL (FROM 60 TO ZERO) →

SPEED CONTROL SEE LITERATURE

Fig. XI. ROCKING BED.

(Courtesy of J. H. Emerson Company, Cambridge, Mass.)
(Photograph by David Wing Nilsson)

and covered with a blanket. This also serves to relieve weight of bedclothes.

The position varies with the type of involvement. These procedures should be known to the patient and to all concerned with his care. A small blanket or towel rolled under the knees and the placement of pillows and sandbags in various positions aid in relieving pressure on muscles and joints. The heel should never rest on the mattress.

Continued and sustained observation of changes in the patient is an integral part of nursing care. These changes are not limited to signs and symptoms of the patient's physical illness but are all-inclusive. They include the emotional reactions of the patient to his illness, his own worries, and the related concerns of his family. The nurse's awareness and recognition of these factors, and a calm, reassuring attitude are vital in promoting recovery of the patient. The nurse should give encouragement to the patient and give supporting answers to his questions. Accurate observation of physical changes during the acute stage of the disease is vital in aiding the physician and in directing the course of treatment. Such observations as changes in rate and depth of respiration should be noted by the nurse. Also signs or symptoms of respiratory involvement should be observed early and promptly called to the attention of the physician.

In communities where the patient remains at home, public health nursing visits are made to give nursing care and to supervise the care given by a member of the family. In large urban centers most cases are admitted to a hospital. When they are discharged from the hospital, the public health nurse visits the home to assist the family in making necessary adjustments, in overcoming fears and anxieties, and in developing wholesome attitudes toward the patient. These plans should be made well in advance to aid the public health nurse in education of the family and patient.

In the school situation the school or public health nurse has an opportunity to interpret medical findings to teachers and to assist the child in muscle re-education and in the maintenance of normal interests and activities. Effort should be made to stimulate abilities and personal qualities which will compensate for physical disabilities.

There are few illnesses that cause so much panic in a community as poliomyelitis. It is, therefore, essential for a program to be carefully worked out in advance so that it may be put into effect as soon as an epidemic threatens. Such a program should include the coordinated activities of the health officer, epidemiologist, public health nurse, private physician, hospital, and social-service agencies. The plan should have the areas of responsibility clearly defined, and the team relationships should be acceptable to all, so that conflicts will not arise even when there is some necessary overlapping.

An interagency referral plan for continuous flow of information from hospital to community nursing agencies is essential for supervision of convalescent care. Follow-up examinations by the doctor or physical therapist are desirable to evaluate improvement in paralyzed muscles.

Physical Therapy. Physical therapy is an important phase of poliomyelitis care. It consists of corrective exercises and whirlpool baths under the direction of physical therapists. The baths lend buoyancy to the weakened body and enable the therapist to limber and exercise unused muscles.

Rehabilitation. The greatest need for expert care in poliomyelitis is in follow-up of patients who have developed disabilities. This is a long-term program which includes orthopedists, physical therapists, public health nurses, and social workers. All play an important part in rehabilitating the patient to his optimal health.

REFERENCES

1. Adamson, J. D.; Moody, J. P.; Peart, A. F. W.; Smillie, R. A.; Wilt, J. C.; and Wood, W. J.: "Poliomyelitis in the Arctic," *Canad. M. A. J.,* **61**:339, 1949.
2. Anderson, G. W., and Skaar, A. E.: "Poliomyelitis and Antigen Injection," *Pediatrics,* **7**:741, 1951.
3. Bodian, D.; Morgan, I. M.; and Howe, H. A.: "Differentiation of Types of Poliomyelitis Viruses," *Am. J. Hyg.,* **49**:234, 1949.
4. Dalldorf, G.: "The Coxsackie Viruses," *Bull. New York Acad., Med.,* **26**:329, 1950.
5. Faber, H.: "Adenotonsillectomy and Poliomyelitis," *Pediatrics,* **3**:255, 1949.
6. Greenberg, M.; Abramson, H.; Cooper, H. M.; and Solomon, H. E.: "The Relation between Recent Injections and Paralytic Poliomyelitis in Children," *Am. J. Pub. Health,* **42**:142, 1952.
7. Greenberg, M.; Siegel, M.; and Magee, M. C.: "Poliomyelitis in New York City, 1949," *New York State J. Med.,* **50**:1119, 1950.
8. Hill, A. B., and Knowelden, J.: "Inoculation and Poliomyelitis," *Brit. M. J.,* **2**:1, 1950.
9. International Poliomyelitis Congress: *Poliomyelitis,* J. B. Lippincott Company, Philadelphia, 1949.
10. Joint Orthopedic Nursing Advisory Service: *Nursing for the Poliomyelitis Patient,* New York, National Organization for Public Health Nursing, 1948.
11. Korns, R. F.; Albrecht, R. M.; and Locke, F. B.: "The Association of Parenteral Injections with Poliomyelitis," *Am. J. Pub. Health,* **42**:153, 1952.
12. Lowman, C. L.: "The Management of Poliomyelitis," *Am. J. Nursing,* **47**:367, 1947.
13. Newton, K.: "The Nurse in Poliomyelitis Care," *Am. J. Nursing,* **47**:370, 1947.
14. Paul, J. R.: "Symposium on Poliomyelitis," *Am. J. Med.,* **6**:537, 1949.

15. Seidenfeld, N.: "Psychological Considerations in Poliomyelitis Care," *Am. J. Nursing,* **47**:369, 1947.
16. Siegel, M.; Greenberg, M.; and Magee, M. C.: "Tonsillectomy and Poliomyelitis," *J. Pediat.,* **38**:537, 1951.
17. Stimson, P. M.: "Some Debated Points in the Treatment of Acute Poliomyelitis," *J. Pediat.,* **36**:704, 1950.

Chapter 26 PSITTACOSIS

General Description

PSITTACOSIS is a viral disease of birds which may be transmitted to man, and which is characterized by a respiratory infection.

The Causative Agent

The causative agent of psittacosis is a large virus intermediate in size between the rickettsiae and the smaller viruses. It is closely related to the virus of lymphogranuloma venereum. It is visible under the ordinary microscope and is found in the cytoplasm of cells in inclusion bodies. It grows readily in tissue culture and in chick embryos and is not readily filterable. It may be inactivated by the usual antiseptics and at 60° C. for 10 minutes. In the frozen state it will maintain its activity for 2 years if held at −70° C. The elementary bodies of psittacosis stain red by Machiavello's method.

The Host

Symptoms

The incubation period is 7 to 14 days. Onset is usually sudden, with fever, anorexia, and headache. Occasionally, the onset is gradual. Fever rises to a level of 102° to 103° F. and remains high, with remissions for 7 to 10 days, and falls gradually to normal. Pneumonic involvement of the lungs occurs early, although neither symptoms nor physical findings are characteristic. There may be a cough at the beginning, but it may not manifest itself until a few days after onset. It is at first dry and irritating. Later, there is thick and mucoid sputum. Respirations are not rapid. Signs in the lungs are few. Localized dullness and crepitant rales may call attention to lung involvement. X rays of the lungs will usually show greater involvement than had been suspected. The pulse is usually slow in relation to the temperature. In severe cases the respiration may be increased, and cyanosis may be present. Insomnia, disorientation, and delirium may occur. The white blood count is of little help; it is usually normal but may show a leukopenia. The fatality rate was thought to be about 20 per cent. The finding of many mild cases in recent years indicates a fatality rate of about 10 per cent.

245

Diagnosis

Patients with pneumonitis who give a history of association with birds should be suspected of having psittacosis. In the early stages of the disease the virus can be recovered from blood and sputum by injection into mice. Virus can also be recovered from the spleen and lungs at autopsy. Laboratory diagnosis may also be made by the complement-fixation test with Lygranum antigen, if lymphogranuloma venereum can be ruled out, since the latter disease also gives a positive complement-fixation reaction. Since individuals exposed to psittacosis virus, such as bird handlers, may also give a positive complement-fixation test for psittacosis, it is essential, for a diagnosis of the disease, to obtain early and later specimens of blood and to show a significant rise in titer.

Immunity

One attack of psittacosis usually confers immunity. However, second attacks have been described. No active immunizing agents are available.

THE ENVIRONMENT

Psittacosis is a disease which is common in birds of the psittacine family. In recent years it has been shown that all birds, including domestic animals, may suffer from the disease or harbor the virus without showing evidence of illness. Meyer has suggested the term "ornithosis" as more appropriate than the older term "psittacosis." Epizootics frequently occur among parrots, pigeons, and ducks While the disease is more common in the winter, it may occur in all seasons and climates and is world wide in distribution.

Human beings of all ages are susceptible, but the disease is more common in middle age and in females, probably because these persons more often come in contact with birds and fowl. Virus is present in the nasal discharges and excreta of ill birds or carriers, so that individuals in close contact with them are easily infected. There is also evidence that the virus can spread by indirect transmission in air. Infection through bites has also been described.

Although the disease is not commonly transmitted from man to man, such spread may occur, and evidence exists of this method of spread in hospitals, particularly to nurses.

Control

The patient should be isolated during the febrile period, and all nasal and mouth discharges should be properly disinfected or burned. It is probably wise for nurses to wear masks when caring for an active case. Contacts need not be quarantined. Investigations should be undertaken to determine the source and if found, the bird should be killed and its spleen examined for virus. If the animal is found in a bird store or aviary, the contact birds should be quarantined until all suspected birds have been removed and the premises cleaned. Several states have instituted laws forbidding the importation or sale of psittacine birds.

MEDICAL CARE PLANS

Treatment

The usual nonspecific measures applicable to lung infections, such as bed rest, sedation for the cough, and proper nutrition, are used. (See pages 141–145.) Penicillin has been shown to be an effective drug in the control of the disease, and there is evidence that the newer antibiotics such as Aureomycin, chloramphenicol (Chloromycetin), and Terramycin are also effective.

Diet

During fever, fluids should be given to replace loss by sweating. As soon as tolerated, a full diet is given.

Supportive Nursing Care

Nursing care is the same as for pneumonia.

If sweating is profuse, sponge baths contribute to general comfort. The position of the patient should be changed frequently.

REFERENCES

1. Armstrong, C.: "Psittacosis; Epidemiological Considerations with Reference to the 1929–1930 Outbreak in the United States," *Pub. Health Rep.*, **45**:2013, 1930.
2. Bedson, S. P.: "Use of Complement-fixation Reaction in the Diagnosis of Human Psittacosis," *Lancet*, **2**:1277, 1935.
3. Flippin, H. F.; Gaydosh, M. J.; and Fittipoldi, W. V.: "Treatment of Human Psittacosis with Penicillin," *J.A.M.A.*, **128**:280, 1945.
4. Heilman, F. R., and Herrell, W. E.: "Penicillin in the Treatment of Experimental Ornithosis," *Proc. Staff Meet., Mayo Clin.*, **19**:57, 1944.
5. Meyer, K. F.: "Ecology of Psittacosis and Ornithosis," *Medicine*, **21**:175, 1942.

Chapter 27 RHEUMATIC FEVER

GENERAL DESCRIPTION

RHEUMATIC fever is an acute disease, the resulting lesions of which are usually chronic. Its cause is unknown, but it commonly follows an infection with Group A, *beta*-hemolytic streptococci. The most common and serious result of acute rheumatic fever is heart disease.

THE CAUSATIVE AGENT

The cause of the disease is not known. An attack usually follows a respiratory infection due to Group A hemolytic streptococci. It is believed that the disease may represent a manifestation of allergy or sensitizaton to the streptococcus. This is based on the fact that there is usually a period of time between infection with the strepto-coccus and onset of the disease, that an attack does not confer immunity but rather predisposes to subsequent attacks, that the disease often has a familial pattern, that antistreptolysin in high titer is found in the blood, and that the disease is not communicable.

THE HOST

Symptoms

An incubation period in its true sense, as the period between infection and onset of symptoms, does not exist in this disease. However, the period between infection with the streptococcus and the later development of rheumatic fever varies from a few days to a few weeks. The onset is usually abrupt, with fever, pains, and tenderness in the joints, discomfort, and sweating. Other common symptoms are chest pain, abdominal pain, and skin rashes. These symptoms vary tremendously in severity and occurrence and are overshadowed by the lesions that occur in the heart in the vast majority of cases. The fever, for instance, may be maintained at a level of 103° to 104° F. in some cases and be low grade in others. The joints may be enlarged, red, swollen and exquisitely tender in some and be only slightly painful in others. Characteristically, the joints are not involved all at one time. Those that are involved early recover, to be followed by involvement in others.

The cardiac manifestations are those of lesions of the endo-cardium, myocardium, pericardium, or any combination of the three. Lesions of the endocardium are usually manifested by mur-murs, those of the myocardium by enlargement of the heart, and those of the pericardium by friction rubs and by evidence of fluid. Signs and symptoms of heart lesions, like the general symptoms, may vary all the way from those in which it is difficult to determine whether a lesion exists at all to those with obvious manifestations of heart failure.

The diagnosis is occasionally strengthened by the finding of subcutaneous nodules. These are more common in patients with severe than in those with mild symptoms of the disease. They occur in the subcutaneous tissue, usually over bony prominences near joints. They are firm, not tender, and may remain for a long time.

Chorea has been considered by many investigators as a manifesta-tion of rheumatic fever. Others believe that while the rheumatic condition may cause changes necessary for the development of chorea, other conditions may also do so, and that it cannot therefore be considered as pathognomonic of rheumatic involvement.

Diagnosis

A diagnosis of rheumatic fever is not difficult in a patient with acute symptoms of fever, migratory joint pains, and evidence of cardiac damage. Difficulty arises in making a diagnosis in those who have had only fleeting general symptoms, insufficient to send them to bed, and then present themselves to the physician with no other manifestation than a heart murmur. Such persons often require careful and prolonged follow-up study before a definite diagnosis can be made.

During the acute symptoms of rheumatic fever there are usually secondary anemia and slight leukocytosis. The antistreptolysin titer of the blood is usually increased. Of considerable assistance is the determination of the sedimentation rate. Although this is a non-specific test, present in most infections, it is usually quite high in rheumatic fever and persists as long as there is active rheumatic involvement. The electrocardiogram may also be of assistance, since it frequently shows a prolongation of the PR interval.

Immunity

There is no evidence of the development of immunity following an attack. On the contrary, susceptibility to further attacks of the disease is definite.

The Environment

The incidence of rheumatic fever is not known, since it is not a reportable disease. However, heart disease is one of the most important causes of death in all ages. In persons under 40 years of age, from one half to three quarters of all such deaths are of rheumatic origin.

The disease is more common in the Temperate Zone than in subtropical areas and is rare in the tropics. The incidence is higher in the winter and spring than in the summer or fall. Children are more susceptible than adults, the average age of a primary attack being 6 years. It is uncommon before this age, but the incidence increases after this age up to about 10 years and then drops slowly. Primary attacks may occur among young adults, especially if they live in crowded quarters, as in barracks. The incidence in girls is higher than in boys. Race and color exert little influence on its occurrence.

Rheumatic fever is more common among the poor than the well to do. The factors responsible for this difference have not been determined. Among these may be crowding, improper food, inadequate sanitation, and a number of environmental factors. Probably the most important relationship is the more frequent occurrence of respiratory infections among the crowded poor than in less crowded homes.

Two relationships of the disease seem to be fairly well established. One is the familial incidence. According to Wilson, the disease is inherited as a Mendelian recessive. The other is its association with infections caused by the streptococcus, which has already been discussed.

Control

No specific measures of control are available. Isolation of the patient is unnecessary, since the disease is not communicable. General measures to improve health and prevent respiratory infections are used. Since a considerable number of the childhood population is crippled by heart disease resulting from rheumatic fever, it is important for communities to organize programs for the proper care of such children.

Medical Care Plans

Treatment

Rest in bed is important. For the acute symptoms the administration of sodium salicylate or acetylsalicylic acid brings prompt and marked relief. The dose depends on the weight of the child. It averages 60 to 80 grains a day. The drug need not be continued after the subsidence of fever and joint pains, since it has no influence on the heart lesions. These have to be treated similarly to heart lesions from any other cause.

Since the discovery of cortisone and ACTH and their beneficial effect in rheumatic arthritis, several studies have been made on the effect of these two drugs in acute rheumatic fever. The results appear to justify the hope of real benefit from their use. It appears that the course of the disease is shortened, the effect on the heart minimized, and a return to the former status is brought about by the use of either cortisone or ACTH. More work will have to be done before an exact appraisal of the value of these drugs can be made.

There is no prophylactic measure of definite value in the prevention of rheumatic fever. Essentially, it depends on the prevention of infection with the *beta*-hemolytic streptococcus. Various measures have been tried, such as sending susceptible individuals to warm climates in the winter and providing proper housing facilities for those who live in cold and damp houses. There is little evidence that tonsillectomy has any value in the prevention of rheumatic fever. With the introduction of the sulfonamides and the antibiotics, attempts have been made to prevent infections in those who have already had an attack of rheumatic fever by the daily administration of one of these drugs. Such a program requires evaluation and is obviously not one to be carried out for a long period of time. It must be confessed that actual prevention must await greater knowledge of the disease.

Diet

The diet should take care of the patient's caloric and protein needs, but overweight should be discouraged. An adequate intake of vitamins should be assured, and if there is anemia, an iron supplement should be given.

Supportive Nursing Care

During the acute illness, the patient is in considerable discomfort and needs good nursing care. The room should be warm and comfortable. Draughts should be avoided, since sweating is a common symptom and chilling may result. Frequent changes of personal clothing and bed linen may be necessary. Flannelette clothing should be worn in cold weather. If the joints are swollen, a bed cradle should be used to relieve pressure of bedclothes, and the patient should be moved as little as possible. Small pillows may be placed under the head, shoulders, and forearms. If sponge baths can be given without disturbing the patient too much, they will add to his comfort.

When chorea is associated with rheumatic fever, padded side-boards may be necessary to prevent the patient from falling out of bed.

After the acute symptoms and fever have declined, the patient continues to stay in bed until there is evidence that rheumatic activity has subsided. This subacute period may last weeks and even months. There are only two requirements for treatment in this stage—rest and diet. Limited activities such as washing the face and hands and self-feeding are permitted.

Educational and occupational therapy need thoughtful considera-tion if the child is to make a satisfactory adjustment to his limita-tions. Bedside instruction by a visiting teacher may be allowed by the physician for 2 or 3 days a week if the local board of educa-tion provides such a service.

Frequent rest periods are essential, particularly before and after meals. The patient should rest before and following meals. On alternate days when there is no teacher, the child may be permitted out of bed in a chair or on a porch, depending upon the weather. As restrictions are lessened, activities are increased.

The healed or arrested period is the most important in the follow-up care program. In communities where a rheumatic fever program has been established, the nursing and medical social-work services are co-ordinated.

The public health nurse makes home visits to cases of rheumatic fever in the acute or subacute stages to give or to supervise nursing care, to instruct in the prevention of acute respiratory infection, to teach good hygienic practices, to indicate ways of improving nutrition, and to assist the family with social and economic adjustments.

Another important responsibility of the public health nurse is case finding. She needs to be well informed about rheumatic fever in order to recognize early signs and symptoms and to refer patients to their physicians for diagnosis and care. In her conferences with teachers, she should be able to interpret medical findings and the rest and play activities which may be permitted.

The school nurse also plays an important role in a community rheumatic fever program. She not only gives guidance to parents and teachers, but, by interpreting the physical limitations of the older child, she acts as a counselor regarding selection of a vocation.

The care of the acute rheumatic child is not the major problem. It is the care and planning for the child whose heart has been crippled by rheumatic fever that takes up much of public health efforts. The problem is a large one and requires the co-operative effort of many agencies in a community—physicians, hospitals, health department, nursing agencies, voluntary agencies, social-service workers, schools, and others. Only through such co-operative programs can the problem be approached and explored in its various ramifications. A number of states and large cities have established programs for rheumatic fever or for handicapped children, a large number of whom are cases of rheumatic carditis.

REFERENCES

1. Coburn, A. F.: *The Factor of Infection in the Rheumatic State,* The Williams & Wilkins Company, Baltimore, 1931.
2. Gibson, Stanley: "Rheumatic Fever and Chorea," in *Brennemann's Practice of Pediatrics,* Vol. II, W. F. Prior Company, Hagerstown, Md., chap. XVIX, 1940.
3. Huse, Betty: "Rheumatic Fever and the Child's Emotions," *Child,* 16:3, 1951.
4. Rutstein, David.: "Rheumatic Fever," in *Top's Communicable Diseases,* 2d ed., The C. V. Mosby Company, Medical Publishers, St. Louis, Chap. XV, 1947.
5. Sadler, Sabra S.: "Nursing the Child with Rheumatic Fever, *Pub. Health Nursing,* 41:489, 1949.
6. Sadler, Sabra S.: *Rheumatic Fever—Nursing Care in Pictures,* J. B. Lippincott Company, Philadelphia, 1949.
7. Sadler, Sabra S., and Seibel, Elizabeth: "The Child with Active Rheumatic Fever and Her Nursing Care," *Am. J. Nursing,* 46:170, 1946.
8. Wilson, May G.: *Rheumatic Fever,* Commonwealth Fund, Harvard University Press, Cambridge, Mass., 1940.

Chapter 28 SMALLPOX (VARIOLA)

GENERAL DESCRIPTION

SMALLPOX is an exanthematous disease caused by a virus and characterized by fever, toxicity, and a vesiculopustular rash.

THE CAUSATIVE AGENT

The virus of smallpox grows readily in man and monkey but not in the lower animals. It can be successfully inoculated on the chorioallantoic membrane of chick embryos, producing pocks, and can then be maintained by serial transfer in the yolk sac. Fluid from smallpox vesicles contains elementary bodies which are small, round structures often referred to as "Paschen bodies," and which are believed to be the virus. They can be stained with a number of dyes.

The virus of smallpox remains alive after drying, so that crusts falling off a patient's skin are contagious. It is readily destroyed by heat but remains alive for long periods if stored at low temperatures or in 50 per cent glycerin.

The virus causes a degeneration of the upper layers of the skin and mucous membranes which produces a pock. Tissues infected with variola virus show cytoplasmic inclusion bodies, known as "Guarnieri bodies." They are large oval or circular structures lying in the cytoplasm close to the nucleus and are acidophilic in stain. Similar bodies are found in vaccinia. They are seen most commonly in the first week of disease but may be seen in the second week. They are believed to be collections of elementary bodies. In addition to the Guarnieri bodies, there are also seen in variola intranuclear inclusion bodies. These do not grow on chick embryos and are not seen in vaccinia. They are usually not found in cells containing Guarnieri bodies. They are not diagnostic, since intranuclear inclusion bodies can be found in other diseases.

If fluid or scrapings from smallpox vesicles are rubbed into the scarified rabbit cornea, the cornea will appear opaque, and tiny vesicles will develop at the scarified areas in 2 or 3 days. If the rabbit is killed and the eye enucleated, and sections are examined under the microscope, Guarnieri bodies will be seen in the cytoplasm of some cells. This is the Paul test; it is positive only in about 50 per cent of cases.

THE HOST

Symptoms

The incubation period is 12 to 14 days, after which symptoms of fever, chills, headache, backache, and prostration follow. These last for a few days, and then a papular rash appears on the face, spreading to the body and extremities. The eruption is symmetrical and is more prominent on the face, forearms, wrists, and hands than on the trunk. It occurs on the palms and soles and on the mucous membranes of the mouth. The isolated lesions are round and deep-seated and appear shotty to the touch. After a few days the papules become vesicular, and after another few days the vesicles become pustular. The pustules then dry and become crusted by the beginning of the third week. By the end of that week the crusts begin to fall off, and desquamation is complete by the fourth to sixth week after onset, leaving pinkish scars which gradually fade but which often leave pitting of the skin. The transitions from papular to vesicular, to pustular, and to crusted stages usually occur at one time on all parts of the body, differing from chickenpox where lesions come out and mature in crops.

With the eruption of the papules the prodromal fever drops, but with the onset of the pustular stage it returns and persists, with toxic symptoms, until the crusting stage. During this period patients appear horribly ill, toxic, often delirious, and stuporous. They have no desire to eat or drink and give off an offensive smell from the discharging pustules. The mortality of smallpox varies from 1 to 40 per cent.

There is a severe, fulminating type of smallpox in which a hemorrhagic rash appears in the first few days of fever. Death usually results within a few days before the appearance of typical symptoms. This is known as *hemorrhagic* smallpox. On the other hand there is a mild type of smallpox known as *varioloid* or *alastrim,* which usually occurs in previously vaccinated persons, in which there are mild prodromal symptoms, a scanty rash, little fever, and no toxicity.

Diagnosis

Smallpox is occasionally confused with chickenpox. While such confusion is not common when the disease is fully developed, it may occur in the early stages. The main differences clinically are that there are no severe prodromal symptoms in chickenpox; that the vesicles are unilocular and superficial, whereas in smallpox they are multilocular and deep-seated; that the lesions appear in crops in chickenpox so that at any one time lesions of different maturation can be seen, while in smallpox all lesions seen at one time are of the same age; that pustulation does not usually occur in chickenpox; and that the distribution of the rash is different in the two diseases, being most prominent on the face and extremities in smallpox and on the trunk in chickenpox.

Several laboratory aids are available in the diagnosis of smallpox:

1. Scraping of cutaneous lesions or fluid from vesicles can be smeared on slides and stained. The finding of elementary bodies or of Guarnieri bodies in cells lends weight to the diagnosis. However, failure to find them does not exclude the diagnosis. Also, the same bodies may be found in vaccinia.

2. The Paul test, described above.

3. A complement-fixation test with serum from the patient and vaccinia virus propagated in chick embryo as antigen. Special skill is required for the performance of the test.

4. A complement-fixaton or a precipitin test done with antigen prepared from the supernatant of vesicles or crusts mixed with saline and centrifuged and serum from rabbits that have been hyperimmunized by repeated injections of vaccinia virus.

5. Isolation on chick embryos of the virus from skin lesions. The virus produces pocks in about 3 days, while varicella does not. Vaccinia virus also produces a pock, but it is different in appearance.

6. A complement-fixation test after isolation of the virus on chick embryos. Antigen consisting of a 10 per cent suspension of infected membrane, cleared by centrifugation, and serum from rabbits that have been hyperimmunized by repeated injections of vaccinia virus are used. A positive test is diagnostic, but further tests are done to differentiate the virus from vaccinia by injecting it into the skin of rabbits. Variola virus does not infect rabbits readily, while vaccinia virus does.

Immunity

One attack of smallpox confers permanent immunity. The presence of antibodies can be demonstrated by precipitin and complement-fixation tests performed with the patient's serum, as described above. Active immunity is obtained by vaccination.

Vaccinia (Vaccination). The process of applying cowpox virus to the scarified skin is known as vaccination and the lesion resulting therefrom is known as vaccinia. There is a close relationship between the viruses of cowpox and smallpox. Whether one is a modification of the other or whether the two are different viruses

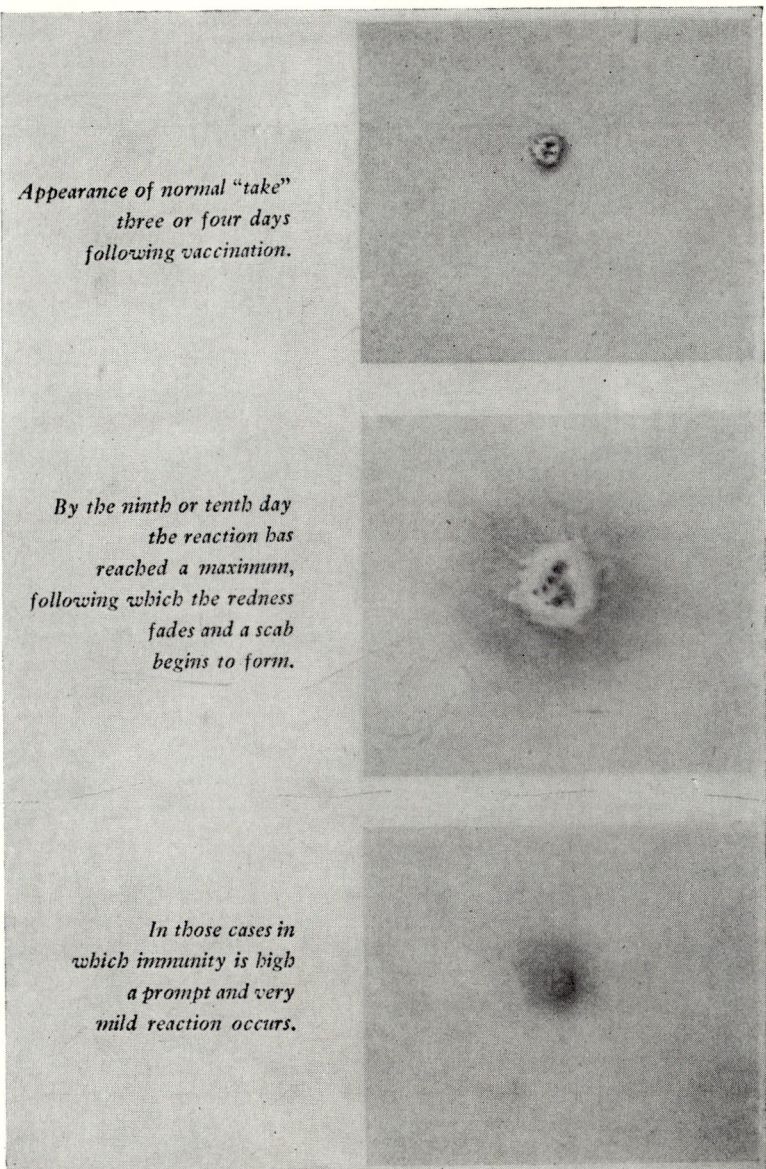

*Appearance of normal "take"
three or four days
following vaccination.*

*By the ninth or tenth day
the reaction has
reached a maximum,
following which the redness
fades and a scab
begins to form.*

*In those cases in
which immunity is high
a prompt and very
mild reaction occurs.*

Fig. XII. SMALLPOX VACCINATIONS.

(Courtesy of Sharp & Dohme, West Point, Pa.)

has not been settled. However, it is definitely known since Jenner's time that an attack of cowpox will immunize against smallpox, and that vaccination with cowpox virus or vaccinia will confer immunity against smallpox.

Vaccine virus is prepared by shaving the skin over the abdomen of calves, and after repeated washings with soap and water, scarifying it superficially with parallel lines and rubbing vaccinia virus into the scarifications. The animals are kept in clean stalls, and after 5 or 6 days the skin is carefully cleaned and the vesicles and contents are removed by scraping. This pulp is mixed with glycerin, frozen, and stored. Later it is titrated, tested for purity, and distributed for use. The virus should be kept at low temperatures to retain its potency.

Virus has been prepared by growing on chick embryos. However, it apparently does not immunize as effectively as calf virus.

Vaccination is performed preferably by the multiple-puncture method. A drop of vaccine is placed on the cleansed skin of the arm. With a needle held parallel to the arm, 20 to 30 puncture marks are made through the vaccine by dipping the point of the needle down to the skin. An alternate method is to make a scratch not more than $\frac{1}{8}$ inch in length, and not deep enough to raise blood, through the vaccine. The excess vaccine should be wiped off and no further precautions taken. Shields are unnecessary and may even be harmful.

Three types of reaction are recognized: (1) primary take, (2) vaccinoid or accelerated, and (3) immune.

A primary take occurs in individuals not previously vaccinated and in those previously vaccinated who have lost their immunity. A papule appears by the third or fourth day after vaccination, changes into a vesicle at the end of a week, and becomes pustular by the ninth or tenth day. By the fourteenth day a firm crust has formed, which falls off in another week or two. At the height of pustulation there is local redness and tenderness of the skin, enlargement of the regional lymph nodes, and often general malaise and fever. Symptoms usually last not more than 1 or 2 days.

A vaccinoid, or accelerated, type of reaction shows a quicker response. The papule appears in 1 or 2 days, turns into a vesicle and then a pustule in another 2 days, and becomes crusted by the end of 1 week.

The immune reaction is the one most difficult to read accurately. A papule forms in 1 or 2 days, does not vesiculate or pustulate, and subsides in another 2 or 3 days. Sometimes a tiny vesicle and crust may form. There should be a firm, indurated area at the site of vaccination within 3 days after vaccination.

Individuals who do not show one of the three reactions should be considered as improperly vaccinated and not as immune, and should be revaccinated with a known potent vaccine.

Immunity resulting from vaccination may last only 1 year or may persist for as long as 20 years. In the presence of smallpox, individuals should be revaccinated yearly. The World Health Organization considers immunity from vaccination valid for 3 years.

The complications that may follow vaccination are postvaccinal encephalitis, generalized vaccinia, tetanus, and other infections. With the care taken in the preparation of vaccinia virus today and the technique used in vaccination no cases of tetanus should occur. Other infections are rare accidents. In 1947, about 5 to 6 million people were vaccinated in New York City. Only one serious infection occurred, and there were no cases of tetanus. The rate of occurrence of encephalitis varies in different countries. In the 1947 epidemic in New York, forty-five cases occurred and four died. Generalized vaccinia occurs almost exclusively in children with eczema. Such children should not be vaccinated, nor should a recently vaccinated person be permitted to take care of them until the vaccination has crusted over. Vaccination of pregnant women is of no risk either to them or to their embryo infants.

The Environment

Smallpox has been known since ancient times. In the Middle Ages numerous epidemics occurred in Europe, with a fatality of about 30 to 40 per cent. Susceptibility is universal among all ages, races, and colors. In the United States smallpox has been reported regularly in fairly large numbers until recent years. In 1950, forty-one cases of smallpox were reported. It is interesting that the states having compulsory vaccination report the lesser numbers while those that do not even have permissive legislation have always reported the larger numbers.

The control of smallpox by vaccination was the first demonstration of the effective use of an immunizing agent. It was introduced in 1798 by Edward Jenner who observed that milkmaids suffering from cowpox did not develop smallpox when exposed to the disease. Previous to that, variolation was largely practiced in Europe. This consisted of inoculation of the scarified skin of healthy individuals with fluid taken from a mild case of smallpox. It was a risky procedure because there was no guarantee that the inoculated individual would not develop a severe case of smallpox and die.

The compulsory vaccination of all children is a necessary public health measure. In many communities there is a law requiring all children to be vaccinated before admission to school and an education law requiring all children between specified ages to attend school. By this combination of efforts all children are vaccinated.

Control

Cases of smallpox should be isolated in a separate room of a hospital, and all individuals in the hospital and entering it should be vaccinated. All contacts to the case, including individuals living in the building where the patient resides, should also be vaccinated, and should be followed for a period of 21 days from the date of first exposure to make sure that no lesions develop. If several cases develop and there have been many exposures, the entire community should be vaccinated. It is true that postvaccinal encephalitis occurs in a certain percentage of vaccinated persons, but this is a risk that must be taken. In New York City, in 1947, the risk was 1 case to 110,000 vaccinated persons.

Individuals arriving from epidemic areas should show evidence of vaccination in the past 3-year period and should be kept under surveillance for 14 days from the date of departure. If smallpox is present on a boat or airplane, the patient should be immediately isolated in a hospital. All passengers should be vaccinated and kept under surveillance for 14 days, and all linens and personal effects should be disinfected.

The nurse taking care of a case of smallpox should be vaccinated. She should wear a gown and cap and practice rigid personal hygiene, especially in hand washing. Care should be taken that no crusts adhere to the shoes. The linen should be boiled. If the patient is in a hospital, the linen should be laundered separately. Nose and throat secretions should be received in paper tissues and deposited in a paper bag fastened to the side of the bed, and then burned. Dressings from skin lesions should be collected in a paper bag and burned.

MEDICAL CARE PLANS

Treatment

There is no specific drug for the treatment of smallpox. Therapy is directed toward the relief of symptoms and the maintenance of nutrition. The skin should be kept clean with mild antiseptic solutions like 1:1,000 bichloride of mercury solution. Itching may be relieved by antihistamines or by applying a 1:10,000 solution of potassium permanganate. Headache and other body aches are relieved by aspirin. Penicillin should be used routinely to prevent secondary infections in the pustular stage.

Diet

Fluids should be given freely. The diet is liquid during the acute stage and is liberalized later.

Supportive Nursing Care

Good nursing care is very important. The patient should be placed in a light and cheerful room and made as comfortable as possible. The room should be well ventilated to provide continuous flow of air. The temperature should be warm and the humidity kept low to lessen odors.

The skin should be kept clean by sponge baths. When pustulation is widespread, the sponge bath may have to be dispensed with in favor of compresses, as outlined above. Lesions frequently occur in the mouth, which should be kept clean with simple mouthwashes of warm saline solution. If conjunctivitis is present, the eyes should be protected from bright light and washed with warm saline solution.

Patients suffering from smallpox often experience feelings of rejection and deep anxieties about the cosmetic effects of the disease. The nurse should reassure the patient and explain that scarring is minimal with modern forms of therapy.

Cases of smallpox are rarely treated at home except in isolated communities. The risk of secondary spread is too great. The public health nurse plays an important part in educating the community in the need of vaccination for the prevention of smallpox. If a localized epidemic occurs and mass vaccination is necessary, the public health nurse assists in setting up vaccination clinics, preparing the sites of vaccination for the physician, instructing those vaccinated in the care of the vaccinated limb, and informing them of the maturation stages of the vaccination.

REFERENCES

1. Dover, C. C.: "Smallpox in the U.S.," *Pub. Health Rep.*, **55**:2303, 1940.
2. Downie, A. W., and Dumbell, K. R.: "Survival of Variola Virus in Dried Exudate and Crusts from Smallpox Patients," *Lancet*, **1**:550, 1947.
3. Greenberg, M.: "Complications of Vaccination against Smallpox," *Am. J. Dis. Child.*, **76**:492, 1948.
4. Greenberg, M., and Appelbaum, E.: "Postvaccinal Encephalitis," *Am. J. M. Sc.*, **216**:565, 1948.
5. Greenberg, M.; Yankauer, A., Jr.; Krugman, S.; Osborn, J. J.; Ward, R. S.; and Dancis, J.: "The Effect of Smallpox Vaccination during Pregnancy on the Incidence of Congenital Malformations," *Pediatrics*, **3**:456, 1949.

6. Leake, J. P.: "Questions and Answers on Smallpox and Vaccination," Reprint No. 1137, *Pub. Health Rep.*, **42**:22, 1927.

7. Parker, R. F., and Muckenfuss, R. S.: "Complement Fixation in Vaccinia and Variola," *J. Infect. Dis.*, **53**:44, 1933.

8. Weinstein, I.: "An Outbreak of Smallpox in New York City," *Am. J. Pub. Health*, **37**:1376, 1947.

9. Wesselhoeft, C.: "The Differential Diagnosis of Smallpox and Chickenpox," *New England J. Med.*, **230**:15, 1944.

Chapter 29 STREPTOCOCCAL INFECTIONS (INCLUDING SCARLET FEVER)

GENERAL DESCRIPTION

THE streptococcal diseases are a group of clinically different syndromes which have the common characteristic of being caused by the hemolytic streptococcus. They include acute tonsillitis, streptococcal sore throat, scarlet fever, erysipelas, and puerperal sepsis.

THE CAUSATIVE AGENT

The streptococci are gram-positive cocci which grow in chains and do not dissolve in bile. They are widely distributed in nature and grow best on blood-enriched mediums. Some are pathogenic and some are not. Certain streptococci produce exogenous substances and toxins which can be obtained from their filtrates. Among these are streptokinase (fibrinolysin) which dissolves fibrin; hemolysin, which dissolves red blood cells; and erythrogenic toxin, which causes the red rash seen in scarlet fever. Streptococci are destroyed by heat and the usual antiseptics.

Streptococci are divided into four divisions, each of which is further subdivided into groups. Division I is made up of the hemolytic streptococci. It is the largest division and includes most of the pathogenic streptococci. Division II consists of the viridans streptococci which produce green-colored colonies on blood agar plates as a result of partial hemolysis of the red blood cells. Division III is made up of the enterococci which are usually not pathogenic. When present in food in large numbers, they may cause symptoms of food poisoning. Division IV is made up of strains of *Streptococcus lactis,* frequently present in milk but not pathogenic as a rule.

The hemolytic streptococci (Division I) were divided into Groups A to E by means of the precipitin test by Lancefield in 1933. Since then, more groups have been added by her and other investigators. Most of the streptococci which are pathogenic for man are found in Group A of the hemolytic streptococci. This group has been further subdivided into a number of different types, by means of the agglutination reaction, by Griffith. The types are designated by

263

numbers. Such typing is of considerable value in epidemiological classification.

The Host

Both man and the lower animals harbor the streptococci and may be made ill by them. Among the diseases in lower animals caused by streptococci are mastitis in cattle, strangles in horses, and genital and respiratory infections in dogs. Group A hemolytic streptococci are responsible for most of the streptococcal diseases in man, although streptococci of other groups of Division I and streptococci in Divisions II and III may also occasionally cause illness in human beings.

The occurrence of disease in man as a result of the seeding of streptococci is influenced by a number of factors among which are personal hygiene, crowding, the state of nutrition, and constitutional factors. The specific diseases commonly caused in the human are discussed below.

The Environment

A number of factors influence the spread of streptococcal infections, particularly those affecting the respiratory tract. Of these, the crowding of people in a closed space is very important. Outbreaks of streptococcal respiratory infections are common in barracks, institutions, schools, and homes, where people are closely congregated. They are more common in the Temperate Zones than in tropical countries and more prevalent in winter than in summer.

Streptococci causing respiratory infections are spread chiefly by droplets or droplet nuclei. Such spread can be partly controlled by allowing sufficient space between seats or beds in schools, hospitals, barracks, etc., and by adequate ventilation. In recent years experiments have been carried on in a number of places on the use of ultraviolet irradiation and disinfectant vapors in the sterilization of air in closed quarters, and on oiling floors, furniture, linen, and bedding for the suppression of dust. The results are not conclusive. The wearing of masks involves so many personal elements that its use as a control measure has not been urged too vigorously.

The distribution of streptococci has been studied extensively by Schwentker, Gordon, and others. The types of streptococci most commonly recovered from persons with scarlet fever and other streptococcal disease in any community at any given time are also found in normal carriers in that community. During nonepidemic periods the streptococci recovered from carriers are of many different types, their prevalence varying greatly. Some are found only occasionally, others make up 10 to 20 per cent of all strains recovered. A type may be rare at one time and then, after months or years, become the prevalent type. Subsequently, it may again recede in frequency, and another type may become prominent. Different groups of streptococci are found in carriers, but group A makes up about 90 per cent of all. The highest carrier rates are usually found in winter.

Streptococcus carrier rates are not influenced by the incidence of the common cold in a community, but they are definitely higher in a community where an epidemic of scarlet fever occurs and also higher where the incidence of tonsillitis and pharyngitis is increased. The carrier rates begin to rise above normal values several weeks before the first cases occur, so that they apparently influence the incidence of these diseases rather than the reverse. The increase in carrier rates is chiefly in the type of organism responsible for the epidemic.

An individual may harbor a virulent streptococcus and not become ill. This is apparently due to his possession of *antibacterial immunity*. This is not measurable at present. The individual's *antitoxic immunity* is measured by the Dick test. At any time in a community a variable number of strains of streptococci are harbored. Most of them are not pathogenic, some are pathogenic but do not produce erythrogenic toxin, and some are pathogenic and also produce erythrogenic toxin. A pathogenic strain widely distributed among carriers will cause more illness than one which occurs only rarely. The resistance of the host and the pathogenicity and distribution of the organism determine the amount and type of illness. If there is antibacterial immunity, no disease occurs; if there is no antibacterial immunity, disease will occur, but the type will be determined by the presence or absence of antitoxic immunity. If antitoxic immunity is absent, scarlet fever results; if it is present, acute tonsillitis or pharyngitis or septic sore throat will result.

Scarlet Fever

GENERAL DESCRIPTION

Scarlet fever is an acute communicable disease caused by the hemolytic streptococcus and characterized by an acute onset, with fever, sore throat, headache, and vomiting, followed by a generalized rash, and ending in desquamation.

THE CAUSATIVE AGENT

The causative agent of scarlet fever is the hemolytic streptococcus, Group A.

The Host

Symptoms

The incubation period is usually 2 to 5 days. The onset is abrupt, with a rise in fever which may reach 103° or 104° F., vomiting, sore throat and headache. The rash usually appears 1 to 3 days later and is first noticed on the chest and back and then spreads to the abdomen and extremities. It is most prominent in the folds. When fully developed, it is bright red in color, and made up of many pin-point macules closely set together. It fades on pressure. The face is usually not involved but is flushed, with the exception of the area around the mouth, giving a characteristic circumoral pallor. The rash usually lasts a few days and then fades. Desquamation may begin then or 1 or 2 weeks later. The peeling is much coarser than in measles and is particularly noticeable on the hands and feet. In former years, desquamation was marked, and large pieces of skin came away at one time. Nowadays it is apt to be much less prominent and often seen only when carefully searched for.

At the onset, the tongue is usually coated. In the next few days the coating clears, first at the edges and then in the center, leaving a surface in which the papillae stand out prominently. This is the so-called "strawberry tongue." The throat and pharynx are infected from the start and feel sore. The tonsils are usually swollen, as in any upper respiratory infection, and may be covered with a slight exudate which rubs off easily. The soft palate and faucial pillars may show bright-red spots, often spoken of as an *enanthem*. The cervical glands are enlarged and tender. The fever usually persists for several days and then declines gradually until it reaches normal in about 1 week.

Scarlet fever was at one time a very serious disease, with evidence of marked toxicity, high and prolonged fever, and frequent complications, particularly otitis media, mastoiditis, and nephritis. Occasionally, there would be an invasion of the blood stream with the hemolytic streptococcus, causing symptoms of generalized sepsis, or there would be a severe toxemia with a marked, bright rash which sometimes was hemorrhagic, and with tachycardia, delirium, coma, and hyperpyrexia. Fortunately, the disease in its severe forms is not frequently seen today. More commonly, fever, sore throat, and rash are so mild as to be overlooked.

The commonest complications are cervical adenitis, which may go on to suppuration, and otitis media, which may develop into mastoiditis. These are probably caused by invasion of the strepto-

STREPTOCOCCAL INFECTIONS

are probably caused by the toxin.

Diagnosis

Clinically, it is not difficult to diagnose a typical case. In mild
cases with little rash and low fever, diagnosis is more difficult.
The laboratory offers little help. The blood count usually shows a
leukocytosis which is also present in other bacterial infections.
The Schultz-Charlton test is usually positive early in the disease
when the rash is marked. A negative test does not rule out scarlet
fever. The test is performed by injecting 0.1 cubic centimeter of
scarlet fever antitoxin or 0.2 to 0.5 cubic centimeter convalescent
serum intradermally in an area where the rash is most marked.
Blanching of the skin surrounding the area of injection occurs in
about 4 to 12 hours. Where there are folds of skin, as in the ante-
cubital and popliteal spaces or in the lower abdomen, dark lines
separating the folds are often seen and are referred to as "Pastia
lines." Cultures from the nose and throat or purulent discharges
will usually grow a hemolytic streptococcus, but since such streptococci may appear in normal individuals, their recovery is not
especially significant. If a Dick test is done early in the disease
or before illness, it is positive; if repeated 1 or 2 weeks later, it
will have become negative. This is presumptive evidence that the
disease was scarlet fever. The test is performed by injecting 0.1
cubic centimeter of scarlet fever toxin intradermally. A positive
test is indicated by the appearance of an area of redness, 1 centimeter or more in diameter, surrounding the site of injection, in
18 to 24 hours.

Immunity

An attack of scarlet fever usually produces immunity against the
rash of scarlet fever but not against the hemolytic streptococcus.
Reinfection with the streptococcus may cause similar illness as in
scarlet fever, except that no rash will occur and that symptoms
referable to the toxin will not appear. Second attacks of scarlet
fever are not rare, but they are probably caused by a toxin-produc-
ing streptococcus of a different strain. Cases of scarlet fever are
usually spread by contact with a case or carrier. Epidemics of sore
throat and scarlet fever may be caused by milk contaminated with
the streptococcus. Those individuals who have never had scarlet
fever before and have a positive Dick test develop scarlet fever,
while those who have had scarlet fever before and have a negative
Dick test develop streptococcal sore throat. The two diseases are

alike in symptoms and possible complications. They differ only in the presence of the rash.

Artificial Immunity—Active. Artificial immunity can be produced in Dick-positive individuals by injections of toxin. About 80 per cent of individuals injected become immune. Injections are begun with a 75 to 100 skin-test dose. They are increased fourfold up to 10,000 skin-test doses, then doubled to 50,000 skin-test doses. Three of the latter are given. The total number of injections given is eight to ten. Different clinics use different amounts and intervals.

Immunity to clinical scarlet fever does not immunize to the streptococcus but only to the erythrogenic toxin. Individuals immunized with the toxin can still be infected with the hemolytic streptococcus and may develop all symptoms except the rash. In view of this and in view of the fact that scarlet fever has become a mild disease in recent years and is amenable to antibiotic treatment, immunization with scarlet fever toxin has been largely abandoned.

Artificial Immunity—Passive. Passive immunity can be conferred on contacts to scarlet fever by injecting them with convalescent scarlet fever serum. A dose of about 20 cubic centimeters is used. Since the serum is not readily obtainable and since the streptococcus is susceptible to the action of antibiotics, the practice now is to treat contacts with sulfadiazine or penicillin or one of the newer antibiotics for 1 or 2 days. This is an effective method of control.

THE ENVIRONMENT

Scarlet fever has been known since ancient times, but it was confused with other exanthematous diseases. In 1675, Sydenham described it accurately and gave it its name.

The disease is present in all countries and climates but is more common in temperate than in tropical countries. In the Temperate Zone it is most prevalent in the winter and least prevalent in the summer. Sex and color are not important factors in the distribution of the disease.

The disease is communicable chiefly by means of droplet infection. However, outbreaks have been reported in which scarlet fever and streptococcal sore throat have occurred as a result of eating contaminated food, especially milk.

Scarlet fever is rarely seen in infants under the age of 6 months. About a fifth of all cases occur in age group 1–4, and about half the cases in age group 5–9. Another fifth occurs in the 10–14 age group. Deaths are more common in the younger age groups, about 50 per cent occurring in the 0–4 age group and 75 per cent under the age of 10 years. Although the incidence from the disease has diminished only slightly, the mortality has greatly decreased in recent years, and the introduction of the sulfonamides and the antibiotics has practically caused the disappearance of complications. In 1935, 14,602 cases were reported in New York City and there were 76 deaths. In 1945, there were reported 8,347 cases and 6 deaths. In 1951, there were 2,144 cases and no deaths.

Control

Cases of scarlet fever are isolated for varying periods of time in different states. In New York City the rules for isolation and quarantine apply equally to other streptococcal throat infections and to scarlet fever. Isolation is enforced until the mucous membranes of the throat are normal but not less than 7 days after onset of the disease. Contacts are not excluded from school or work.

If an outbreak of scarlet fever occurs in an institution for children, the cases are isolated and treated. All contacts are given full doses of sulfadiazine by mouth every 4 hours for a few days. Outbreaks are rapidly brought under control by this method.

MEDICAL CARE PLANS

Treatment

Mild cases of scarlet fever require little treatment. The moderate and severe cases should be treated adequately. In former years reliance was placed on the use of convalescent scarlet fever serum. A few years ago, gamma globulin was tried in some hospitals, and the reports indicate that it has equal value with convalescent serum. In recent years the antibiotics have been used with considerable success. Sulfadiazine or the soluble sulfonamide, Gantrisin, may be employed, or penicillin can be used by injection. The newer antibiotics, Aureomycin, chloramphenicol (Chloromycetin) and Terramycin are all effective against the streptococcus and have the advantage that they can be administered by mouth. The use of these drugs has cut down the severity of scarlet fever and eliminated the complications.

Scarlet fever antitoxin is of no value in the treatment of the bacterial infection. It is of value, however, in combating the toxicity caused by the exogenous toxin of the streptococcus, and may be used if the patient shows toxic symptoms.

The general medical and nursing treatment of scarlet fever is the same as for any upper respiratory infection. The patient is kept in bed as long as there is fever and evidence of acute inflammation of the throat. Fluids are given freely. Sponge baths with alcohol and water are used for the patient's comfort and to reduce the fever. Salicylates, especially aspirin in 5-grain tablets, are usually administered to soothe the soreness of the throat, relieve the general aches and pains and reduce fever if it is very high. If the throat is very sore, hot saline irrigations are comforting. An ice collar around the neck is also often soothing. If the lips are dry, cold cream or a simple ointment should be applied. The rash is usually not itchy and desquamation is not bothersome, so that no special care is needed for the skin.

Diet

Food is liquid in the febrile stage. As the patient improves, cooked cereals, vegetables, and fruits are added, and a general diet is gradually resumed.

Supportive Nursing Care

The practice of home visits by the public health nurse to cases of scarlet fever in the home varies in different communities. In some communities this has been abandoned. In others, visits are still made. The public health nurse gives or demonstrates nursing care procedures to a responsible member of the family and assists with prescribed treatments. She gives instruction on nutrition and assists the family with other health problems.

Acute Upper Respiratory Infection

The most common way in which the streptococcus enters the human body is through the nasopharyngeal passages. As a result, infection of the mucous membranes of the nose and pharynx occurs. An inspection at this time shows a reddened and turgid nasal mucosa, reddened pharynx and reddened and enlarged tonsils. The cervical glands are usually palpable and tender. Fever is commonly present. In children, particularly the younger ones, it is apt to be high, but in adults it frequently does not rise above 99° or 100° F.

The infection may spread from the nose to the nasal sinuses, causing a sinusitis, with its attendant pain and discharge of purulent material into the nose. The infection may also pass from the nasopharynx by way of the eustachian tube to the middle ear, causing a catarrhal otitis media which may become purulent. Such an infection may extend to the mastoid cells and cause a mastoiditis. This complication is a serious one because it usually requires operative intervention and because, in its turn, it may be complicated by sinus thrombosis, meningitis, brain abscess, and septicemia.

Acute Tonsillitis

In children an acute upper respiratory infection involves all parts of the nasopharynx, and a general inflammation results, as described above. In adults the infection is apt to be localized in the tonsils, resulting in the condition known as acute follicular tonsillitis. The tonsils increase in size, are very congested, and the follicles are studded with grayish membrane which may coalesce, giving the appearance of a diphtheritic membrane. However, in contradistinction to diphtheria, it wipes off easily without leaving bleeding spots. At the height of an attack of tonsillitis the patient feels quite miserable, with high fever, rapid pulse, headache and backache, and severe pain in the throat, which is particularly intense when swallowing. The cervical glands are usually enlarged and tender.

There may be some swelling of the tissues around the tonsils, and now and then the inflammation may localize there and form an abscess, popularly known as "quinsy" but technically known as "peritonsillar abscess." Surgical intervention is necessary to evacuate the pus. Sometimes the tissues in the posterior pharynx become sufficiently involved to break down and form an abscess, spoken of as a "retropharyngeal abscess." A patient with peritonsillar abscess tends to keep his jaws closely approximated, simulating lockjaw, and one with a retropharyngeal abscess holds his head retracted and his neck stiff, simulating meningitis.

MEDICAL CARE PLANS

Treatment

The treatment of streptococcal disease of the nasopharynx or tonsils does not differ from the treatment of scarlet fever and is discussed on page 269. Otitis media is an uncommon complication since the advent of the sulfonamides and the antibiotics. When it does occur, it is usually catarrhal and clears up rapidly. During the acute stage, however, there are pain and restlessness. If antibiotics have been started, they should be continued; if not, they should be begun. In the interim, application of a hot-water bag or an electric pad to the ear and the use of aspirin will relieve the pain.

If the infection has gone on to the purulent stage and the drum has ruptured, antibiotics should be used. In addition, local treatment consists of cleansing the outer ear frequently and applying a paste or ointment, such as zinc oxide or Lassar's, to the skin to prevent irritation from the discharge.

Diet

A liberal fluid intake is given during fever and gradually changed to a soft diet.

Supportive Nursing Care

The public health nurse and the nurse in school should be aware of the possible results of chronic middle-ear infections. Impairment of hearing may result from neglect or improper treatment. The importance of medical care should be stressed to the family, and the patient should be referred for treatment. Following recovery, an audiometer test should be made, either at the school or at an agency, to determine if there is a hearing loss.

Erysipelas

Erysipelas is a skin disease caused by the hemolytic streptococcus. The infection usually starts as a small raised and reddened area and usually progresses. The skin is red, brawny, thickened, and tender and sharply demarcated from the adjacent normal skin. The lesion spreads peripherally for about 1 week and then subsides. Sometimes, localized abscesses result which have to be incised. Constitutional symptoms are marked during the spread of the skin lesion. The patient usually has high fever and appears very toxic. With the subsidence of the skin lesions, the fever and toxicity abate.

Although the infection of the skin probably occurs through a crack in the epidermis, this is not always obvious. Erysipelas was at one time a frequent complication of wounds. It was always considered a serious illness, particularly in the very young and very old in whom the mortality was highest.

The introduction of the antibiotics has lessened the seriousness of the disease. It yields readily to the sulfonamides and to penicillin. Children who develop erysipelas should be given sulfadiazine in a dose of 1½ grains per pound of body weight per day. Penicillin may be used instead, in a dose of 100,000 to 300,000 units of the aqueous suspension twice a day. Adults receive sulfadiazine in a dose of 4 grams a day or the higher dose of penicillin. Aureomycin, Chloromycetin, and Terramycin are also effective in treatment.

Puerperal Infection

Puerperal fever is an infection of the genital tract of women following the puerperium. The infection may be limited to the uterus or may extend to the peritoneum, causing a peritonitis, or to the blood stream, causing general sepsis. The infection is due to the contamination of raw surfaces with streptococci on hands or instruments or in the nasopharynx of doctors or nurses, from contaminated dressings, or from pre-existing contamination of the genital tract.

Puerperal sepsis used to be a most dreaded disease. Oliver Wendell Holmes called attention to its contagiousness in 1842, but his views were opposed by the medical profession. Semmelweis, in 1847, sent a communication to the Vienna Medical Society pointing out that the rates of childbirth fever were highest in hospitals where the women were attended by students coming from the dissecting room without washing their hands. He insisted on scrupulous washing of hands, and the mortality immediately declined. The medical profession was not convinced, however, and ridiculed and persecuted him. He died at 47 years of age in an insane asylum.

Great strides have been made in the reduction of deaths from puerperal sepsis as a result of infrequent examinations of women during their pregnancy, care in keeping doctors and nurses with infections out of the delivery room, and taking the same aseptic precautions in a delivery as in an operating room. The successful use of antibiotics in streptococcal infections has added another effective tool in the reduction of deaths from sepsis. It is undoubtedly due to such measures that the maternal mortality decreased 70 per cent in the United States from 1930 to 1945. This decrease was due largely to the decrease in deaths from puerperal sepsis, which declined during the period from 24.4 per 10,000 to 7.3.

Control

The great decrease in puerperal infections that has been brought about in the United States has been due to the advances made in the care and the delivery of pregnant women. Most obstetricians make only one antepartum vaginal examination. Progress during labor is judged by symptoms, and if necessary, by rectal examination. The procedures followed in the delivery room are similar to those used in operating rooms. As is true in operative procedures, physicians and nurses with respiratory or skin infections are not permitted to assist or even to be present in the delivery room. If the pregnant woman has an infection prior to delivery, she is treated intensively with antibiotics.

The patient is isolated to prevent infection of other women under obstetrical care. Dressings and soiled napkins are placed in paper bags and burned.

MEDICAL CARE PLANS

Treatment

The treatment of puerperal sepsis is mainly prophylactic. If puerperal infection occurs, specific treatment with antibiotics is undertaken. Penicillin is the drug of choice. Antipyretics are employed to reduce excessive fever.

Diet

The diet is fluid at first and is increased as the patient improves, until a full diet is permitted.

Supportive Nursing Care

The primary factors to consider in nursing care are the emotional needs and comfort of the patient. Since patients are usually tense and apprehensive, the surroundings should be cheerful and comfortable. Some obstetricians place the patient in Fowler's position to facilitate drainage. Tepid sponge baths may be given when the temperature is high.

In her work with expectant mothers, the public health nurse should stress the importance of early prenatal care, and refer patients to their physician or to a proper agency for medical care. The hygiene of pregnancy should be included in all plans for individual and group instruction. The assignment of public health nurses to many hospital prenatal clinics for individual conferences with expectant mothers is a forward step in modern practice of obstetrics.

REFERENCES

1. Coburn, A. F.: "Prevention of Respiratory Tract Bacterial Infections by Sulfadiazine Prophylaxis in the United States Navy," *J.A.M.A.*, **126**:88, 1944.
2. Dublin, L. I.: "Maternal and Infant Mortality in the United States—A Forecast Fulfilled," Proceed. 3d Amer. Congress of Obstetrics, 1947, pp. 348 to 352.
3. Griffith, F.: "The Serological Classification of Streptococcus Pyrogenes," *J. Hyg.*, **34**:542, 1934.
4. Lancefield, R. C.: "Serological Differentiation of Human and Other Groups of Hemolytic Streptococci," *J. Exper. Med.*, **57**:571, 1933.
5. Meads, M.; Flipse, M. E., Jr.; Barnes, M. W.; and Finland, M.: "Penicillin Treatment of Scarlet Fever," *J.A.M.A.*, **129**:785, 1945.
6. Schwentker, F. F.; Janney, J. H.; and Gordon, J. E.: "The Epidemiology of Scarlet Fever," *Am. J. Hyg.*, **38**:27, 1943.
7. Shank, R. E.; Maxwell, R. W.; and Bozalis, G. S.: "Sulfonamides in Treatment of Erysipelas," *J.A.M.A.*, **117**:2238, 1941.

Chapter *30* TUBERCULOSIS

Pulmonary Tuberculosis

GENERAL DESCRIPTION

TUBERCULOSIS is a disease caused by *Mycobacterium tuberculosis* and characterized by the formation of tubercles which may undergo necrosis and spread, causing destruction of local tissue.

THE CAUSATIVE AGENT

The tubercle bacillus is a rod-shaped organism which is acid-fast; i.e., it is not decolorized by acid alcohol as most other bacilli are. There are three principal strains of tubercle bacilli, the human, bovine, and avian. Humans are susceptible to the human and bovine strains, but not to the avian which is, in the natural state, infectious in birds only. *Mycobacterium tuberculosis* does not grow readily on ordinary culture mediums but grows on specially devised culture mediums. It is readily destroyed by heat but not by the usual antiseptics. To disinfect sputum containing tubercle bacilli an exposure of 12 hours is needed for 5 per cent phenol or 2 per cent cresol solution. In dried sputum or feces, the bacillus may survive for long periods. The human, bovine, and avian strains can be differentiated by cultural characteristics as well as by injection into guinea pigs and rabbits, since the former are susceptible to the human and bovine strains but not to the avian, and the latter can be infected artificially with the bovine and avain strains but not the human.

In man the human strain is usually found in pulmonary tuberculosis, while in bone and gland tuberculosis the human and bovine types are found. Pasteurization of milk, which destroys the bacillus, has greatly reduced the incidence of the latter.

When tubercle bacilli are grown in glycerin broth for several weeks and the bacilli are then removed by filtration and the filtrate is evaporated to one tenth its volume, a clear brown, sirupy liquid results. This is known as "old tuberculin" and is used, in proper dilutions, to test for the presence of tuberculous infection. In recent years synthetic mediums have been used in place of glycerin broth in order to get a preparation as free as possible from nonspecific substances. The filtrate from such cultures, after purification, is known as P.P.D. (purified protein derivative) and is replacing old tuberculin for diagnosis of tuberculous infection.

THE HOST

When tubercle bacilli are inhaled by a susceptible host, an acute inflammation occurs in the lung where the bacilli lodge. There is an exudate into the alveolar spaces and the reaction, which may be very small or quite large, resembles pneumonia. This lesion may heal by resolution. The bacilli cease to multiply, they are destroyed, and the tissue heals completely. More often the lesion changes from the exudative to the productive type. There is a diminution in exudate, and mononuclear phagocytes appear. Then cells of a different type, known as "epithelioid," appear and multiply. After a few weeks fibroblasts and lymphocytes appear around the periphery and surround the old lesion, where giant cells are now seen in the center. The entire structure is known as a tubercle and consists of one or more giant cells in the center, a zone of epithelioid cells around them, and a capsule of fibroblasts, lymphocytes, and other cells as a peripheral zone. Several such tubercles may coalesce and form a macroscopic tubercle. Necrosis may occur in the center of the lesion, with the formation of a cheesy material. Calcium may be deposited in the caseous material, and as a result a healed lesion is obtained which can be identified on an X ray plate. This is known as a "first infection" or "childhood type" of tuberculosis. While this process of primary tuberculous infection goes on, the infecting tubercle bacilli spread by the lymph vessels to the regional lymph glands where growth and multiplication go on. The bacilli may spread from one gland to its neighboring one. In the glands, too, tubercles are formed, which may caseate and then heal by calcium deposition.

Primary lesions are, as a rule, comparatively small and benign. They lead to a sensitization of the body tissues which can be demonstrated by a positive tuberculin test. Such sensitization plays an important part in determining the types of lesions that will occur if the individual is reinfected later.

Occasionally, a caseous tubercle in the lung or mediastinal lymph node does not heal but invades a lymph vessel or a vein. As a result there is a hematogenous spread, and tubercles develop in various organs of the body, particularly the lungs, liver, spleen, and kidneys. This is known as "miliary tuberculosis" and is a very serious, septic type of tuberculosis with a high fatality rate. Some of the tubercles may form in the brain and meninges, giving rise to tuberculous meningitis.

Sometimes the first infection does not resolve and does not go on to form a calcified primary lesion but undergoes necrosis, often involving a large area; bacilli may be discharged from such a necrotic area or from a caseating lymph gland into the trachea or a bronchus and then be aspirated into another part of the lungs. As a result, an acute tuberculous pneumonia results. This is usually a serious condition with severe symptoms and widespread inflammation. Cavities may form, and such cavities often discharge infected material which is aspirated by the bronchi, causing other lesions in different parts of the lung and larynx, and if swallowed, in the intestines.

Primary, or first infection, or childhood type of tuberculosis is the most common type of tuberculosis when tubercle bacilli are first inhaled. Individuals with a healed primary lesion who become reinfected or whose primary lesion becomes reactivated develop reinfection or adult type of tuberculosis. It should be pointed out here that in a healed primary lesion the bacilli are usually not dead but dormant.

The adult or reinfection type of tuberculosis differs from the primary type in many ways. It usually has its origin near the apex of the lung. The progress is a very slow one and spreads down through the bronchi. There is no tendency to spread by the lymphatics or blood stream. Tubercles are formed, and they frequently caseate and result in cavities which may heal with scar formation or remain as cavities for long periods of time. The lymph nodes are hardly ever affected, as in the primary form. As a result of the discharge of infected material, aspiration into bronchi may result, causing lesions in other parts of the lungs. Tuberculous material may also be swallowed and cause infection of the intestinal tract.

The essential difference between the primary and the reinfection types of lesion is that the former spreads to the neighboring lymph glands by the lymphatics, has a tendency to heal and become calcified, and causes the development of sensitization to the tubercle bacillus in the tissues of the body. Only under unusual circumstances does the primary lesion spread locally and involve neighboring tissue or break into the circulation and invade different organs. The reinfection type, on the other hand, is quite destructive locally and has a tendency to spread by contiguity. Although destruction of tissue goes on, there is also a tendency by the body to resist invasion by the formation of enveloping capsules and by the attempt to obliterate cavities and destructive lesions with scar tissue. The outcome of the tuberculous lesion of the reinfection type depends on a continuous struggle between the attacking tubercle bacillus and the resistance of the host's immunizing mechanism. The treatment used is largely an attempt to bolster the host's resistance. If the defense mechanism is sufficiently good the lesion will heal, scar tissue will replace infected tissue, a balance will be struck between agent and host, and recovery will ensue. If the tubercle bacilli are too virulent for the defensive powers, extension of the tuberculous process will follow.

The terms "childhood type" and "adult type" are used because the first-infection type occurs most commonly in children and the reinfection type in adults. This is not, however, an inflexible rule. The childhood type may occur in adults and the adult type in children. What determines whether one or the other will occur is the existence of a previous infection. Adults who have never before had a tuberculous infection will develop the first infection or childhood type of lesion, while those who have already developed a childhood type of infection will develop the adult type. In essence, the development of a reinfective or adult type of lesion depends on previous sensitization by a primary or childhood type of infection. The period between the healed primary type of tuberculosis and the occurrence of the reinfection type may be many years. As long as tuberculin sensitivity exists, the tuberculosis which develops will be of the reinfection type.

Symptoms

The childhood or first-infection type of tuberculosis usually does not give any symptoms and is discovered roentgenographically. Only rarely, when the consolidation is massive, or when the enlarged regional lymph nodes cause pressure on trachea or bronchi, do symptoms occur. Onset of reinfection type of pulmonary tuberculosis is usually insidious. There may be no symptoms or there may be fatigue, loss of weight, and a general feeling of not being up to par. These symptoms often persist for a long time without any concern on the part of the patient. If he gradually becomes aware that he is not in his usual health and takes his temperature he will find a slight rise in the afternoon, and there will be loss of appetite. A slight cough may have been present for some time, and a tinge of blood may have appeared now and then in the sputum. Sometimes the bleeding is more profuse. Occasionally, the first symptom noticed by the patient is pain in the side of the chest, and examination may reveal a definite pleurisy. If the lesion progresses the feeling of weariness increases, loss of weight becomes more pronounced, fever in the afternoon is fairly high, and sweating, especially at night, is bothersome. There is a secondary anemia, the pulse is rapid, and the patient looks gaunt. Cough is now a very troublesome and exhausting symptom, expectoration is profuse, and blood in the sputum is a fairly common occurrence. The course is downhill, with increase in all the symptoms, and the development of others, such as laryngitis, pain in the chest, frank hemoptysis and dyspnea, and not infrequently, symptoms of tuberculosis in other parts of the body.

A physical examination in the early stage of reinfection tuberculosis may give no signs, or there may be some dullness at an apex with bronchovesicular breathing and rales. An X ray is very important, for it will usually show clouding or mottling in the suspected area. The advanced stage of pulmonary tuberculosis gives a variety of signs, depending on the underlying lesions. The X ray, likewise, presents a variety of pictures, depending on whether there are consolidation, cavitation, fibrosis, pleurisy, etc.

Diagnosis

Tuberculosis is an insidious disease, and in its early stages resembles many of the other respiratory infections. It is, therefore, important to examine a patient for tuberculosis whenever he presents such symptoms as a persistent cough, hemoptysis, loss of weight, pain in the chest, persistent fever, or other vague symptoms of malaise.

The blood count and sedimentation rate are only of general assistance. The former is normal in the early stage but may show a leukocytosis when there is fever and considerable destruction of the lung. The sedimentation rate is increased.

There are three specific aids in the laboratory diagnosis:

Tuberculin test. An individual infected with the tubercle bacillus develops an allergy to its products. If tuberculin or P.P.D. is applied to the broken skin, a reaction will occur. There are three methods of making the test:

1. In the *scratch* or *von Pirquet test,* two scratches about ⅛ inch long are made in the skin of the forearm. Into one, old tuberculin is rubbed with a sterile toothpick. The other is used as control. In 48 to 72 hours the sites are examined. A positive reaction is indicated by induration and an area of redness, from 1 to a few centimeters in diameter, around the inoculated site.

2. In the *intracutaneous* or *Mantoux test,* either old tuberculin or P.P.D. is injected intradermally. If old tuberculin is used it is usual to start with a dilution of 1:10,000 and inject 0.1 cubic centimeter, which is equivalent to 0.01 milligram of tuberculin. If no reaction occurs after 72 hours the test may be repeated with 0.1 cubic centimeter of a 1:1000 dilution, which is equivalent to 0.1 milligram. If P.P.D. is used, the first test is performed with a dilution giving 0.00002 milligram in 0.1 cubic centimeter and the second with 0.005 milligram in 0.1 cubic centimeter. If the test is positive with the weaker dilution, the stronger one should not be used. A positive reaction is indicated when there is an induration 5 cubic centimeters or more in diameter.

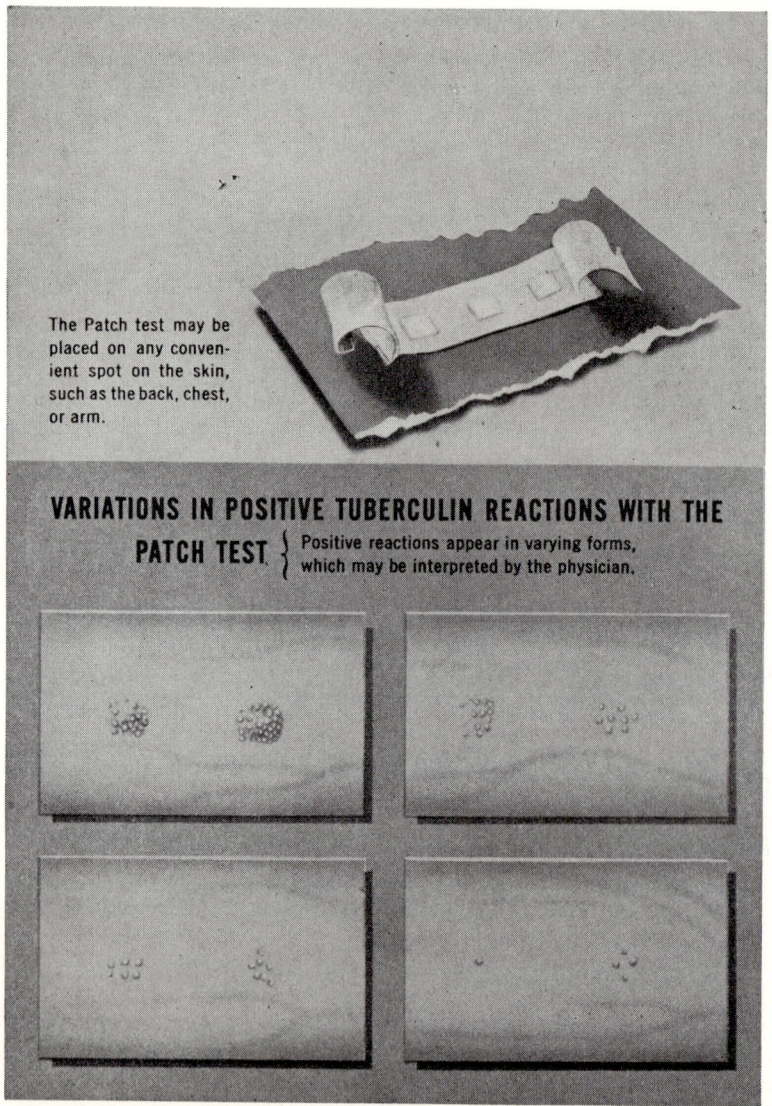

Fig. XIII. PATCH TEST IN TUBERCULOSIS.

(Courtesy Lederle Laboratories, Pearl River, New York)

3. A patch, which consists of a strip of adhesive tape to which three pieces of gauze are attached, is used in the *patch test*. The upper and lower gauze pieces have been saturated with tuberculin and allowed to dry. The middle piece is untreated and acts as a control. The patch is applied to the skin. It is removed after 48 hours, and the test is read after another 48 hours. A positive test is indicated by infiltrated red areas, usually surrounded by small vesicles, at the sites of the treated pieces of gauze. No reaction is present at the site of the untreated control.

Of the three tests, the intradermal is the most accurate and should be performed in a suspicious case if the scratch or patch tests are negative. The patch test is used by many physicians for its convenience. The scratch or von Pirquet test was the first to be introduced but has been largely discarded for the Mantoux test.

It is important to start with a weak dilution of tuberculin in performing the intradermal or Mantoux test, because constitutional reactions may occur in an individual with tuberculosis, and a dormant focus may even be lighted up.

A positive tuberculin test indicates an infection with the tubercle bacillus. It does not indicate its location or its activity. An individual with a completely arrested lesion or with a calcified primary focus will still give a positive tuberculin test. However, an individual with a primary lesion which has completely healed may lose his sensitivity to tuberculin. The test does not become positive until about a month after primary infection with the tubercle bacillus. Occasionally, allergy is lost during an overwhelming infection, and the tuberculin test is then negative. This is an unusual occurrence, and the test later becomes positive again. The tuberculin test indicates the presence of infection but not active illness. If the tuberculin test is negative, tuberculosis can be ruled out. If it is positive, determination must still be made of the activity of the disease. This is done by symptoms and physical examination and confirmed by X ray and by the bacteriological examination of the sputum or gastric contents.

Bacteriologic tests. Examination of the *sputum* is made by the Ziehl-Neelsen technique which indicates acid fastness. The following four methods are in use:

1. The sputum is smeared on a slide, stained, and examined under a microscope. This is called a *direct smear*.

2. If the direct smear is negative the sputum is digested with a chemical which liquefies mucus, and is centrifuged. The *concentrated* sediment is then smeared, stained, and examined.

3. If the two tests are negative, the sputum is liquefied by a chemical which destroys contaminants but does not harm the tubercle

bacillus. It is then centrifuged, and the sentiment is *cultured* on an appropriate medium.

4. The material is prepared as for culture and is injected into guinea pigs—*animal inoculation*. The animals are tested with tuberculin at intervals for several weeks. If a positive reaction develops, the animal is sacrificed and examined for tuberculosis.

When sputum is not obtained, *gastric contents* may be obtained by stomach tube and tested as for sputum. The presence of tubercle bacilli in the stomach is due to the fact that they are frequently swallowed with the saliva.

X Ray. The use of the X ray for diagnosis of tuberculosis has become more and more popular. The advantage of the X ray over tuberculin testing in surveys is that it does not require a second visit for reading, that the films can be taken by technicians, that the film indicates activity or inactivity, and that it can be stored as a permanent record. Positive X ray findings should be confirmed by the other laboratory tests.

Immunity

A tuberculous individual usually shows the presence of precipitin, agglutinin, and complement-fixing antibodies in his blood, but there is no evidence of antibodies that destroy the tubercle bacillus. He also develops an allergy to the tubercle bacillus and its products, which is indicated by the fact that reinfection tuberculosis tends to be slow and limited and chronic, in contradistinction to the rapid advance of a primary lesion.

The *Koch phenomenon* demonstrates the presence of allergy in animals. If a guinea pig is injected with tubercle bacilli an ulcer develops in about 2 weeks, the tubercle bacilli spread to the lymph glands, and the pig may die as a result of general tuberculosis. If a tuberculous guinea pig is similarly injected, an indurated area occurs at the site of inoculation. This undergoes necrosis, with formation of an abscess which ulcerates and subsequently heals. The lymph glands do not become infected, and the tuberculosis does not spread.

The relationship between allergy and immunity in tuberculosis has been studied extensively but is still not quite clear. What can be stated as a generally accepted fact is that tuberculin-negative individuals appear more apt to contract progressive tuberculosis when exposed to a case than do tuberculin-positive individuals. It is this observation which has encouraged the use of BCG for immunization.

Immunization with BCG—Bacillus Calmette-Guérin is a vaccine of living, attenuated, bovine tubercle bacilli which has been used in different parts of the world for many years to immunize tuberculin-negative individuals. It has been found to be perfectly safe. In this country it has not been widely used because most of the experiments abroad were not well controlled and the results not clear cut. The dose is one injection of 0.1 cubic centimeter BCG intradermally, or by multiple puncture with a special instrument.

When BCG is introduced into the skin of an individual with a negative tuberculin, a primary tuberculous lesion results, similar to the primary focus that occurs naturally in the lungs. The difference is that the lesion is in subcutaneous tissue and is caused by a non-virulent bovine strain. It does not expose the injected person to the risks involved when the lesion is in the lungs and is caused by a virulent human strain. The regional lymph glands may become enlarged, as happens in a primary lesion in the lungs. Within about 1 month to 6 weeks, the injected individual becomes sensitive to the tubercle bacillus and develops a positive tuberculin test. He is now in the same immunologic position as a person with a primary pulmonary lesion. It is not unusual for the bacilli in the artificially induced primary lesion to die out. As a result, the tuberculin test again becomes negative. How frequently immunized individuals should be tested and whether and how often they should be reinjected with BCG are questions the answers to which await further investigation.

The question whether a primary lesion predisposes or offers resistance to exogenous reinfection has not been completely resolved. There are still competent individuals who accept the former thesis. Unfortunately, when BCG was first introduced, its use was so poorly planned and the results so poorly controlled that a critical judgment of its value could not be made. In recent years carefully controlled experiments in infants exposed to tuberculous mothers, in nurses exposed on tuberculosis wards, and in individuals such as the American Indian, living in communities where prevalence is high, have convinced most people that immunization with BCG appears to offer some protection against clinical tuberculosis.

Experiments are being carried on at present by the Federal Public Health Service and by selected health agencies to test its value under carefully controlled conditions in larger groups of individuals whose exposure to tuberculosis is more than average. In the meantime the production and distribution of BCG is rigidly controlled, and commercial manufacture has not been sanctioned.

THE ENVIRONMENT

Tuberculosis has occurred as far back as there is historical evidence. Bone tuberculosis was apparently present among the Egyptians, as evidenced by examination of mummies. The term "phthisis" was used by the early Greeks. The relationship of the various types of tuberculosis and their common causation was not definitely established until Koch discovered the tubercle bacillus in 1882.

Tuberculosis has a world-wide distribution and does not appear to be much influenced by climate or season. It is prevalent in the Esquimos in Alaska and in the diamond-mine workers of South Africa. Although there has been a consistent reduction in mortality in the United States and in several other countries, the rates in some countries are still very high. The accompanying table, taken from the World Health Organization's epidemiological reports, gives the rates for 1947 in some American, European, and African countries:

Death Rates from Tuberculosis per 100,000 Inhabitants, 1947

Africa	
Egypt	65
America	
Canada	43
United States	34
Chile (1946)	237
Europe	
Austria	85
Belgium	64
Czechoslovakia (Bohemia, Moravia, and Silesia)	96
Denmark	30
England and Wales	54
Finland	143
France	79
Germany United States	56
British	65
French	66
Hungary	106
Ireland	122
Italy (Rome)	138
Netherlands	37
Norway (1946)	65
Portugal	153
Scotland	80
Slovakia	104
Spain	124
Switzerland	67
Sweden	51

Occupation plays an important role in determining mortality from tuberculosis. Those occupations in which exposure to silica dust is unavoidable have a high rate. Mortality from tuberculosis is lowest in agricultural workers and highest in miners. It is also high among metal grinders and stonecutters.

A comparison of death rates according to economic status indicates a higher rate among those with a low income. The rate among skilled laborers is about half that in unskilled laborers, and the rates in the intermediate classes lie between the two. The factors of malnutrition and crowding are always bound up with economic status. After World Wars I and II, tuberculosis attained high levels in the central European countries. It was especially noticeable in the displaced persons' camps following World War II. It is difficult to separate the two factors and determine which played the greatest part in the increase, but there is little doubt that malnutrition alone and crowding alone contribute to the prevalence and mortality of tuberculosis.

The incidence of infections is higher in diabetics than in other individuals. This is true of tuberculosis as well as of pyogenic infections. It is important, therefore, in the care of diabetics, to be on the alert for the occurrence of symptoms and signs of tuberculosis.

Pregnancy was considered, at one time, as a complication in tuberculosis. Therapeutic abortions were frequently advised. In recent years there has been a change in this attitude. The general opinion is that tuberculous women can usually go through a pregnancy without adverse effect.

The influence of genetic factors and of constitution on the development of tuberculosis is difficult to gauge since other factors enter. In animals it is possible to breed strains which are much more resistant than others. In humans it has been shown that if one of monozygotic twins develops the disease, the other is apt to get it even if exposed to a different environment; this is not equally true of dizygotic twins.

The influence of race is also difficult to gauge. Quite uniformly, deaths from tuberculosis are three to five times as high in nonwhites as in whites in the United States, both in the American Indians and in Negroes. It is difficult, however, to separate race from socioeconomic factors. Both Indians and Negroes live under much more unfavorable conditions than do whites, and it is hard to separate the racial from the other factors. Even when comparable groups are examined, such as soldiers in the Army, the difference in mortality rates is found, but even here one cannot positively exclude environmental factors. What does seem impressive is that the rapidly spreading type of pulmonary tuberculosis is much more often seen in young Negroes than in whites of similar ages.

The factors of age and sex are much more clear cut since they

apply equally to different races and different environmental conditions. Although the tuberculosis death rate has fallen in all age
groups, the mortality rate in infants and very young children has
fallen proportionately more than in other age groups. In 1870 and
1880 this age group had the highest mortality rate, whereas today
it has next to the lowest rate. The lowest rate, now as well as in
previous years, is in the 5–14 age group. Above the age of 15 there
has been a consistent shift in age specific mortality since 1900 from
the younger to the older age groups. In 1900 the highest rates were
reached at 30 to 35 years, in 1910 at 40 to 45, in 1920 at 50 to 55,
and in 1950 at 65 years and over.

The rate for females has shown a different distribution than for
males in both whites and nonwhites. In males, after reaching a low
at ages 5 to 14, the curve of mortality rises gradually until it attains
its maximum at ages 65 to 75 when it begins to decline. In females,
after the low rate at the 5–14 age level it rises to reach its peak at
ages 25 to 30 and then gradually falls until the age of 50, when it
begins to rise again to approach the male curve at very advanced
ages. At all ages and in both sexes the mortality rates for nonwhites
greatly exceeds that of the whites.

The reduction of mortality from tuberculosis in the United States
since 1900 has been phenomenal. The rate, then, was about 200 per
100,000 population. Today it is 30, a reduction of about 85 per
cent. Yet one must remember that in some other diseases, such as
typhoid fever, an even greater reduction in mortality has been
made. Today, tuberculosis still ranks among the ten leading causes
of death in this country, and in the 15–34 age group it ranks second.
The fight against tuberculosis has not yet been won.

The factors influencing mortality from tuberculosis also influence
the occurrence of the disease, but not necessarily in the same way.
It is true that a low socioeconomic level, poor nutrition, over-
crowding, and certain occupations influence adversely not only
mortality but also the acquisition of a tuberculous infection. Yet
they do not necessarily do it to the same extent. That communities
with large aggregations of population cause greater exposure and a
larger percentage of infections than rural communities has been
shown by tuberculin surveys. The most potent determining factor
in infection is exposure to a case of open tuberculosis. Individuals
exposed to tuberculosis are infected from three to five times as often
as those not known to have been exposed to a definite case.

Age is an important predisposing cause of tuberculous infection.
All surveys indicate that the numbers of infected individuals increase with advance in age. The difference between 30 years ago
and today is enlightening. Then, students in medical schools were

taught that it was hardly worth while to do a tuberculin test on children above the age of 5 since practically all were positive. Today, negative tests are obtained in a large percentage of children and young adults. While the figure for the population as a whole is not known, it is estimated that about 50 per cent have a negative reaction.

Strange as it may seem from the discussion of mortality, tuberculin surveys do not show marked differences in the incidence of infection between the sexes nor between whites and nonwhites. The explanation of the variations in morbidity and mortality by age and color must be that young adult women develop a more active and rapid tuberculous process than males do, and die more rapidly, and that this is even more true of Negroes as compared with whites.

It has already been stated that most primary lesions of tuberculosis tend to regress and heal and become calcified. In young infants the prognosis of a primary lesion is worse than in older children and adults, because not infrequently it breaks into a vein and is disseminated to give a miliary tuberculosis and tuberculous meningitis. It is therefore highly important to keep infants away from anyone with an active lesion. In older people tuberculosis is apt to be of the reinfection type, which is chronic and prolonged. Whether such lesions are the result of an exogenous reinfection or whether they are the result of the lighting up of an old, endogenous focus has been much discussed by specialists in the field. Whichever it may be, there is no reason to dispute that control of tuberculosis rests in segregating open cases of tuberculosis, treating them properly, and keeping people generally, and especially those who have been exposed, as well housed, well fed, and under as good hygienic conditions as possible.

Control

Measures for the control of tuberculosis have been well standardized in this country and have undoubtedly been potent factors in the reduction of morbidity and mortality. They are discussed below:

Elimination of extrahuman sources. The control of tuberculosis in cattle has made this country unique in the eradication of certain forms of extrapulmonary lesions. Milk-giving cattle are tuberculin-tested and, if positive, are not used as milk producers. The pasteurization of milk, widely used in this country, is an added aid, since it destroys tubercle bacilli that have inadvertently been introduced.

Case finding. Since there are few, if any, symptoms in early tuberculosis, the only way to pick them up and treat them is by intensive case-finding procedures. These have been along two dissimilar lines: by tuberculin testing and by routine X ray examination of the lungs. The former method requires expert personnel for testing and reading, needs more than one visit, occasionally requires retesting, causes a certain amount of pain, and requires a follow-up X ray plate of the lungs if the test is positive. X ray examination requires only one visit, is painless, takes less time, is fairly cheap, can be done by technicians, and gives a permanent record which can be stored for later comparison. Since the introduction of sensitized paper and the use of a 70-millimeter size, the cost has been greatly reduced, and mass surveys are practicable. The large 14-by 17-inch film on celluloid is reserved for questionable cases.

Since it is not possible to survey the entire population, various recommendations have been made about the precedence that should be accorded to different groups in the population. Experience has shown that the lowest incidence of tuberculosis is in preschool and school children. It is, therefore, not profitable to make surveys in this group. Contacts to tuberculosis are the first to be X rayed. They usually develop lesions within the first 2 years of contact; it is therefore not important to follow them for more than 5 years. Surveys among noncontacts should be made in the more susceptible groups. By age, these are under 5 and over 15 years. Of the racial groups, the nonwhites are more susceptible than the whites. In economic groups, those with a low income and those employed in industry should be chosen by preference. A routine X ray of the chest for all admissions to hospitals and of all schoolteachers is also recommended.

Isolation of cases. Cases of tuberculosis admitted to general hospitals should be isolated in a private room or on a ward reserved for them. Wards should be so arranged that there is minimal traffic through them. The patient should be taught the method of spread of disease and his part in its control. These include scrupulous personal hygiene, conscientious hand washing, avoidance of kissing or close contact, especially with young children, and the use of paper tissues to cover the mouth when coughing and to receive respiratory discharges. The tissues should be deposited in a paper bag pinned to the side of the bed and disposed of by burning, if possible. If there is excessive expectoration, a paper sputum cup may be necessary. This should be stoutly constructed and held in a metal ring or frame. The cups should be collected once or twice daily, depending on need, and the patient should learn how to remove the cup properly from its holder and how to place it in a paper bag for disposal. The wrapped cups are placed in a proper cardboard receptacle and are then removed by an attendant for incineration. Cup holders should be collected two or three times a week, washed with soap and water, and boiled.

Dishes are cared for as in other communicable diseases. In a general hospital, trays from tuberculous patients should be cleaned last. Leftover food is scraped from the dishes and placed in a paper

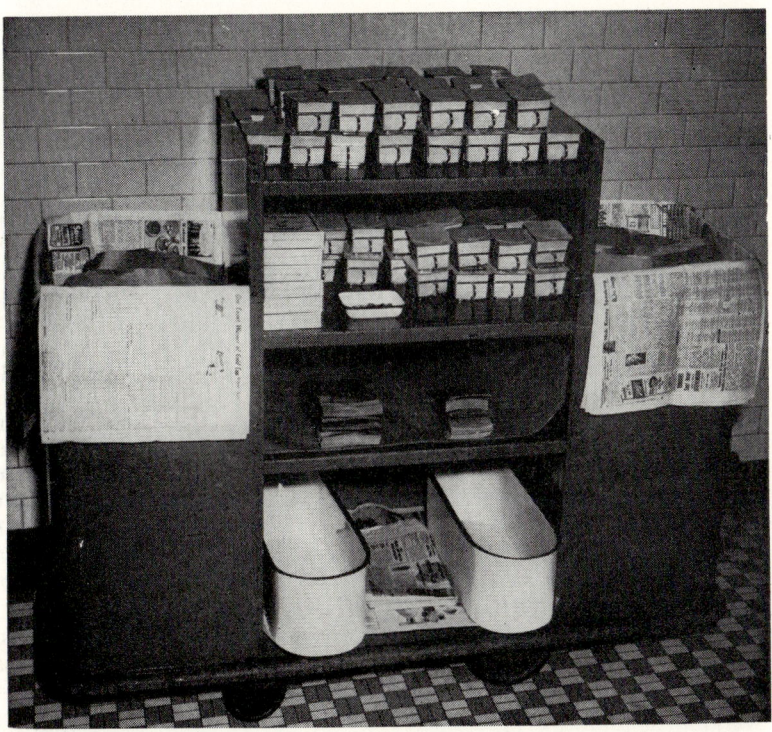

Fig. XIV. UNIT FOR DISTRIBUTION AND COLLECTION OF MATERIALS FOR SPUTUM CONTROL.

(Triboro Hospital)

bag or newspaper and secured for incineration. The dishes are rinsed, then scalded with boiling water or boiled and allowed to dry in the air. They are assembled on a tray and placed on a separate shelf that is properly labeled. If a mechanical dishwasher is used, scalding with hot water is unnecessary.

Basins and other utensils should be cleaned after use and then boiled in a large basin sterilizer for 5 minutes. They can then be placed on a shelf in the utility room and distributed to patients when needed.

Medicine can be dispensed in calibrated paper cups, which are discarded after use.

Linen is placed in a mesh bag at the bedside and then in a clean canvas bag. The nurse giving care keeps a record of the linen that is to go to the laundry and submits it to the head nurse. Sorting and counting are not done in the laundry until after the linen is washed. In general hospitals, linen from tuberculosis wards should be washed last. In the home, linen from tuberculous patients should be washed separately. Mattresses and pillows should be protected with rubber coverings.

Thermometers should be properly cleaned. Routine temperatures are not necessary for ambulant patients. The thermometer tray should be equipped with a covered receptacle containing enough thermometers for each patient, a receptacle containing green soap, a jar of cotton pledgets, lubricant, and a pad and pencil for recording. Temperatures are taken either orally or rectally. After taking the temperature, the nurse places the thermometer in the receptacle with the soap solution. When all temperatures have been taken, the tray is carried to the utility room, and each thermometer is cleaned with a cotton pledget, using friction and a rotary movement. All thermometers are then rinsed under cool, running water, dried, and placed in a clean receptacle. Cresol, 2 per cent solution, is poured over them, and they are allowed to remain in the receptacle for at least 5 minutes. After this, they are washed under running water, dried, and placed in a clean receptacle. They are then ready for use.

Gowns offer protection to the nurses if they are left on the ward when the nurses leave. They should be discarded at the end of the day and sent to the laundry. Masks, properly constructed, may offer protection to the nurse. If masks are worn, they should be changed frequently, and especially when they get wet. A better protection to the nurse, with much less discomfort, is to mask the patient adequately when giving nursing care. Careful hand washing should be observed by the nurse before and after caring for each patient.

Specimens of sputum required for bacteriological examination are best obtained early in the morning. The patient is given a sputum cup, such as is provided by most health departments, properly labeled, and instructed to cough into it. The cup is then sent to the laboratory, accompanied by the proper slip. If the patient is at home, the cup and slip are given to the patient at the time of the nurse's visit, and he is instructed to bring the specimen to the clinic or mail it to the health department.

Terminal disinfection is done in the usual manner. Utensils are boiled, linen is laundered as described, mattresses and pillows are exposed to the sun. The room is well aired.

BCG vaccination. The use of BCG as an immunizing agent has already been discussed. Since nurses face a special hazard, its use in those working on tuberculosis wards has been recommended.

MEDICAL CARE PLANS

Treatment

Until the discovery of the antibiotics, treatment was nonspecific and depended chiefly on rest and proper diet for long periods of time. Rest is particularly important when there are toxic symptoms such as fever, sweats, and rapid pulse. It should be as complete as possible, with confinement to bed. The importance of bed rest is that the lessened activity allows the body metabolism to come close to basal requirements. There is less wear and tear of tissue, less need of an active circulation and of increased respiratory activity, and a lesser opportunity for the development of dyspnea or cyanosis. Loss of weight is often arrested, and a sense of improvement may replace the feeling of malaise, weakness, and tiredness from which the patient suffered before. As the patient improves, modifications from complete bed rest may be introduced.

When only one lung is involved, or when the lesion in the other lung is slight, *pneumothorax* is frequently employed. It consists in the introduction of clean air into the pleural cavity through a hollow needle. This allows the lung to collapse and thus aids it in healing. Treatment is continued for several years in order to ensure healing. The lung is then permitted to re-expand. Another method of resting the lung is to introduce air into the peritoneal cavity, or *pneumoperitoneum.* Still another method is to crush the branch of the phrenic nerve on the side of the affected lung. This will cause temporary paralysis of half the diaphragm and thus rest the lung.

Two other surgical procedures are sometimes used when there is extensive cavitation in one lung. One is *thoracoplasty,* in which sections of several ribs are removed, resulting in a collapse of the tissue overlying one lung and allowing the walls of the cavity to approximate so that fibrosis and healing result. The other is *lobectomy* or *pneumonectomy,* in which a lobe or an entire lung is removed surgically. These are major operations and are undertaken by competent surgeons only in well-selected cases.

Since the introduction of antibiotics, extensive experimental work has been done in animals, first with sulfonamide derivatives and then with streptomycin. Penicillin appears to be ineffective. *Strepto-*

mycin, however, offers promise, particularly in miliary tuberculosis and in tuberculosis meningitis. It has to be given over a prolonged period of time and must be carefully watched, since toxic symptoms are common. It is given either alone or combined with such drugs as sulfadiazine, Promin, Promizole or para-aminosalicylic acid (PAS). In pulmonary tuberculosis the choice of patient to be treated with these drugs must be carefully made. The choice of patient, the drugs used, and their amount and frequency are still in the investigative stage. The treatment in miliary tuberculosis and in tuberculosis meningitis is somewhat more standardized and is discussed elsewhere.

Isonicotinic acid hydrazide. The most recent drug to be introduced in the treatment of tuberculosis is isonicotinic acid hydrazide, which is marketed under several names, such as Nydrazid, Rimifon, and Marsilid. It is a synthetically produced chemical related to nicotinic acid. In the test tube it is bacteriostatic against the tubercle bacillus in low concentrations. In animals it has given promising results in arresting the course of experimentally induced tuberculosis. In humans it has been used in a dose of 3 to 5 milligrams per kilogram of body weight per day, orally in two or three divided doses. In advanced cases of pulmonary tuberculosis its use has caused reduction in fever and cough, gain in appetite and weight, and some clearing of the lesion, as indicated by X ray. Favorable response to the drug has also been observed in nonpulmonary tuberculosis and in tuberculous meningitis.

The results so far achieved have been encouraging, but much more work will have to be done to determine its exact usefulness. Among the problems that still require solution are the exact mechanism of the drug's action, its toxicity when used over a long period of time, the optimal dosage, the length of time treatment should be carried on, the possibility of drug resistance of the tubercle bacilli, the need of ancillary measures of treatment, and the results that can be achieved in ambulant treatment.

The level of toxicity of the drug is fortunately low, and the cost of its manufacture is not excessive. Its administration is simple and, since it can be taken by mouth, there are none of the disadvantages that arise with parenteral injections. The final evaluation of isonicotinic acid hydrazide in the treatment of tuberculosis will not be made until patients have been followed for a considerable period of time.

Symptomatic treatment will depend on the patient's symptoms and complaints. Insomnia may be due to the strange surroundings, to nervousness, to discomfort, or to a number of other causes. Psychotherapy often helps. It may be necessary to prescribe barbiturates for a while. Cough is often a distressing symptom. When severe, it gives the patient little rest. A spell of coughing is apt to be prolonged and tiring in the early morning after waking. Patients should be taught how to suppress nonproductive coughs and how to help themselves by various changes in posture. A warm drink will sometimes alleviate the condition. If necessary, sedatives should be prescribed. Sudden pulmonary hemorrhage is a frightening event to the patient. He should be reassured and made comfortable, with his head low. Sedatives are often necessary. Fluids may be given in small sips or in the form of cracked ice. Bleeding is rarely severe enough to cause fear of a fatal result. The blood and secretions may be emptied directly into a water-flushed toilet. If this is not available, they should be received in a basin and a solution of 10 per cent cresol should be added.

Diet

The diet is a general, well-balanced one, of sufficient caloric value to make up for the extra catabolism that results from fever and tissue destruction. Supplementary vitamins should be added to the diet. Although cod-liver oil has been a standard drug in tuberculosis for many years, the tendency is not to use foods or drugs with high fat content, since these often cause digestive disturbances. Fortunately, concentrated vitamin preparations are now available in pill or soluble form, are easy to take, and cause no digestive upsets. The anemia which is common in tuberculosis, as in all chronic infections, can be combated with a proper diet. Occasionally, soluble hematinics are added as accessory drugs.

Supportive Nursing Care

One of the important determinants in effective recovery is the adequacy of nursing care. Poor nursing is not excusable in any illness, but it has a devastating effect on individuals with chronic diseases. When a patient is admitted to a hospital or sanatorium he is tense, apprehensive, and morose. He is disturbed not only by knowledge of his disease and its chronicity but by the separation from family and friends. If he is the support of parent, wife, or child, the economic catastrophe that promises to overwhelm him becomes almost unbearable. The first person with whom he comes into close and prolonged contact is the nurse. If she is cheerful and understanding she can put him at ease, minimize his fears, and diminish his tensions. A warm, friendly approach and a permissive informality will enable him to talk more freely. The nurse explains ward routines and visiting hours and assures him that his social and economic needs will be properly taken care of. She guides him to a clearer perception of his disease, answers his questions intelligently, and adapts her replies to his level of comprehension. She reassures him and tries to instill a feeling of optimism by reference to the many cases that have made good recoveries. In her daily contacts with the patient she teaches him facts about tuberculosis, dispels the false rumors about the disease that the patient has picked up, and discusses treatment and measures necessary for readjustment.

It is difficult for normal people who are confined for long periods of time in a comparatively small place to remain sweet and cheerful. It is understandable that on a tuberculosis ward tensions will arise, resentments against other patients or personnel will occur, complaints about food and physical care will be expressed, and a general feeling of unhappiness will result. The nurse should utilize every opportunity to smooth over difficulties, to allay hurt feelings, and to act as general counselor. This can be accomplished by maintaining a cheerful attitude and advising and assisting the patient in a variety of ways. In so doing, the nurse is encouraging the harmonious state so essential to recovery.

The temperature and humidity of the room should be comfortable and the ventilation adequate. Bed covering should be light in weight but warm. The bed should be comfortable. Pressure of bedclothes on the toes and feet should be avoided. It can frequently be obviated by placing a board across the bed between the foot and the mattress. Change of the patient's position from time to time should be encouraged. Comfort in the side position is often enhanced by small pillows placed under the back.

Daily sponge baths ensure cleanliness, improve the circulation of the skin, and have a freshening and tonic effect. If fever is high, alcohol sponge baths contribute to general comfort. The care of the hair in female patients is often difficult if it is long. Women with long hair should be encouraged to have it cut and thus conserve energy in its care.

The combined efforts of all health and welfare workers in the community who are concerned with tuberculosis are essential for rehabilitation of the patient. The formulation of a comprehensive plan for nursing care which integrates the inpatient, outpatient, and home care or health supervision is essential to co-ordinate instruction to the patient and family and to eliminate confusion. Continuity in medical and nursing care is achieved when mutual understanding and agreement on policies among all community workers are maintained. Under such a plan the best practices in nursing care are utilized, and a unified concept is projected. To implement such a program, periodic conferences with all workers and wider use of interagency referral devices should be incorporated into a community nursing program.

A home visit is generally made by a public health nurse to all reported cases of tuberculosis. As in the hospital, the first contact between the nurse and the patient in the home is an important one psychologically. Usually this visit follows shortly after the diagnosis has been established and the patient has not fully recovered from the shock. An effective working relationship and skill in counseling the patient at this critical period in his life often determine the productiveness of the home visit. The public health nurse should listen attentively to the expression of the patient's feelings regarding diagnosis and recovery, and what the disease will do to him in terms of family relationships. She should be sensitive to the feelings of the family toward tuberculosis and toward the patient and his general fears and anxieties. She should help the patient to understand his disease, teach him its hopeful aspects, and aid him in accepting the diagnosis. Before giving any detailed instruction on precautionary measures, she should determine the readiness of the patient for learning at this stage. Intensive home visiting is essential at this point, because the family and the patient are most receptive to instruction, and positive action usually follows.

The hospital or sanatorium offers the most satisfactory method of segregating the infectious case from the family and community and for educating the patient. This is frequently recommended by the physician. Where hospital facilities are limited, placement on a waiting list may defer hospital care until a vacancy occurs, and the patient temporarily remains at home.

The public health nurse may provide nursing care under the direction of the physician or she may demonstrate and supervise nursing care given by the family or relatives. Precautionary measures for open infectious cases in the home are the same as in the hospital. A gown should be worn by the family member when giving care to the patient. The instructions to the family should be simple and easily understood. All household members should be referred for X ray examination to their physician or to a clinic. The importance of periodic examination must be emphasized. If the family requires help with social and economic problems, the nurse should be familiar with community resources and be able to make referrals to the agency best suited to meet the family's needs. If hospital or sanatorium care has been recommended, she should be familiar with the policies of and care at the institution and be able to interpret them intelligently. A summary of home visits with the findings should be sent to the attending physician or to the hospital where the patient will receive care.

For effective supervision of the patient and family, the nurse should have a knowledge of tuberculosis and the sanitary-code regulations for management of home care. Many nurses have fears and obsessions about tuberculosis, and these feelings are sometimes transferred to the patient and family. Lack of scientific information and insecurity contribute considerably to antagonisms which may arise in future contacts with patients.

Preparation of the family for the return of the patient from the hospital contributes to wholesome family relationships. The nurse making the home visit should follow through on the physician's recommendations and assist the family with the necessary adjustments. Instruction in precautionary measures to be observed in the home will depend upon the progress of the lesion. If arrested, no isolation is required, but periodic medical checkups to control reactivation are vital.

Selection of a room in the home setting is often a difficult problem. A light, well-ventilated room through which other members of the family will not pass and one with a southern exposure is most desirable. The room should be cheerful, attractively furnished, and have all necessary conveniences for the patient's comfort. Children should be discouraged from entering the room, and visitors should be limited.

Unattached men and women have great difficulty locating suitable living quarters on account of the community's fear of and repugnance to the disease. Suitable arrangements can frequently be made with social-work agencies.

The nurse should make every effort to provide recreational activities for the patient and further aid in readapting him to his normal role in the community. If he returns to his former occupation or obtains a new one, he will need help in making an adjustment.

The public health nurse's major role in the community tuberculosis program is case finding and education of the patient and family. She assists with mass surveys of selected community groups and works co-operatively with a team of other professional workers.

Rehabilitation. In a chronic disease like tuberculosis, the term most commonly used for a recovered patient is "arrested" rather than "cured." This indicates that the possibility of recurrence must be kept in mind, and that the patient's way of life must be altered, if necessary, to remove strains that are known to increase the possibility of tuberculosis. Important among these is that of occupation. Tuberculous patients who become arrested and whose previous employment was one in which there were no unusual physical or emotional strains can go back to their work. Many, however, were employed in occupations requiring unusual exertion. Such patients must learn other skills. The readjustment is often difficult and involves economic and emotional strains. The time to begin indoctrinating the patients is not when their treatment has been completed but right at the beginning. It is a gradual indoctrination, carried on over a considerable period of time. It avoids the shock and disappointment resulting from the sudden knowledge that one must not do what one has been accustomed to. Also, it gives the patient, the family, and the medical, nursing, and social-service attendants ample opportunity to work out a plan of rehabilitation, so that the patient can become economically useful as soon as permitted by his physician.

Extrapulmonary Tuberculosis

Not infrequently, tuberculosis spreads from the lungs to adjacent tissues. Among those occasionally involved are the larynx and the intestines. Tuberculosis of the larynx is seen, as a rule, only in advanced cases. As a result of involvement of the vocal cords, the voice may become hoarse or husky. Pain is a common symptom. Diagnosis is made by laryngological examination. Until recently, treatment was unsatisfactory. The introduction of streptomycin has been of distinct help in the treatment of this complication.

Intestinal tuberculosis also occurs most commonly in advanced pulmonary cases and is apparently due to infection from swallowed sputum. The lower part of the small intestine and the adjacent areas are usually involved. Symptoms may be mild, with slight abdominal pain and occasional diarrhea. In advanced cases diarrhea may be persistent and troublesome. Ischiorectal abscesses and fissures may occur.

Pleurisy with effusion is said to be one of the most benign forms of tuberculosis. It may occur without any other pulmonary lesion. Symptoms may be absent, especially in the early stage. However, pain in the side, low fever, and general malaise frequently occur. Sometimes the pain is quite sharp and may require codeine for relief. If the fluid accumulates rapidly, there may be dyspnea and cyanosis. Usually, however, the accumulaton is slow and no great discomfort is felt. Aspiration of fluid should be done for diagnostic purposes. Frequent aspiration is inadvisable because of the danger of secondary infection and because reaccumulation occurs. Rest in bed is essential. Symptomatic treatment should be used as needed. With proper care the disease may be arrested at this stage. The fluid is gradually absorbed.

Tuberculosis of bones and joints occurs usually without manifestation of tuberculosis in other parts of the body. Certain bones and joints seem to have a predilection over others. The bodies of the vertebrae and the hip joint are two of the commonest locations. In tuberculosis of the spine there are frequently no symptoms early in the disease. Later there may be back pain or deformity. Occasionally, there are no symptoms referrable to the back, and the first sign noted is a swelling in the inner aspect of the thigh which is caused by an abscess that developed in the vertebrae and that has traveled down between the sheaths of the back muscles. Diagnosis is usually established by X rays. Treatment consists of complete rest, with splinting of the back by means of braces or casts.

In tuberculosis of the hip there is also destruction of bone, with pus formation. Here, too, there are few symptoms. Usually, lameness is the presenting sign. There is a limp, and the affected limb is favored. Examination may show spasm of the muscles about the affected joint, and there may be shortening of the limb. The diagnosis is made by X ray. The treatment of this condition is also complete rest, which is usually brought about by orthopedic appliances. Surgical procedures are often used to fix joints.

Bone and joint tuberculosis has decreased very much in recent years. This is due to the elimination of bovine tuberculosis in many communities by the slaughter of tuberculous cows and the pasteurization of milk. There is evidence to indicate that bone and joint tuberculosis was caused largely by bovine tubercle bacilli. This is also true of tuberculosis of lymph glands which was a much more common disease in previous years than it is today.

Tuberculosis of the kidney may also occur as a solitary lesion. If not diagnosed and treated early, the urinary bladder may become secondarily infected. There are no symptoms early in the disease. When the bladder is infected, pain and difficulty in urination may result. Early signs of renal tuberculosis are persistent pus or blood in the urine. This always requires careful investigation by a urologist. X ray of the kidney with contrast dye helps in the diagnosis. Ureteral catheterization with examination of sediment from each kidney separately is usually necessary. The sediment should be examined directly for tubercle bacilli and by culture and guinea-pig inoculation. If only one kidney is affected, nephrectomy will usually prevent spread and bring about a cure.

Tuberculous meningitis is one of the most serious forms of meningitis. It occurs chiefly in young children who are intimately exposed to an individual with tuberculosis, often in their homes. The onset is usually insidious, with headache, malaise, and drowsiness. There may be vomiting and paralyses of muscles supplied by the cranial nerves. Not infrequently, convulsions occur. The temperature is elevated, and there is an increase in the pulse rate.

Examination reveals an acutely ill child with retracted head. The Kernig and Brudzinski tests are positive. The pupils may be unequal, and there may be strabismus. A spinal tap yields clear fluid under pressure. The protein content is increased, and there is a decrease in the percentage of sugar as well as of chlorides. There is an increase in cells, numbering several hundred, as a rule. These are chiefly mononuclears, although polymorphonuclears may predominate at first. If the fluid is allowed to stand, a pellicle forms. This can be floated onto a glass slide and stained for tubercle bacilli. It is also possible to demonstrate tubercle bacilli by centrifugation of the spinal fluid and staining the sediment.

A careful examination of the child will usually indicate the presence of tuberculosis elsewhere. Usually, miliary tuberculosis is present and can often be seen in a roentgenogram of the chest. Even when miliary tuberculosis is not seen definitely on the chest plate, evidence of pulmonary involvement is usually found.

The progress of an untreated case of tuberculous meningitis is downhill to a fatal termination. The child becomes progressively weaker, the stupor changes into coma, breathing becomes irregular, emaciation becomes extreme, and death ensues. This was the picture of practically all children with tuberculous meningitis prior to the introduction of the antibiotics. A considerable change has occurred since then.

The antibiotic that has been used most extensively in the treatment of tuberculous meningitis is streptomycin. It has been given both intramuscularly and intrathecally. The Medical Research Council of Great Britain reported on 105 cases after a minimum observation of 4 months after treatment. It found that 64 per cent had died and 28 per cent were making good progress. A British report of a follow-up of 54 cases that had been observed for at least 2½ years indicated a survival of 30 per cent. Of these, 2 were mentally retarded, 2 were deaf, 1 had hemiplegia, and 2 developed nonmeningeal tuberculosis which was under control. It is obvious that the results of treatment in tuberculous meningitis are not nearly so brilliant as the results with antibiotics in other types of infection. Nevertheless, a survival rate of about 30 per cent, even with sequelae, in a disease that was formerly almost 100 per cent fatal, is a considerable accomplishment. The dosage usually used is 1 gram daily of streptomycin intramuscularly for 3 to 6 months and 0.1 gram in 5 to 10 cubic centimeters of saline solution intrathecally daily for about 1 month. Some investigators have added other drugs, particularly the sulfones such as Promizole and Sulphetrone, to the streptomycin treatment.

The use of isonicotinic acid in tuberculosis has been discussed on pages 292–293.

REFERENCES

1. Aronson, J. D., and Palmer, C. E.: "Experience with BCG Vaccine in the Control of Tuberculosis among North American Indians," *Pub. Health Rep.* **61**:802, 1946.
2. Birkhaug, K.: "BCG Vaccination in Scandinavia," *Am. Rev. Tuberc.*, **55**:234, 1947.
3. Bryant, Z.: "Tuberculosis Case Finding in General Hospitals, *Pub. Health Rep.*, **65**:710, 1950.
4. Bryant, Z., and Jones, G. S.: "Community-wide Chest X-ray Surveys, II. Nursing," *Pub. Health Rep.*, **65**:1573, 1950.
5. Cady, L. L.: *Nursing in Tuberculosis,* W. B. Saunders Company, Philadelphia, 1948.
6. Calman, W. L.; Rubie, J.; and Mohun, A. F.: "Tuberculous Meningitis," *Brit. M. J.*, **1**:794, 1951.
7. Chadwick, H. D., and Pope, A. S.: *Modern Attack on Tuberculosis,* Commonwealth Fund, Harvard University Press, Cambridge, Mass., 1946.
8. Chadwick, H. D., and Zachs, D.: "Incidence of Tuberculosis Infection in School Children," *New England J. Med.*, **200**:332, 1929.
9. Edwards, H. R.: "Tuberculosis Case Findings: Studies in Mass Surveys," *Am. Rev. Tuberc.*, **41**:3, Suppl., 1940.
10. Geiser, P. B.: "Role of the Nurse in Research," *Pub. Health Rep.*, **65**:1860, 1950.
11. Guralnick, L., and Glaser, S.: "Tuberculosis Mortality in the United States, 1948," *Pub. Health Rep.*, **65**:468, 1950.
12. Hartz, J.: "Human Relationship in Tuberculosis," *Pub. Health Rep.*, **65**:1292, 1950.
13. Hetherington, H. N., and Eshleman, F. W.: *Nursing in Prevention and Control of Tuberculosis,* G. P. Putnam's Sons, New York, 1950.
14. Hilleboe, H. E., and Morgan, R. H.: *Mass Radiography of the Chest,* Year Book Publishers, Inc., Chicago, 1945.
15. Holm, J.: "BCG Vaccination in Denmark," *Pub. Health Rep.*, **61**:1298, 1946.
16. Joint Tuberculosis Nursing Advisory Service: *Safer Ways in Nursing to Protect against Tuberculosis,* National League of Nursing, New York, 1948.
17. Levine, M. I.: "An Evaluation of the Use of BCG in the Prevention of Tuberculosis in Infants and Children," *Am. J. Pub. Health*, **37**:1089, 1947.
18. Lincoln, E. M., and Krimse, T. W.: "The Diagnosis and Treatment of Tuberculosis Meningitis in Children," *Am. J. M. Sc.*, **219**:382, 1950.
19. Long, E. R., and Ferebee, B. A.: "A Controlled Investigation of Streptomycin Treatment in Pulmonary Tuberculosis," *Pub. Health Rep.*, **65**:1421, 1950.
20. Medical Research Council: "Streptomycin Treatment of Tuberculous Meningitis," *Lancet,* **1**:582, 1948.
21. Pinner, M.: *Pulmonary Tuberculosis in the Adult,* Charles C Thomas, Publisher, Springfield, Ill., 1945.
22. Rosenthal, S. R.; Blahd, M.; and Leslie, E. I.: "Ten Years' Experience with BCG," *J. Pediat.*, **26**:470, 1945.
23. South, J.: *Tuberculosis Handbook for Public Health Nurses,* National Tuberculosis Association, New York, 1950.
24. Taylor, Ruth B.: "Social Services for the Tuberculous and Their Families," *Pub. Health Rep.*, **65**:279, 1950.

25. Teague, R. E.: "Study of Tuberculosis Control in Philadelphia," *Pub. Health Rep.*, **65**:269, 1950.
26. Tucker, W. B.: "An Evaluation of Streptomycin Regimens in the Treatment of Tuberculosis," *Am. Rev. Tuberc.*, **60**:715, 1949.
27. *United States Summary of Vital Statistics*, National Office of Vital Statistics, Public Health Service, Washington, D.C., 1948.
28. Walgren, Arvid: *Tuberculosis and Other Problems in Pediatrics*, The Williams & Wilkins Company, Baltimore, 1950.

Chapter 31 WHOOPING COUGH (PERTUSSIS)

General Description

WHOOPING cough is an acute communicable disease caused by *Hemophilus pertussis* and characterized by spasmodic attacks of coughing.

The Causative Agent

The causative agent is a small, nonmotile gram-negative bacillus possessing a capsule. It does not grow well on ordinary mediums but grows readily on special mediums. Several forms of colonial growth occur on artificial mediums. These have been designated as Phase I, which is the virulent form, Phase IV, which is avirulent, and Phases II and III which are intermediate in virulence. Only Phase I organisms are used in the preparation of vaccines.

The organism is destroyed by heat, the usual antiseptics, and ultraviolet light. It dies when desiccated, but it may remain alive in expectorated sputum for several hours. It grows on the epithelium of the respiratory tract but does not invade the blood stream. In nature, whooping cough is found in man only.

The Host

Symptoms

The incubation period is 7 to 10 days. The symptoms can be divided into three stages: (1) catarrhal, (2) paroxysmal, and (3) convalescent. The first stage is indistinguishable from an upper respiratory infection—there are running nose, sore throat, slight fever, and beginning cough. This lasts from 1 to 2 weeks. Unless the child has been exposed to whooping cough, there is usually no suspicion of the disease.

Toward the end of the catarrhal stage, the cough becomes persistent. Gradually, it assumes a spasmodic character, with free intervals. When the paroxysmal stage is fully developed, the child usually has no fever and appears normal. However, without any warning, the child gets a paroxysm of coughing, which consists of a number of short, tight coughs during an inspiration followed by a prolonged drawing in of breath and a crowing sound, or "whoop." During the paroxysm the child appears to be in great distress, with its face red or even blue, and its eyes popping. Frequently, the child vomits immediately after a spell and expectorates some thick, glairy mucus. It may then remain free and apparently normal until the next spell. Occasionally, several paroxysms follow each other with little rest between. They occur more frequently at night and more often indoors than outdoors. The number and severity of attacks vary. They may be so frequent and so severe as to exhaust the child, or they may occur infrequently and be so mild as not to disturb the child unduly. As a result of a lack of desire for food and of the vomiting, the child's nutrition suffers, and there may be considerable weight loss.

The paroxysmal stage may last only 1 or 2 weeks in the mild cases or may be prolonged to 1 or 2 months in the severer ones. Usually, the paroxysms become milder toward the end of the siege. The severe paroxysmal attacks, with their concomitant disturbance of nutrition and rest, are often quite serious in young infants. Paroxysms may be so mild in some children, particularly if they have previously been immunized, as to make the diagnosis doubtful. During this stage, examination of the lungs shows surprisingly few signs.

The convalescent stage follows. There is still some cough, but it tends to be less spasmodic and not so frequent or so disturbing. The child gradually improves, but occasional spells of coughing may continue to occur for months. It is not unusual, even after complete recovery, when a child gets an upper respiratory infection and cough, for the latter to take on the characteristic paroxysmal character of whooping cough. This often disturbs parents, who think their child is getting another attack of the disease.

The commonest complications are hemorrhages in the conjunctivae or skin and pneumonia as a result of plugging of a bronchus. The latter is a frequent complication in young infants and usually the cause of death. In young infants, convulsions may occur during the paroxysmal stage.

Diagnosis

In the presence of a typical cough and whoop the diagnosis is not difficult. The milder cases are the ones that offer difficulty. The white count in the catarrhal stage usually shows a leukocytosis of 15,000 to 20,000 or even higher, with a preponderance of lymphocytes. Bacteriological diagnosis is made by a pharyngeal swab or a cough plate. In the former, a swab is passed through the nares to the pharynx and then cultured on Bordet-Gengou medium; in the latter, a Petri dish containing the medium is held about 6 inches from the patient's mouth during a coughing spell. After growth, the colonies are picked and identified. About 75 per cent positive cultures are obtained in the catarrhal stage and approximately 60 per cent in the paroxysmal stage. Hardly any positives are obtained in the third stage.

A skin test has been tried experimentally but has not been sufficiently developed for routine use. Antibodies do not appear in the blood until convalescence, so that their demonstration is of limited value in diagnosis.

Immunity

One attack of whooping cough usually confers a permanent immunity. However, there is little passive transfer of immunity from mother to child. Unlike in measles, small infants are quite susceptible to whooping cough and make up the bulk of fatal cases.

Complement-fixing, neutralizing, and agglutinating antibodies appear in the blood during convalescence. Their determination is frequently used to measure the effectiveness of vaccines.

In recent years there has been increasing evidence of protection offered to children by the use of a vaccine made from killed *Hemophilus pertussis,* Phase I organisms. A fluid vaccine is available, which is given in three doses, in a total of 80 billion organisms. Since the vaccine contains 20 billion organisms per cubic centimeter, the first dose is 1 cubic centimeter and the second and third doses $1\frac{1}{2}$ cubic centimeters each, given subcutaneously or intramuscularly. If alum-precipitated vaccine is used, the total dose needed is 45 billion organisms per cubic centimeter. Recently there has been a tendency to combine whooping cough vaccine with diphtheria toxoid or with diphtheria and tetanus toxoids. This saves extra injections. Furthermore, there is evidence that both the pertussis and the diphtheria stimulation is enhanced by the combined mixture. It is put up in an alum-precipitated mixture, so that 0.5 cubic centimeter given three times at monthly intervals will complete the immunizations.

The question of the optimum age for beginning injections is important, since about one half of all deaths occur in the first 6 months of life and about 75 to 80 per cent in infants under 1 year of age. It is therefore important to start immunization as early as possible. There is evidence to indicate that very young infants do not develop antibodies for whooping cough and diphtheria as a result of stimulations of antigen as well as older infants and children do. Investigations in the laboratory and the field indicate that an adequate immunization can be conferred if injections are started at 3 to 4 months of age. It is advisable to give a booster dose 6 months to 1 year following completion of injections.

Children who are exposed to whooping cough and have been previously immunized should receive a booster dose of fluid pertussis vaccine of 1 cubic centimeter. If they have not been previously immunized against whooping cough, they should receive an injection of 20 cubic centimeters of hyperimmune pertussis serum or of 2.5 cubic centimeters hyperimmune pertussis gamma globulin made from such serum if they are under 5 years of age. This confers a passive immunity which lasts about 3 to 4 weeks. The serum is obtained from normal persons who give a history of whooping cough and who have been hyperimmunized with a pertussis vaccine. When their blood shows a high titer of immune bodies, it is drawn and processed for use.

THE ENVIRONMENT

Whooping cough exists in all parts of the world. It is commoner in thickly populated areas. It usually occurs endemically, but epidemics are occasionally reported. Unlike the other respiratory diseases, the incidence is fairly evenly distributed throughout the year, with some peaking in the winter months. Both morbidity and mortality are higher in females than in males. Negroes are equally susceptible with whites, but the mortality is higher among them.

Unlike measles, whooping cough may occur in very young infants. Approximately 15 per cent of cases occur in infants under 1 year, and more than half the cases occur in children under 5 years of age. Most of the deaths occur in infants. About half the deaths are in infants up to 6 months of age, about three quarters in infants under 1 year of age, and almost all in children under 5 years. It

Cases and Deaths from Whooping Cough
New York City, 1911–1949

YEARS	AVERAGE CASES PER YEAR	AVERAGE DEATHS PER YEAR	CASE FATALITY, PER CENT
1911–1914	3,888	353	9.1
1915–1919	5,560	456	8.2
1920–1924	5,633	302	5.4
1925–1929	4,575	222	4.9
1930–1934	7,449	148	2.0
1935–1939	7,401	67	0.9
1940–1944	5,706	43	0.6
1945–1949	2,616	11	0.4

is obvious that efforts at immunization should be stressed for infants and very young children.

Whooping cough is second only to measles in the number of people attacked. By age 16, about 80 per cent of people in urban communities have had whooping cough, as against 90 per cent for measles. The incidence of the disease has not declined appreciably, but the deaths have, as may be noted from the accompanying table. In 1947 the number of deaths from whooping cough in the United States was 1,954, approximately the same as the number of deaths from measles, diphtheria, scarlet fever, and poliomyelitis, combined.

Control

Cases of whooping cough should be isolated for a period of 3 weeks after the onset of the whoop. Since there are no true carriers of the disease, there is no reason for the quarantine of contacts. However, these should be kept under observation and isolated at the beginning of the catarrhal stage.

All infants should be actively immunized at the age of 3 months or as soon thereafter as possible, and a booster dose should be administered 1 year after the completion of the injections.

Children under 5 years who have previously been immunized and are exposed to whooping cough should receive a booster dose, and those who have not been previously immunized should receive a prophylactic injection of hyperimmune pertussis serum or hyperimmune pertussis gamma globulin.

MEDICAL CARE PLANS

Treatment

Mild cases should be kept in bed during the catarrhal stage, particularly while they have fever, but may be permitted moderate activity thereafter. It is advisable to keep them in the fresh air, but rigid precautions must be taken not to allow them to come in contact with other children. Severe cases, particularly in infants, require meticulous nursing care.

Nonspecific therapy is directed toward keeping up the child's nutrition, avoiding paroxysms, and minimizing their effects if they do occur, combating anoxemia, and keeping the child quiet and comfortable by means of physical procedures and drugs.

In infants, the thick mucus which cannot be coughed up may cause obstruction to respiration. It is then necessary to aspirate it immediately. In hospitals treating many cases, an aspirating apparatus, electrically driven, is standard equipment in a whooping cough ward or room. Where this is not available, a simple suction bottle can be easily made by using a widemouthed bottle closed with a cork through which two holes are punched. Through each of the holes bent glass tubes are inserted. To one of the tubes a rubber catheter, size 10 or 12 F, is attached. This is inserted into the pharynx through the mouth or nose. Suction is maintained by drawing on the other glass tube. If this simple apparatus is not immediately available and signs of obstruction occur, the infant should be held up by its legs and gently patted. A good deal of exudate may drain out in this way.

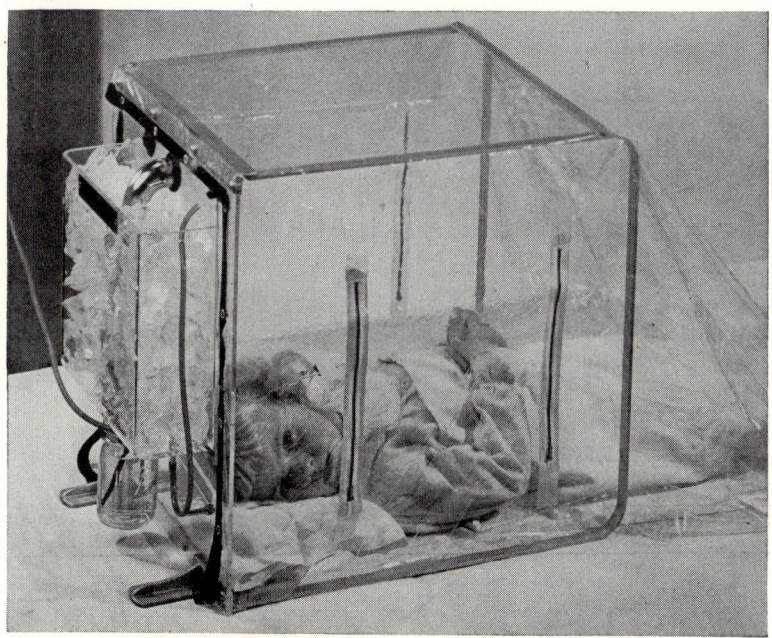

Fig. XV. OXYGEN CROUP TENT.

(Courtesy of Air-Shields, Inc., Hatboro, Pa.)

Anoxemia occurs frequently in whooping cough. To some extent, it is due to partial obstruction of respiratory passages and may also be due to pneumonia. It is indicated chiefly by cyanosis. The best treatment is oxygen. In infants and children the use of nasal catheters or a mask for administration of oxygen is extremely difficult. The children fret and are unhappy and pull at the apparatus. On the other hand, they quiet down as soon as they are placed in an oxygen tent. A simple tent is now made which consists of a hood placed over the child's head and neck, leaving the rest of its body free. Oxygen content can be maintained at 60 to 70 per cent, and the temperature in the hood can be kept at about 70° F.

Drugs should be used sparingly. They are needed chiefly to help relieve the cough. Barbiturates act as valuable sedatives. Morphine should not be given, since it depresses the respiratory center. Tepid sponge baths also have a sedative effect. Support of the abdomen with a binder helps to minimize the discomfort in a severe coughing spell.

Specific therapy consists of the antibiotic drugs and hyperimmune serum. Penicillin is of little value. Streptomycin appears to be of some value. The antibiotics of broader spectrum, Aureomycin, chloramphenicol, and Terramycin appear to be of value when given in fairly large doses, but results from their use are not dramatic. Hyperimmune pertussis serum or hyperimmune pertussis gamma globulin is administered in doses of 20 to 60 cubic centimeters of the serum or 2.5 to 7.5 cubic centimeters of the gamma globulin. The dosage may be repeated for the next 1 or 2 days.

Diet

It is important to maintain the nutritional needs of infants and children who have whooping cough. The prolonged coughing and the exhaustion resulting from it, the vomiting and lack of sleep depress the child's appetite, and feeding becomes a major problem. In the case of infants, simple formulas should be given, and the child should be held while feeding. Bottles should not be propped up in the crib. Older infants should get the solid food between bottle nursings so as not to overfill the stomach. Young children should be given small meals at shorter intervals than is customary in the usual three-meals-a-day pattern. The usual amount of fluid intake is sufficient. If a child has had improper nursing care and is admitted to a hospital in a state of dehydration, intravenous glucose solution or plasma should be administered.

Supportive Nursing Care

Skilled and constant nursing care is required for infants and young children. Paroxysms of coughing occur more frequently if a child is overactive or is emotionally upset. It is part of good nursing care to keep a child with whooping cough quiet and peaceful. This may require considerable ingenuity in providing games, simple reading matter, and various amusements. If paroxysms do occur the baby, if small, should be picked up and held in the nurse's arms or lap. Raising the arms above the head is of no assistance. Occasionally, lowering the head and chest may aid in expelling mucus. If this is thick and tenacious, it may be removed by the nurse's finger wrapped in gauze. Older children can usually manage a paroxysm well enough if left to their own devices.

The psychologic aspect of the nursing care of children with whooping cough is important. The onset of a coughing spell with its unpleasant after results is frightening to a child. He must be reassured and quieted and given the necessary assistance. The child's morale is not aided if its mother looks and acts anxious and gets upset whenever a spasm occurs. Children who are hospitalized have an added psychologic trauma in the sudden separation from their homes, parents, and familiar surroundings. They feel lost and abandoned. An impersonal attitude on the part of the nurse aggravates the feeling of rejection. The nurse must be pleasant and cheerful and try to gain the child's confidence and friendship. Frequent visiting by parents should be encouraged.

In some communities home visits to cases of pertussis are made by the public health nurse if the cases are unattended medically and are under 2 or 3 years of age. The purpose of the home visit is to instruct the family about the importance of medical care, demonstrate nursing care and isolation procedures, and arrange for immunization of susceptible contacts under 3 years of age. The number of visits needed is determined by the nurse. She should stress the nutritional and the psychologic aspects of the patient's needs. If the child has a severe case of the disease, and especially if it is very young, hospitalization should be urged so that proper therapy can be instituted.

The public health nurse also participates in the educational programs of community groups to teach prevention of the disease. In elementary and nursery schools, the nurse gives teachers information on methods of early detection of whooping cough and interprets the health department's regulations.

REFERENCES

1. Anderson, G., and Arnstein, M.: *Communicable Disease Control*, 2d ed., The Macmillan Company, New York, pp. 240–243, 1948.
2. Bell, J. A.: "Pertussis Immunization," *J.A.M.A.*, **137**:1276, 1948.
3. Bell, J. A.; Pittman, M.; and Olson, B. J.: "Pertussis and Aureomycin," *Pub. Health Rep.*, **64**:589, 1949.
4. di Sant' Agnese, P. A.: "Combined Immunization against Diphtheria, Tetanus and Pertussis in Children over Three Months of Age," *J. Pediat.*, **31**:25, 1947.
5. Kohn, J., and Olson, E.: "Whooping Cough," *Am. J. Nursing*, **50**:723, 1950.
6. Lapin, J.: *Whooping Cough*, Charles C Thomas, Publisher, Springfield, Ill., 1943.
7. Payne, E. H.; Levy, M.; Zamora, G. M.; Villarroel, M. S.; and Canelas, E. Z.: "Pertussis Treated with Chloramphenicol," *J.A.M.A.*, **141**:1298, 1949.

8. Pullen, R. L.: *Communicable Diseases,* Lea & Febiger, Philadelphia, 1950.
9. Sako, W.: "Studies on Pertussis Immunization," *J. Pediat.,* **30**:29, 1947.
10. Wanamaker, L. W.; Kohn, J. L.; and Weichsel, M.: "Streptomycin in Treatment of Whooping Cough," *Am. J. Dis. Child.,* **78**:201, 1949.

Chapter 32 FOOD AND WATER-BORNE DISEASES

GENERAL DESCRIPTION

THE diseases that are transmitted by food or water frequently occur in epidemic form, since the source of supply is usually the same for a number of persons. Water is used for drinking, washing, and bathing. It is a solvent for food substances, drugs, and chemicals and is also employed in waste disposal. It therefore has frequent opportunity to carry disease. It may transmit poisonous substances such as cholera, typhoid, or dysentery. Bathing in polluted water may cause Weil's disease, schistosomiasis, or infectious hepatitis. A trace of iodine is necessary in drinking water to prevent goiter. An excess of fluorine may cause mottled tooth enamel, but a lack of it may predispose to caries.

A water supply may be contaminated at the source, as when there is gross pollution of a stream, reservoir, or well; in transit, as when there is a break in water mains or a breakdown in a treatment plant; or in the consumer's home, as a result of cross connections or improperly made repairs. The size of the outbreak will depend on the number of people using the water supply and on the pathogenicity of the agent.

Outbreaks of disease resulting from the ingestion of infected milk or other food are apt to be more explosive than those caused by water. This is due to the fact that organisms grow in food, so that the source is more heavily seeded than is water. As a rule, contamination of food does not extend over so long a period as pollution of water, so that food-borne epidemics tend to have a sharper rise and come down more promptly than do water-borne outbreaks. Milk-borne epidemics may be quite extensive, however, if the supply covers a large territory, and if the contamination continues over a long period of time. Milk-borne outbreaks are uncommon with a pasteurized supply, unless there is a breakdown in the pasteurization or there is improper handling later.

THE CAUSATIVE AGENT

The causative agent may be (1) an inorganic substance, often a heavy metal, like lead, cadmium, or arsenic; (2) an organic toxin like botulinus or muscarine; (3) a living organism like the typhoid bacillus or the virus of Q fever; (4) a protozoan like *Endamoeba histolytica;* or (5) a metazoan, like fish tapeworm. Some of these are carried chiefly by water, some by milk, some by other foods, and some by all of these.

The viability of the agent is an important factor in transmission. Living agents can multiply in the medium, whereas nonviable toxic substances tend to be diluted. Multiplication of living agents is much greater in food than in water. In the latter the agent survives longer if the water is raw than if it is treated. However, even in raw water, viability is influenced by certain factors, such as variations in temperature, the presence of organic matter and chemicals, the acidity or alkalinity, and the natural resistance of the organism.

In foods the agent is frequently affected by the method of treatment or preservation. Chemicals or heavy metals are usually not affected, while living organisms are. Heating is a common method of preparing food and destroys most bacteria if the heat is sufficiently high. Spores require an exceptionally high temperature over a long period of time to be destroyed. Smoking of meat or fish depends to a considerable extent on heat and kills most bacteria, yet some may survive. Outbreaks of salmonellosis from smoked fish and of trichinosis from smoked pork have been described. Drying and evaporation likewise depend on heat. Refrigeration will destroy trichinae and tapeworms if the temperature is low enough and if the holding time is sufficiently long. Salting and pickling depend on a high concentration of salt to destroy living organisms. Chemical preservatives, in the amounts permitted by law, have little effect on the viability of the agent.

THE HOST

Symptoms

The incubation period varies with the causative agent. It is extremely short in the case of inorganic poisons, is usually of several hours' duration in the case of organic toxins, and in the case of living organisms may last from 12 to 24 hours in salmonellosis, 1 or 2 weeks in typhoid fever, and 1 month or more in infectious hepatitis. The symptoms in many of the diseases that are food or water-borne are gastro-intestinal. In some of the diseases, as in trichinosis, other symptoms supervene. In still others, gastro-intestinal symptoms may play a very minor part or no role at all. The symptoms may be those of a general toxemia, as in typhoid, or predominantly neurologic, as in botulism, or chiefly pulmonary, as in Q fever.

Customs and Habits

The customs and habits of a community determine to a considerable extent the chances of illness resulting from food or water Trichinosis is more apt to occur if hogs are fed raw garbage than if fed grain. Where night soil is used to fertilize gardens, the chances of typhoid are greater. A community that uses a pasteurized milk supply has much less chance of illness than one using a raw supply. People who are accustomed to refrigerate perishable food that is kept for some length of time run less risk of illness than do those who are not so accustomed.

In the case of water, too, there are varying habits and customs. Some drink large quantities of water; others do not. Many people have their liquids almost exclusively in boiled water, as tea or coffee. Among some nationalities plain water is rarely used for drinking; some other beverage, like wine or bottled spring water, is used extensively. The manner of excreta disposal may have considerable influence on the purity of the water supply. If care is taken to protect the water source and to treat it properly, the chances of contaminating it are minimized.

The body of the host attempts to defend itself against the entry of harmful substances. The sense organs rebel against water or food which does not look, taste, or smell right. If this barrier is passed, the stomach will rebel against irritating substances by attacks of nausea and vomiting; if this barrier, too, is passed, the intestinal tract will attempt to eliminate the undesirable food or water by diarrhea; and finally, if some of the substance is absorbed, the liver is able to strain out and detoxify many obnoxious agents. If living agents pass all these barriers and enter the blood stream, the body still has left the biological method of defense—phagocytosis and specific immunity.

THE ENVIRONMENT

The physical environment often determines the food and water supply of a community. If rain water is used, the supply is pure, but care must be taken in its storage. Surface waters, such as rivers and streams, vary considerably in their purity, depending on the terrain they traverse. They are subject to pollution and should always be suspected. Ground water, obtained from springs or wells, is relatively purer than surface water, since the soil acts as a filter. Wells should, however, be protected from surface contamination.

The kind of food that is produced and eaten also depends to a great extent on physical environment. Certain soil is good for truck gardening, other kinds for grazing. People living on coastal land use a good deal of fish.

The season and climate play a considerable part in eating habits. In the summer and in hot weather, more water and milk are drunk and more dairy foods are eaten. There is greater need for refrigeration and greater opportunity for spoilage in hot than in cold weather.

The social and economic habits are also factors in the occurrence and spread of food and water-borne diseases. A hog-raising country is apt to have more trichinosis than a beef-raising one, and both will have more undulant fever than a coastal community that lives largely by fishing. The failure to use privies and the practice of going barefoot may contribute to the spread of hookworm and ascarides infections. Socially and politically, advanced communities are more apt to have good housing, a good water supply, pasteurization of milk, proper refrigeration, a good sewage-disposal method, and an overseeing health department, all of which are conducive to a cleaner and purer water, milk, and food supply and to a lessening of opportunities for the spread of disease transmitted by water and food.

Medical Aseptic Techniques

Gowns and Caps

In giving nursing care to patients ill with diseases transmitted by food or water, emphasis should be placed on the prevention of spread of the disease to others. This requires that the nurse observe meticulous hand-washing techniques and that she take adequate measures for the disinfection or destruction of remains of meals and of excreta, and for the sterilization of equipment used by the patient. The wearing of a gown is not necessary if proper hand washing, cleaning of fingernails, and concurrent disinfection are rigidly observed. If aseptic techniques are faulty, the gown offers no assurance against the spread of infection.

Concurrent Disinfection

Spread in this group of diseases is chiefly through fecal discharges. Stools, urine, and vomitus may be flushed down the toilet without treatment. Remains of soft and liquid foods may be disposed of in the same way. Remains of solid food should be wrapped in a paper bag and placed with other garbage. Bedpans and urinals should be sterilized after use, either by boiling or in an autoclave. If the bedpan or urinal is not used for any other patient, it may be cleaned with soap and hot water after use and sterilized after the patient's recovery. Bed linen may be laundered with other linen.

Terminal Disinfection

After the patient has recovered and has been discharged, the room or unit should be aired and thoroughly cleaned with hot water and soap or other detergent. Utensils and equipment should be cleaned and sterilized.

Chapter *33* BRUCELLOSIS
(UNDULANT FEVER)

BRUCELLOSIS is a disease caused by one of the *Brucella* organisms and characterized by fever, a prolonged course, and frequently by recurrences.

THE CAUSATIVE AGENT

The *Brucella* organism is a nonmotile gram-negative bacillus which grows well on ordinary laboratory mediums. Primary isolation from man or animals, however, requires special mediums and carbon dioxide for optimal growth. Three species are known: (1) *Brucella melitensis,* the cause of undulant fever, which affects goats, (2) *Brucella abortus,* the cause of Bang's disease, which affects cows, and (3) *Brucella suis,* which affects hogs. All three cause the same disease in man. Brucellae are readily destroyed by heat and disinfectants and do not survive pasteurization, but they remain alive in slaughtered animals for some time. Although the three species cannot be distinguished one from the other by staining properties and appearance under the microscope, they can be differentiated by suitable cultural techniques.

THE HOST

Symptoms

The infection in man occurs as a result of drinking milk or eating milk products from infected cows or goats, or from handling infected animals. After entering the body, the organisms are spread through the lymph channels to the reticulo-endothelial system and blood and can be found in lymph glands, liver, spleen, bone marrow, and other structures.

After an incubation period of 2 to 3 weeks, the patient complains of fatigue, headache, backache, and general malaise. Fever steadily rises to a height of 102° or 103° F. and may be maintained for several weeks, during which the chief symptoms are a general sense of ill-being, chills and sweats, headache, backache, and pains in the joints. There are no localizing symptoms, and the disease resembles other general infections such as typhoid fever and sepsis. Relapses after a period of normal temperature are not uncommon, and a chronic stage with vague symptoms of bone and joint pains and emotional instability may follow. The chronic stage is a very unhappy one. The patients have no specific symptoms. They feel miserable, depressed, and sick. They have a poor appetite, sleep poorly, and feel unable to work. They frequently complain of pains in the joints and muscles. They may have an occasional bout of fever, but in the interim their temperatures are normal or only slightly elevated. They frequently become neurotic and are considered as pests by their relatives and friends.

Diagnosis

The white blood count is usually normal or somewhat reduced. The most important laboratory confirmation is the isolation of the organism from the blood, which may be done very early in the disease and often as late as several months after onset. Agglutinins appear in the blood by the end of the second week, and the titer gradually rises. Blood taken at intervals of a week or more should show the rise. Low titers frequently occur in normal bloods, and too much signficance should not be attached to them. A third confirmatory test is the skin test. Either heat-killed vaccine or an extract of the organisms may be used; o.1 cubic centimeter is injected intradermally. Readings are made at the end of 24 to 48 hours. A positive test is shown by redness and induration. A fourth diagnostic test, the opsonocytophagic test, depends on the increased opsonic index in the blood and is not too reliable. Of the four diagnostic aids, the recovery of the organism from the blood is the only true evidence of infection with *Brucella*. Positive cultures have also been obtained from bone marrow, bile, and suppurative lesions, if they occur.

Immunity

There is no method in use for vaccinating humans against brucellosis, nor is there any serum for passive immunization. A live vaccine of attenuated *Brucella abortus* is used to immunize cows. The presence of infection in a herd is determined by the Bang test, a skin test similar to the one used for diagnosis in man.

The Environment

Undulant fever was first reported in the Mediterranean area in the nineteenth century and was known as "Mediterranean fever" or "Malta fever." It was thought to be a disease of goats and man only. Bruce isolated the causative organism in 1886. Bang isolated an organism which caused abortion in cows, and this became known as Bang's bacillus. Traum recovered a bacillus from swine which had characteristics similar to Bang's bacillus. In 1918 Alice Evans proved that *abortus* and *melitensis* were different species of the same organism and all were placed in one genus, *Brucella*. They are referred to as *Brucella melitensis, abortus,* and *suis* or the caprine, bovine, and porcine types of brucellosis.

All three affect man. *Brucella melitensis* affects primarily goats and sheep but may also infect cattle and swine. *Brucella abortus* affects cows chiefly and is the cause of infectious abortion in this animal. However, it can also infect horses, goats, sheep, dogs, fowl, and rats. *Brucella suis* affects swine primarily but may also infect cattle, horses, dogs, and fowl.

Adults are more commonly infected than children. This may be due to the fact that the disease is, in a way, an occupational one, affecting farmers, butchers, slaughterers, and others that handle cattle, goats, and swine. Man is infected chiefly by drinking milk from infected animals or by handling them. There is no communicability from man to man. The organism enters the body through the gastrointestinal tract or the skin. In the United States very little brucellosis occurs in large urban centers. The disease is quite common, however, in the hog- and cattle-raising states, particularly the former. Its transmission by milk can be readily avoided by pasteurization, which destroys the organism. Its control in cattle has been attempted, by testing and eliminating all positive reactors, and by vaccinating uninfected cattle. However, its presence in swine and the readiness with which these infect cattle make the problem difficult.

Control

Cases of brucellosis need not be isolated since they are not infectious to others. Infection occurs only as a result of drinking milk from, or handling, infected animals. Pasteurization kills the *Brucella* organisms, and a community can readily avoid this source of infection by insisting that all milk should be pasteurized.

The control of the disease in animals is a more difficult problem. In cattle, it depends on (1) blood testing of animals by the agglutination technique before introducing them into a herd, and selling the positive ones for slaughter; (2) the vaccination of calves with *Brucella* vaccine to immunize them; and (3) the practice of careful sanitation and hygiene in the herd. Cleanliness, frequent testing, and isolation of positive reactors and use of maternity stalls are all helpful.

The control of the disease in hogs depends on similar measures, but these are more difficult to carry out. In essence, the problem is not really a medical or veterinary one, since adequate measures can be organized. It is largely an economic and social one.

MEDICAL CARE PLANS

Treatment

Until recently, only asymptomatic treatment was available. Penicillin has been given a fair trial, with negative results. The introduction of the antibiotics active against gram-negative organisms and particularly those with wider spectrums of therapeutic effect have raised the hopes of undulant fever patients.

Reports of trials indicate beneficial effects of streptomycin given alone or combined with sulfadiazine. Favorable results have also been obtained with Aureomycin and chloramphenicol, particularly with the latter. There are indications that Terramycin is also effective.

When the disease has become chronic the results are not so brilliant as in the acute stage. It should be pointed out that a diagnosis of chronic brucellosis is difficult to make and is occasionally made without adequate basis. The difficulty lies in the fact that there are no specific symptoms or signs. Temperature is normal, sedimentation rate is not elevated, while blood count may be low but is often normal, and the symptoms are extremely vague—nervousness, headache, lack of appetite, vague joint pains, insomnia. The laboratory is of little help, since blood cultures are usually sterile and the agglutination test may show a low titer or be negative.

A variety of methods has been used to treat chronic cases. These include bed rest, drugs, vaccines of *Brucella* organisms, antibrucellar serums, immune blood, convalescent serum, transfusions, and psychotherapy. Where so many therapeutic procedures are used, there is usually none that stands out as specific. Recently Aureomycin and particularly chloramphenicol appear to have given fair results in chronic as well as in acute cases.

Diet

Fluids are given freely during the febrile period to offset fluid loss during perspiration. The diet should be well balanced with essential nutrients. The emphasis should be on proteins, carbohydrates, and supplementary vitamins. The menu should be varied, and the food should be served as attractively as possible to stimulate the appetite.

Supportive Nursing Care

Nursing care in brucellosis is dependent upon the severity of symptoms and the course of the disease. Many patients are ambulatory and able to work. Only a small proportion of those with acute symptoms receive hospital care.

During the acute stage the patient remains in bed and receives care similar to that given in other acute infections. The surroundings should be cheerful, and the room temperature should be constant to prevent chilling. Daily bathing is essential, as the patient perspires profusely, and there is a strong sweet odor to skin excretions. Frequent sponge baths and change of linen may be necessary for the general comfort of the patient.

When joint pains are present, support of affected parts and the use of a bed cradle to ease pressure of bedcovers may be necessary. Rubbing the joints with oil of wintergreen may be prescribed by the physician.

Since the illness tends to be a long one, the psychological management of the patient becomes very important. Satisfactory interpersonal relationships and techniques are essential in guiding patients to recovery and in giving continuous support. There is a tendency for the patient to become a chronic invalid. Too much emphasis on rest should be avoided, since fatigue and depression are characteristics of the disease. The nurse should select and plan activities which are interesting and require little concentration. These should contribute to mental well-being and may include radio, television, handicrafts, games, light reading, or short walks.

Nursing care of the patient at home may be very difficult. While the constant activity and contact with different people in a hospital environment lessens anxiety, the patient remaining at home may be very morose and apprehensive. A housewife ill with brucellosis may become very anxious about the management of the household during her illness. She may find fault with everything, no matter how well others perform the tasks. To lessen preoccupation with her disabilities, the nurse should help the family plan recreational activities.

The public health nurse gives or demonstrates nursing care of the patient to a family member. In rural areas the nurse should emphasize the importance of using pasteurized milk and milk products. She should be able to recognize symptoms which are obvious and refer individuals for medical care to prevent complications and chronic disability.

REFERENCES

1. Brennan, F.: "Brucellosis," *Am. J. Nursing,* **50**:358, 1950.
2. Dalrymple-Champney's, Sir Weldon: "Undulant Fever—A Neglected Problem," *Lancet,* **258**:429, 1950.
3. Evans, A. C.: "Brucellosis in the United States," *Am. J. Pub. Health,* **37**:139, 1947.

4. Harris, H. J.: "Aureomycin and Chloromycetin in Brucellosis," *J.A.M.A.*, 142:161, 1950.
5. Harris, H. J.: *Brucellosis,* 2d ed., Paul B. Hoeber, Inc., New York, 1950.
6. Ralston, R. J., and Payne, E. H.: "Treatment of Chronic Brucellosis with Chloramphenicol and Aureomycin," *J.A.M.A.*, 142:159, 1950.
7. Smadel, J. E.: "Clinical Use of the Antibiotic Chloramphenicol (Chloromycetin)," *J.A.M.A.*, 142:315, 1950.
8. Smith, R. W.; Birch, R. R.; Bishop, C. P.; Donham, C. R.; and West, R. L.: "What Is Known about Brucellosis," *Proceedings, 52d Annual Meeting, U.S. Livestock Sanitary Assn.,* Oct., 13–15, 1948.
9. Spink, H. W.; Brande, A. I.; Castaneda, M. R.; and Goytia, R. S.: "Aureomycin Therapy in Human Brucellosis," *J.A.M.A.*, 138:1145, 1948.

Chapter 34 CHOLERA

GENERAL DESCRIPTION

CHOLERA is a disease caused by the cholera bacillus and characterized by an acute onset, profuse diarrhea, and marked prostration. The case fatality is high (30 to 80 per cent).

THE CAUSATIVE AGENT

The organism, frequently referred to as the cholera vibrio, is comma-shaped, possesses a single polar flagellum, and is very mobile. It is gram-negative. It grows well on the usual culture mediums in the presence of oxygen. It is readily destroyed by acids, heat, and the usual disinfectants and by drying. The cholera vibrio does not attack animals other than man.

THE HOST

Symptoms

There is an incubation period of 2 to 3 days, rarely as long as 5 days. Then there is an acute onset, with diarrhea and abdominal pain. The diarrhea may become very severe, with numerous evacuations which at first may contain some solid material and have a yellow color but later look like turbid water. The term "rice water stools" has been applied to them. Diarrhea is often followed by vomiting. As a result of the loss of fluid, the blood becomes concentrated, the skin is clammy and cyanotic, and the eyes are sunken. There is evidence of dehydration, and the patient goes into collapse. There is a fall in blood pressure, and the pulse becomes imperceptible. Death may occur within a matter of hours after onset or after several days. In the patients who recover there is a gradual lessening of the diarrhea, the stool begins to show solid matter, the dehydration is overcome, toxicity disappears, and recovery ensues.

Diagnosis

The clinical diagnosis can be confirmed by growing the organism from the stools in culture mediums. The organism does not invade the blood stream as in typhoid. The patient's serum agglutinates cholera vibrios, and this reaction can be used as a corroborating test.

Immunity

Immunity follows recovery from cholera, but its duration is not definitely known. Prophylactic immunization is performed with a vaccine of killed cholera vibrios, 8 million per cubic centimeter. Two inoculations are given, 1 week apart, the first 0.5 cubic centimeter and the second 1 cubic centimeter. Immunity lasts for about 6 months to 1 year, and a booster dose of 1 cubic centimeter should then be given.

THE ENVIRONMENT

India may be considered as the original home of cholera, and the disease is still prevalent there. Early in the nineteenth century it began to travel in epidemic waves to other places, reached Europe about 1830, and soon after spread to America. It created havoc in Europe in the nineteenth century, and it was not until Snow's classic studies that the true method of spread by water was demonstrated. Even after this careful demonstration, it took years to convince the medical profession of its truth. Cholera was finally wiped out in America about 1890 and in Europe in 1925. At present it is found chiefly in Asia. India still reported more than 200,000 cases in 1944, and epidemics have occurred in recent years in China, Burma, Thailand, and Indo-China. In 1947, an epidemic occurred in Egypt, but it was controlled within a comparatively short time.

Method of Spread

Cholera is spread chiefly by poor water supplies. In few other diseases does the role of environmental sanitation play so large a part in control. The cholera vibrio can survive in water for 2 weeks or more. Under poor hygienic conditions where sewage from cholera patients has access to a water supply, contamination will occur, and if the water is not purified prior to use, an epidemic will result. There are other methods of spread, such as by eating contaminated food or by handling soiled linen. This may even transfer the organisms mechanically from feces to food. It must also be remembered that there are carriers of cholera who may contaminate food and thus spread the disease. Carriers of cholera, however, do not persist for long periods of time like typhoid carriers and are therefore not so great a hazard. All these other methods of spread, while important, are completely overshadowed by the importance of water as a medium. All the famous epidemics of cholera were caused by bad drinking water.

The London Cholera Epidemic of 1854—In 1854, cholera was epidemic in London. John Snow, a doctor with a mind that reasoned sharply, noted that the cases were focused around Broad Street where one of the city pumps was located. The cases became very numerous toward the end of August. Snow investigated all of them and showed that almost all had drunk water from the Broad Street pump. On the other hand, a workhouse with a population of 535 had only 5 deaths from cholera, although it was surrounded by houses where cholera occurred in large numbers. The workhouse, however, had its own well. Similarly, a brewery in Broad Street had no cases, but the employees were permitted to drink beer and there was a separate well. In a cartridge factory, however, some distance from the Broad Street pump, drinking water from that pump was regularly brought and kept in tubs for use. Eighteen deaths from cholera occurred. Snow pointed out many other single instances incriminating the water from this pump. He was able to convince the Board of Guardians of the Parish, and the handle of the pump was removed on September 8th. The outbreak soon came to a close. However, it already had begun to wane, so Snow widened his investigation to the rest of London. He noted that many cases occurred along the river front, and he reasoned that they probably arose as a result of the use of that water, which was grossly polluted. There were two water companies serving London, one of which, the Southwark and Vauxhall, got its supply from the lower Thames, which was grossly polluted. The other company, the Lambeth, had moved its waterworks to the upper Thames, which was relatively free of pollution. The pipes of the two companies ran together but supplied different houses. Snow obtained lists of deaths from cholera from the Registrar and systematically investigated every house where a death had occurred and inquired about the water supply. At the end of the investigation he was able to draw up this table:

	NUMBER OF HOUSES	DEATHS FROM CHOLERA	RATE PER 10,000 HOUSES
Southwark and Vauxhall	40,046	1,263	315
Lambeth	26,107	98	37
Rest of London	256,423	1,422	59

This was the first example of the use of rates in epidemiological investigation and clearly indicated the connection between deaths from cholera and the lower Thames water supply.

Other epidemics of cholera have been studied since the famous London one, but none is more dramatic. When it is recalled that Snow proposed his advanced views of the method of spread at a time when the nature of the infectious process was not known and when the bacterial causation of disease had not yet been accepted, his acumen seems all the more remarkable.

Control

The control of cholera is largely a problem of sanitation. It requires a safe water supply and proper disposition of excreta. These are measures which are used widely in this country so that their introduction in endemic areas is qualified solely by the need of adequate funds. Individual precautions consist of careful washing of one's hands after contact with a patient. An additional precaution is immunization with cholera vaccine.

MEDICAL CARE PLANS

Treatment

Specific therapy has not been clearly established in cholera. Reports on the sulfonamides indicate that they are of value, but to what extent is not clear. Penicillin is apparently without effect. Streptomycin and the broader spectrum antibiotics—Aureomycin, chloramphenicol, and Terramycin—have not had sufficient trial. Bacteriophage has been used by many workers, but its value is still in doubt.

Nonspecific therapy consists of maintaining a fluid balance, keeping up the patient's nutrition, and making him comfortable. The first of these is most important, because death is due largely to dehydration. Since vomiting and diarrhea are outstanding symptoms, fluid must be given intravenously. This is usually given in the form of 5 per cent glucose in saline or Ringer's or Hartmann's solutions. It must be given regularly to make up the body's loss and to combat acidosis. As soon as vomiting ceases, fluid can be given by mouth.

Drugs are used symptomatically. If cramps are severe, atropine is given by injection. Morphine should be avoided.

Diet

Food is withheld in the early acute stage. As soon as the patient is able to retain food, liquids and then simple solids are given. As the appetite improves, the patient is served a well-balanced diet containing essential nutrients, supplemented with vitamin concentrates and minerals.

Supportive Nursing Care

The patient suffering from cholera is usually irritable, depressed, and severely prostrated. The room or ward in which the patient is isolated should have adequate hand-washing facilities, and all windows should be tightly screened against flies.

Skilled nursing care is fundamental to recovery of the patient. Recovery of the patient is dependent upon his general physical health.

External heat should be applied to the body, as the temperature is below normal and the patient has severe muscular cramps.

The pulse and blood pressure should be taken at regular intervals, and the patient should be observed for changes in symptoms and collapse.

The position of the patient should be changed at periodic intervals. Because dehydration is pronounced, the skin is dry and may be very sensitive. Special attention should be given to fissures and pressure areas.

The nurse must follow a rigid technique to prevent contamination of her hands. The care of the patient's linen and of his stool is similar to that in typhoid fever. (See pages 383–384.) The nurse caring for a cholera patient should be immunized.

In outbreaks, public health nurses may be required to give nursing care to patients and to assist with immunization of the general population. It may also be necessary, in the event of an epidemic, for nurses to assist with epidemiological investigations under medical direction.

In the teaching of families, the nurse should stress boiling of all drinking water, good practices in personal hygiene, and immunization of contacts. The use of insecticides for flies, proper measures for isolation, disinfection of stools, and terminal disinfection should also be included in the nursing plan.

REFERENCES

1. Napier, L. I.: *Principles and Practice of Tropical Medicine,* The Macmillan Company, New York, 1946.
2. Pullen, R. L.: *Communicable Diseases,* Lea & Febiger, Philadelphia, 1950.
3. Schousha, A. T.: "Cholera Epidemic in Egypt, 1947. A Preliminary Report," *Bull. World Health Organization,* 1:354, 1948.
4. Snow, J.: *On Cholera,* Commonwealth Fund, Harvard University Press, Cambridge, Mass., 1936.

Chapter *35* DYSENTERY, AMEBIC

GENERAL DESCRIPTION

AMEBIC dysentery, or amebiasis, is a disease caused by a protozoan and characterized in its severe form by an ulcerative colitis which causes diarrhea with blood and mucus and which tends to become chronic. Milder cases tend to have recurrent diarrhea, abdominal pain, and vague constitutional symptoms.

THE CAUSATIVE AGENT

The infective agent is the *Endamoeba histolytica,* a protozoan inhabiting the large bowel. It occurs in two forms, one of which is the *trophozoite* or motile form, which invades tissues. This form is readily destroyed, so that when it is passed in the stool it is not infective; if swallowed, it is destroyed by the gastric juice. The second stage is the *cyst* which is found in the feces of patients and carriers. The cyst is resistant to destructive agents and, when swallowed, survives in the stomach and passes to the gut where it hatches and becomes attached to the wall of the colon.

THE HOST

Symptoms

The incubation period is variable. Persons may harbor the organism for months before showing symptoms, which are chiefly those of diarrhea and abdominal cramps. In most cases the diarrhea is not severe, but occasionally it may be severe and accompanied by cramps and tenesmus. In addition, there are poor appetite, loss of weight, and a feeling of malaise. If not treated, the disease has a tendency to become chronic and may continue for years. The most serious complication, in such cases, is the development of a liver abscess. This lesion occasionally occurs early in the disease and as an isolated manifestation.

Carriers of amebic dysentery are quite common. Since the symptoms of the disease are often extremely mild, a sharp line cannot be drawn between the case and the carrier. It is becoming more and more common to speak of infected individuals as suffering from amebiasis rather than to separate them into cases and carriers. Surveys of normal populations in the United States have indicated fairly high percentages of symptomless carriers, the percentages varying from 5 to 25 per cent, depending on the community, the number of stools examined, the type of stool examined, and other factors.

Diagnosis

The diagnosis is made by the finding of trophozoites and cysts in the stools. Examinations should be made in a laboratory properly equipped, and by trained personnel. Other protozoa occur in the stool and may be confused by the inexpert with the *Endamoeba histolytica*. For a definitive diagnosis several specimens, both cold and fresh, should be examined at intervals of time.

A complement-fixation test has been recently devised, but there has been insufficient experience with it to make it a valuable tool in diagnosis.

Immunity

An attack of amebic dysentery does not confer immunity. On the contrary, second attacks and relapses are quite common. There are no available means of immunizing, actively or passively, against the disease.

The Environment

Amebic dysentery is more common in tropical countries than in Temperate Zones, but it is chiefly due to improper sanitation. Since it is spread largely by the contamination of foods by cases and carriers, it is common among groups whose hygienic habits are poor. It is frequently found in mental hospitals. Large water-borne epidemics are uncommon, but some of these have been reported. A notable one was the epidemic in Chicago during the World's Fair in 1933, when it was traced to a single hotel and was believed to be due to cross connections between the water and sewer lines. When an outbreak occurs, control depends on discovering cases and carriers and treating them, on removing such cases and carriers from food-handling occupations, and on the enforcement of strict hygienic procedures.

Control

As in bacillary dysentery, outbreaks are commonest in jails and insane asylums or other institutions where people are crowded and sanitation is poor. Control depends on the institution of adequate washing and toilet facilities, elimination of crowding, and avoidance of the use of people with substandard mentality as food handlers. Cases should be isolated and treated. Contacts should have their stools examined and, if positive, should also be isolated and treated. The instruction of all residents of the institution in personal hygiene in order to avoid the disease is a function of the nurse.

MEDICAL CARE PLANS

Treatment

Most cases can be cured if treated promptly and effectively. The difficult cases to cure are those that have developed extensive bowel ulcerations and liver abscesses. For treatment, compounds of iodine and arsenic are the drugs of choice. The former is used in Diodoquin, which is administered in tablets of 0.2 gram (3.2 grains) ten to twelve tablets a day for 20 days; or in chiniofon (Anayodin), in tablets of 0.25 gram (4 grains) three to four tablets three times a day for 8 to 10 days. The most commonly used arsenic preparation is carbarsone, in gelatin capsules or tablets of 0.25 gram (4 grains), one capsule twice a day for 10 days. In cases with severe bowel ulceration or liver abscess, emetine may be used in 0.06 gram (1 grain) daily doses subcutaneously for about 5 to 10 days. It is a toxic drug and must be used with caution.

Since the advent of the broad-spectrum antibiotics, trials of their effectiveness have been made. Aureomycin, in the usual doses, appears to give as good results as Diodoquin. Relapses appear to be as common, however. Cases of amebiasis should not be discharged until they have been followed for long periods of time with examination of freshly passed as well as casual stools.

Nonspecific treatment is symptomatic. If the diarrhea is profuse, sedative drugs have to be used. A bland ointment should be applied to the sore buttocks. Abdominal pain is relieved by applicaton of a hot-water bag or electric pad.

Diet

A nutritious bland diet containing basic nutrients is given.

Supportive Nursing Care

Many patients are ambulant and under medical treatment by a physician or clinic. The nurse in the clinic is responsible for administering medications, giving instruction in personal hygiene, and the collection of stool specimens for microscopic examination. Stool examinations need to be warm and are usually examined in laboratories attached to parasitology clinics. The patient is also instructed to bring all household contacts for stool examination. Those engaged in food-handling occupations are informed to discontinue work until they have been pronounced cured.

In the acute stage, the patient is on bed rest, and nursing care is symptomatic. The nurse should observe careful hand-washing techniques after giving care to patients.

The public health nurse is responsible for case finding and for referral for medical care of individuals who have disturbances in their bowel pattern. When follow-up nursing visits are requested by a physician or clinic the public health nurse should instruct the family in rigid hand-washing techniques before meals and after use of toilet and should refer all household members for stool examination. When the water supply is contaminated, boiling water for drinking is essential.

REFERENCES

1. Birnkrant, W. B.; Greenberg, M.; and Most, H.: "Amebiasis in a Hospital for the Insane," *Am. J. Pub. Health*, **35**:805, 1945.
2. Bundesen, H. N.; Connolly, J. I.; Rawlings, I. D.; Gorman, A. E.; McCoy, G. W.; and Hardy, A. V.: *Epidemic Amebic Dysentery, The Chicago Epidemic, 1933*, Bull. No. 166, Government Printing Office, Washington, D.C., 1936.
3. Craig, C. F.: *Amebic Dysentery and Amebiasis*, Charles C Thomas, Publisher, Springfield, Ill., 1934.
4. Craig, C. F.: "A Suggested Program of Control of Amebiasis by Health Departments," *Am. J. Pub. Health*, **28**:187, 1938.
5. Craig, C. F., and Faust, E. C.: *Clinical Parasitology*, Lea & Febiger, Philadelphia, 1943.
6. Hughes, J. D.: "Treatment of Amebiasis with Aureomycin," *J.A.M.A.*, **142**:1052, 1950.
7. Most, H.; Miller, J. W.; and Grossman, E. J.: "Treatment of Amebiasis with Bacitracin and Other Antibiotics," *Am. J. Trop. Med.*, **30**:491, 1950.
8. Thompson, P. E.; Dunn, M. C.; Bayles, A.; and Reinertson, J. W.: "Action of Chloramphenicol (Chloromycetin) and Other Drugs against Endameba Histolytica in Vitro and in Experimental Animals," *Am. J. Trop. Med.*, **30**:203, 1950.

Chapter 36 DYSENTERY, BACILLARY (SHIGELLOSIS)

General Description

BACILLARY dysentery is an acute infectious disease characterized by severe diarrhea, often bloody, and slight fever.

The Causative Agent

The causative agent is known as *Shigella,* which is the group
name. The types of *Shigella* recognized are *Shigella dysenteriae
(Bacillus shigae); Shigella paradysenteriae (Bacillus flexneri);
Shigella sonnei; Shigella ambigua (Shigella schmitzii).* All cause
similar symptoms, although *Shigella dysenteriae* infections are more
severe than the others. The commonest types prevalent in the
United States are *Shigella paradysenteriae* and *Shigella connei.
Shigella ambigua* is occasionally encountered, and *Shigella dysenteriae* is practically never found here. All the types look alike and
cannot be distinguished by cultural characteristics, but only by fer-
mentation tests and by their antigenic structure.

The *Shigella* is a slender, nonsporeforming, gram-negative rod,
nonmotile and nonencapsulated. It grows in ordinary mediums,
but selective mediums aid in its identification. It is readily destroyed
by heat and disinfectants but may survive in water for several
days. It does not survive long in the stool.

The Host

Symptoms

The incubation period is short, usually not more than 24 to 48
hours. Onset is sudden, with abdominal cramps followed by
diarrhea which is accompanied by straining and tenseness. The
stools are liquid and contain mucus and blood. Fever may be high
or only moderate in degree. Symptoms last for 1 or 2 weeks, and
recovery is the rule. Mild cases of the disease manifest few symptoms
besides a slight diarrhea. In the severe cases, particularly those of
the *shiga* variety, fever may be quite high, toxic and nervous symptoms may be prominent, and death may result. The mortality in
this country varies. In the Northern states there is practically no

mortality from the disease. In the South and Southwest, the case fatality varies from 2 to 10 per cent.

Patients recovering may carry the bacillus and excrete it in their stools. While convalescent carriers are the rule, chronic carriers are not known. In most instances carriers clear themselves in a few days or weeks. Occasionally, a carrier will continue to shed bacilli for several months.

Diagnosis

The laboratory diagnosis rests on the recovery of the organism from the stool or the rectal wall. If the stool is used for culture, it should be fresh. If it is necessary to delay the examination, the stool should be preserved in 30 per cent neutral glycerin. Best results are obtained by swabbing the rectum and streaking the swab on culture medium at the bedside.

Although the *Shigella* stimulates the production of agglutinins, the occurrence of many types and the frequent presence of agglutinins in normal bloods make the agglutination test of limited value. The recovery of organisms from the stool is so simple that it is a preferable as well as a more exact method. *Shigella* does not enter the blood stream and cannot, therefore, be recovered in a blood culture.

Immunity

The disease does not confer long-lasting immunity. Recurrences are not uncommon. Vaccines have not been used for immunization, because they are toxic and they do not seem to offer much protection. Dependence should be put on avoiding the disease and on treatment with sulfonamides.

The Environment

Bacillary dysentery is world wide in distribution, but it is more common in tropical countries. The *shiga* type, *Shigella dysenteriae,* is found almost exclusively in India, the Far East, and the Near East. The *flexneri* and *sonnei* types are the most widely distributed and the most common types found in America. Dysentery has accompanied all wars and is a constant companion of jails, insane asylums, and institutions for defective children. It affects both sexes and all ages and occurs in all seasons, although it is commoner in summer. The source of the disease is always man, since animals are not susceptible.

Epidemics of bacillary dysentery which are due to contaminated water supplies have been reported. They are usually not so extensive nor so long-lasting as typhoid epidemics, presumably because the bacilli are less resistant to destruction. Outbreaks caused by flies have also been described. In most outbreaks in institutions, spread has been the result of contamination of foods by the hands of cases or carriers. The possibility of spread is enhanced by the use of inmates as food handlers, since their practice of hygienic measures is inferior to that of normal individuals.

Control

The control of dysentery is largely one of environmental sanitation. A properly protected or treated water supply and pasteurization of milk are of some help, but these rarely cause outbreaks. Proper sanitation in orphan asylums, old people's homes, institutions for defectives or the insane, and jails is very important in control. This means the elimination of crowding, adequate washing and toilet facilities, proper excreta disposal, and elimination of the practice of using people with substandard mentality as food handlers. If diarrhea occurs, all cases and contacts should have rectal swabs taken for culture. Positive cases should be isolated and treated until cured. Contacts should be given a prophylactic dose of 1 gram of sulfadiazine daily for a period of 4 to 5 days.

Ambulant cases should be given instruction by the nurse in personal hygiene. Special attention should be paid to the emptying of the bedpan into water-flushed and sewer-connected toilets or else disinfecting the stool in the bedpan with 5 per cent solution of chloride of lime before disposing of the contents. The bedpan should be sterilized after use. The patient should wash his hands carefully after stool and before eating. Soiled diapers should be laundered separately. Patients who are food handlers should not be permitted to return to work until two successive stool specimens, obtained not less than 24 hours apart, are negative for *Shigella*.

MEDICAL CARE PLANS

Treatment

Specific treatment consists in the administration of sulfonamides. They have been shown to exert a favorable effect on cases as well as on carriers. Strangely enough, the absorbable sulfonamides, particularly sulfadiazine, are more effective than the unabsorbed ones like sulfaguanidine, even when the latter are given in doses five times as high as the former. Sulfadiazine is given in a daily dose of 4 grams for adults and 0.2 gram per kilogram of body weight for children. Penicillin is of little value.

General treatment is directed toward correcting the dehydration, minimizing the diarrhea, and making the patient comfortable. The loss of fluid by rectum requires its replacement, which may be done by mouth or, if there is vomiting, by vein. The diarrhea can be eased by sedative drugs. Some form of opium is frequently required.

Diet

Usually the vomiting and diarrhea preclude the feeding by mouth. As these symptoms subside, liquids may be given cautiously. If they are retained, soft foods can be added, and the patient then may be gradually introduced to a regular diet.

Supportive Nursing Care

Plans for nursing care are dependent upon the severity of the infection. The patient is confined to bed in the acute stage of illness.

In severe attacks there is profuse sweating, and frequent change of bed linen may be necessary. The bed covering should be warm and light to minimize weight over a painful abdomen. Tepid sponge baths may be given to relieve high elevations in temperature and for general comfort.

The application of hot flannel stupes, an electric pad, or hot-water bottle may be prescribed by the physician for abdominal discomfort.

The bowel evacuations are fluid and contain mucus, blood, and pus. They are very frequent and produce great distress to the patient. He may remain on the bedpan continuously or refuse to release it from his bedside. To obviate fears of having accidents, large Cellucotton pads under the buttocks may be helpful. Soiled pads require careful handling and should be wrapped in newspapers, tied securely, and burned. The frequency, color, consistency, and odor of stools should be observed by the nurse or attendant and recorded on the patient's chart.

The application of a bland ointment or zinc stearate powder to the perianal region after washing with soap and water may ease irritation and prevent excoriations.

Home visits are made by public health nurses to give or to instruct the family in nursing care procedures. The nurse should be acquainted with the procedure for collection of stool specimens and give accurate information to the patient. Co-operation with laboratory technicians is essential.

The public health nurse can assist in the case finding of dysentery. In the presence of an epidemic, emphasis should be placed on personal hygiene, and families should be instructed to boil drinking water and to use measures for controlling flies to a minimum. In elementary and secondary schools, any unusual absence of students because of gastro-enteritis should be reported to the health officer.

School children suffering from dysentery should be excluded until they have had sufficient treatment.

REFERENCES

1. Felsen, J. B.: *Bacillary Dysentery, Colitis and Enteritis,* W. B. Saunders Company, Philadelphia, pp. 90–119, 239–290, 1945.
2. Gorman, J.: "An Outbreak of Dysentery Due to *Shigella Sonne,*" *M. Officer,* 83:241, 1950.
3. Halpern, S. R.: "Bacillary Dysentery in Children," *Am. J. Nursing,* 50:320, 1950.
4. Hardy, A. V.: "Studies of Acute Diarrheal Diseases, Further Cultural Observations on the Relative Efficacy of Sulfonamides in Shigella Infections," *Pub. Health Rep.,* 60:1037, 1945.
5. Hardy, A. V.; De Capito, T.; and Halbert, S. P., "Studies of the Acute Diarrheal Diseases—Immunization in Shigellosis," *Pub. Health Rep.,* 63:685, 1948.
6. Hardy, A. V., and Watt, J.: "Study of Acute Diarrheal Diseases, Clinical Observations," *Pub. Health Rep.,* 60:521, 1945.
7. Mayo, M.: "Nursing Care in Bacillary Dysentery," *Am. J. Nursing,* 50:304, 1950.
8. Watt, J., and Lindsay, D. R.: "Diarrheal Disease Control Studies," *Pub. Health Rep.,* 63:1319, 1948.

Chapter 37 EPIDEMIC DIARRHEA OF THE NEWBORN

General Description

EPIDEMIC diarrhea of the newborn is an acute communicable disease affecting newborn infants in nurseries and characterized by diarrhea which may be of such severity as to result in dehydration and death. The causative agent is not known.

The Causative Agent

No specific etiologic agent has been found. Cultures of the nose and throat have yielded the usual flora found in newborn infants. Cultures of the stools have likewise yielded only organisms commonly found in normal babies. Light and Hodes obtained a filterable agent from the stools of cases of epidemic diarrhea of the newborn which produced diarrhea in calves. This work requires confirmation.

The Host

Symptoms

The incubation period is from 2 to 21 days. The main symptom is diarrhea, which may be mild at first but rapidly becomes profuse. There are loss of appetite, irritability, loss of weight, and, occasionally, vomiting. The stools are frequent, watery, without mucus or blood. Fever is absent or low grade. Gradually, symptoms of dehydration supervene, with depressed fontanel, loss of tissue turgor, sunken eyes, ashen-gray color, and evidence of circulatory collapse. There is marked loss of weight. The infant may go into coma and die. If treated early and vigorously, recovery occurs, with decreasing frequency of stools, improvement in tissue turgor, and increase in weight. Mortality varies from zero to 50 per cent in different epidemics.

Diagnosis

There are no laboratory aids to distinguish epidemic diarrhea of the newborn from other types of diarrhea in the newborn period. The diagnosis is based on clinical and epidemiological findings.

Immunity

Susceptibility to the disease is general in newborns. Since the disease is limited to the newborn period, little can be said about the acquisition of immunity.

THE ENVIRONMENT

The disease was first described in New York City in 1937. Since then, outbreaks of the disease have been reported chiefly in the Temperate Zones. They occur in all seasons of the year and are not limited to infants of any race or color. The disease is limited to the newborn period but attacks the two sexes equally. There is little question that it is more readily spread in nurseries where the nursing care is poor or inadequate and where babies are crowded.

Control

Recognition of the disease is one of the essentials in control. All infants suspected of diarrhea in a nursery for newborns should be placed by the nurse in an observation unit. If the diagnosis is definitely established by the physician, the baby is removed to the isolation nursery and treatment is begun immediately. If the isolation unit is an integral part of the obstetrical service, it should be staffed by separate personnel. In some hospitals the isolation unit is attached to the pediatric service.

Nurses on duty should wear short-sleeved dresses specially designated for use in the nursery. Gowns, caps, and masks are not essential and only give a false sense of security. Rigid hand-washing technique should be carried out before and after handling an infant. No nurse should be permitted in a nursery if she has a respiratory, enteric, or skin infection. Nurses assigned to the nursery should not be assigned for duty in any other part of the hospital. A physical examination including a chest X ray should be done every 6 months on all employees working in a nursery, and positive action should be taken on physical findings.

Visitors should not be permitted in the nursery. Personnel other than regularly assigned nurses, such as porters and maids, who must enter the nursery, should wear clean gowns, caps, and masks and should remain there only long enough to perform their duties. There should be no dry dusting.

All infants should be examined by a physician when they enter the nursery and prior to discharge. Interim examinations are unnecessary unless there is a specific indication. The doctor should wash his hands and arms with soap and water and then put on a clean gown, cap, and mask before the examination. Examinations should be made in an examination room adjacent to the nursery, with instruments reserved to this room. All equipment and supplies coming in contact with newborn infants must be scrupulously clean. This includes sterilization of basins, tongue depressors, otoscopes, stethoscopes, and all supplies used in the nursery.

Formulas should be prepared in a specially equipped formula room which should have two sections, one reserved for the thorough cleaning of bottles and the other for the preparation of the formulas and the filling of the bottles. After the nipples have been applied and the bottles have been capped, they are terminally sterilized in an autoclave or in flowing steam.

Proper nursing procedures in the nursery are of great importance. In many hospitals the practice of bathing or oiling the infant daily has been abandoned. No skin care is given from the time the infant leaves the delivery room until he goes home, other than removing excess vernix and cleaning the buttocks after a stool. This practice minimizes skin infections and allows additional nursing time for more important duties. Babies are weighed only two or three times a week routinely, and temperatures are taken only when indicated. Infrequent handling of infants minimizes the risk of infection. The practice of dressing, undressing, and giving other nursing care to the infants in a nursery on a common table is discouraged. Each infant receives a daily bundle of sterilized clothes and supplies, which is kept near its crib. Clothing, including diapers, is laundered separately, using mild soap. Sterilization by autoclave is not practical.

Infants should be held while being fed. This duty may be safely assigned to the mothers. The nurse should instruct mothers to wash their hands thoroughly before handling the baby and particularly after changing the diaper. No visitors should be permitted during feeding hours. The custom of propping bottles in the infant's crib is a pernicious one. The bottle often rolls down from its prop, and the nipple is pulled out of the infant's mouth. Milk is spilled over the baby and in the crib, the baby is unfed, and the opportunities for malnutrition and for infection are increased.

Experience has indicated that if the precautionary measures outlined are observed, epidemics of diarrhea rarely occur. However, if an epidemic of diarrhea does, for one reason or another, occur in a nursery, the best method of limiting its spread is to close the nursery to further admissions. All infants with diarrhea are isolated and treated. The nursery is quarantined until all infants have been evacuated to their homes and the nursery thoroughly cleaned.

Medical Care Plans

Treatment

The treatment of infants with epidemic diarrhea does not differ from the treatment of other diarrheas in newborn infants. Essentially, it consists of measures to check the diarrhea, to supply the necessary fluids, to combat acidosis if present, and then to supply sufficient food for growth.

Diet

The best measure for checking diarrhea is to withhold food by mouth for 24 to 48 hours. The fluid needs are made up by parenteral injection of a physiologic solution, such as 5 per cent glucose in saline or Hartmann's solution. This may be given as a slow, continuous, intravenous drip or slightly more rapidly as an intravenous infusion two or three times a day or as combined intravenous and subcutaneous injections. The addition of water and then of modified milk by mouth is begun cautiously and is increased only as rapidly as the baby can take it without aggravation of the diarrhea. In the meantime, the difference in fluid requirements between what the baby needs and what it obtains by mouth is made up by parenteral injections. In some hospitals, a transfusion is given after the first 24 to 48 hours. As the infant improves, the formula is strengthened until it meets the baby's food requirements. There are no effective drugs.

Supportive Nursing Care

Nursing care procedures are based on ideal control practices in nurseries for newborns. Daily bathing of infants with soap and water, weighing, umbilical cord dressings and binders, and all unnecessary routine nursing procedures are discontinued. Care of the infant is individualized, and all routine care is given to the baby in its own bassinet.

All infants *must* be held by the nurses or by the mother when fed formulas. In feeding infants, a new formula is used if the nipple becomes clogged. Nipples *should not* be removed from bottle and changed.

Because of early ambulation, many mothers are discharged from hospitals within 5 to 7 days following delivery. Susceptible infants often develop symptoms of diarrhea after they arrive home and may be visited by public health nurses. When infants under 1 month old are discovered to have diarrhea, the nurse instructs the mother to discontinue all feedings and to obtain prompt medical care for the baby. The family is referred to a physician or hospital. The nurse also obtains the name of hospital, date of delivery, and name and address of infant and telephones this informatoin to the local district health officer as soon as possible for epidemiological investigation.

REFERENCES

1. Cummings, G. D.: "Epidemic Diarrhea of the Newborn," in *Top's Handbook on Communicable Diseases*, 2d ed., The C. V. Mosby Company, Medical Publishers, St. Louis, Chap. XXXV, 1947.
2. Frant, Samuel, and Abramson, Harold: "Epidemic Diarrhea of the Newborn," in *Brennemann's Practice of Pediatrics*, Vol. 1, W. F. Prior Company, Hagerstown, Md., Chap. XXVIII, 1948.
3. Light, J. S., and Hodes, H. L.: "Isolation from Cases of Infantile Diarrhea of a Filterable Agent Causing Diarrhea in Calves," *J. Exper. Med.*, 90:113–135, 1949.
4. Smith, F. R.; Finley, R. D.; Wright, H. J.; and Laner, E. A.: "Terminal Heating of Infant Formula. Bacteriological Investigation of Low-pressure Technique," *J. Am. Dietet. A.*, 24:755, 1948.

Chapter 38 FOOD POISONING

GENERAL DESCRIPTION

FOOD poisoning is a general term which refers to illnesses caused by eating contaminated or infected food. A number of different agents may be causative factors. Used in its widest sense, the term "food poisoning" should include diseases like typhoid fever and trichinosis. By custom, however, the term has come to mean disease caused by one of a number of specific types of agents. These are listed below.

The term "ptomaine poisoning" is frequently used incorrectly to denote the syndome of food poisoning. Ptomaines are alkaloids that occur in putrefying matter. There is little evidence that they are poisonous. Putrefied food is not infrequently eaten with knowledge aforethought. It is often considered a delicacy and causes no harm. Examples are putrefactive cheeses like Limburger or Camembert; rotten eggs, considered a delicacy by the Chinese; rotten fish and meats eaten by people in Arctic countries. Such foods do not cause illness. Furthermore, outbreaks of disease are often caused by fresh food which has been accidentally seeded by bacteria or contaminated by chemicals. The term "ptomaine poisoning" should be discarded.

Three types of food poisoning can usually be differentiated by symptoms and incubation periods:

1. Food poisoning caused by inorganic chemicals (cadmium, arsenic, fluoride, nitrites, etc.)
2. Food poisoning caused by organic toxins
   a. Poisonous plants or animals (mussel poisoning, mushroom poisoning, ergotism, favism, etc.)
   b. Bacterial toxins (staphlococcus enterotoxin; botulinus toxin, etc.)
3. Food poisoning caused by bacteria (salmonellosis)

The incubation periods and symptoms differ somewhat in the three types and they will, therefore, be considered separately.

Food Poisoning Caused by Chemicals

THE CAUSATIVE AGENT

This type of food poisoning is caused by the accidental or purposeful introduction of harmful chemicals into food. Among the common chemicals that occasionally contaminate food are antimony, arsenic, cadmium, fluoride, lead, mercury, and nitrites.

THE HOST

Symptoms

The incubation period of chemical food poisoning is characteristically short. Symptoms often begin within a few minutes after the food is eaten. It is rare for symptoms to begin more than 1 hour after eating. Furthermore, the symptoms are chiefly upper gastrointestinal. Nausea and vomiting are common. Abdominal cramps may occur, and occasionally there is some diarrhea. As a result of the vomiting, the stomach empties itself, and recovery rapidly sets in. Only if a large quantity of the poison is ingested do constitutional symptoms occur.

Diagnosis

The laboratory diagnosis of chemical food poisoning is made by finding excess quantities of the chemical in the food. Tests for excess quantities in the blood or urine of the affected individuals are possible for some of the chemicals.

THE ENVIRONMENT

Arsenic and lead poisoning have resulted from eating raw fruit from recently sprayed trees. However, poisoning from these metals occurs more commonly in industry as chronic poisoning. Cadmium poisoning is usually due to the drinking of a liquid which has been stored in a cadmium-plated container. If the liquid is slightly acid, the cadmium dissolves in it. A number of cases have occurred in New York as a result of placing slightly acid drinks or desserts in cadmium-coated ice trays. As a result, the Sanitary Code was amended to prohibit the use of cadmium in coating utensils used for the storage of food.

Fluoride poisoning is caused, as a rule, by the careless dusting of insecticides in kitchen cupboards and refrigerators. In one such instance, four persons became ill, and a chemical examination of the crust of veal chops which they ate showed that it contained 0.64 per cent fluoride.

Mercury poisoning is not common as a result of contamination of foods, but the symptoms are similar and may be mistaken for food poisoning. In one instance a group of employees in a thermometer factory complained of vomiting and diarrhea which they ascribed to the sandwiches they ate for lunch. The investigation proved conclusively that they were poisoned by fumes of mercury which was heated in open pots over a gas flame.

Nitrite poisoning is somewhat distinctive because, in addition to the gastro-intestinal symptoms, cyanosis and faintness occur. An outbreak of such poisoning occurred in a cafeteria in New York City as a result of the careless addition of curing salt containing a large percentage of sodium nitrite instead of table salt to a batch of oatmeal.

MEDICAL CARE PLANS

Treatment

Although nausea and vomiting may be quite distressing, the stomach empties itself and thus cures the patient. He may feel fairly exhausted but, as a rule, convalescence is rapid. After the vomiting has subsided, liquids may be administered in small quantities at frequent intervals. Simple food may be given a few hours after cessation of vomiting. A general diet is cautiously introduced. Other symptoms are treated as they arise.

Food Poisoning Caused by Organic Toxins

This type of food poisoning results from eating poisonous plants or animals or food containing bacterial toxins.

Poisonous Plants or Animals

Food poisoning may result from eating such foods as poisonous mussels, mushrooms, ergot, or fava bean. Poisoned mussels occur on the West Coast between the months of May and October. The mussels are apparently poisoned by eating poisonous plankton. Mushroom poisoning results from eating poisonous mushrooms. They contain an alkaloid, muscarine, which causes the symptoms. Poisoning hardly ever occurs from eating cultured mushrooms. It usually results from eating fresh mushrooms gathered in the field by a member of the family or a kind friend who has mistaken the inedible kind for one he was familiar with. Ergot poisoning is not common in this country. It is caused by eating spoiled rye. Favism results from eating the fava bean or smelling its blossoms. It occurs chiefly among Italians living in this country who cultivate the bean. Apparently, not all people are susceptible. It is believed that only those who are allergic to the plant are affected.

Poisonous types of mushrooms can be identified by a trained mycologist. Tests for mussel poisoning are made by injecting mice with an alcoholic extract of mussel liver. Spoiled ergot can be recognized by a botanist.

Bacterial Toxins—Staphylococcus Food Poisoning

GENERAL DESCRIPTION

The second group of organic toxins is more important as a cause of food poisoning. Botulism has such a characteristic symptomatology and epidemiology that it is considered separately. Staphylococcus food poisoning is one of the most important types of food poisoning from the point of view of the frequency of its occurrence.

THE CAUSATIVE AGENT

The staphylococci elaborate several toxins, but only the enterotoxin causes symptoms. Not all strains produce the enterotoxin, and there is no bacteriologic method of telling in advance which strains will and which will not produce the toxin. It is extremely heat resistant; boiling for 1 hour does not completely destroy it. It is also resistant to acids and alkalies and survives storage in the refrigerator. It can be produced in food contaminated with staphylococci in as short a period as 5 hours.

THE HOST

Symptoms

The incubation period in food poisoning caused by organic toxins is from 1 to 8 hours, usually 2 to 4 hours. There are nausea, vomiting, abdominal cramps, and diarrhea. There may be a low-grade fever, or the temperature may be normal. The severe vomiting and diarrhea may leave the patient quite exhausted and prostrated, and the loss of fluid may cause dehydration. However, recovery usually sets in after a few hours and goes on to completion in from 1 to several days.

Diagnosis

The diagnosis of staphylococcus food poisoning is made by the symptoms in the affected individuals and the finding of large numbers of staphylococci on culture of the suspected foods. The Dolman test is used for enterotoxin: Filtered material of the suspected food or filtrates of staphylococci grown from the food are placed in boiling water to destroy *alpha* and *beta* toxins. It is then injected intraperitoneally in 0.5-cubic-centimeter amounts into 6-to-8-week-old kittens. After a short incubation period the kittens get nauseous and vomit. The test is not pathognomonic, since sterile broth alone may cause similar symptoms in kittens.

THE ENVIRONMENT

Many foods have been involved in staphylococcus food poisoning. Custard and cream-filled pastries are common offenders. Other foods frequently involved are minced meat, cheese, chicken gravy, milk, sausage, and hollandaise sauce. Foods containing the enterotoxin do not necessarily appear spoiled and may have no offensive taste.

MEDICAL CARE PLANS

Treatment

Treatment depends on the severity of symptoms. Mild cases require little treatment. Severe cases may require bed care for the prostration and parenteral fluids for the dehydration.

Diet

During the period of vomiting nothing should be given by mouth. Later, fluids may be given repeatedly in small quantities. If unable to retain them, the patient should be given an intravenous injection of 5 per cent glucose solution. When symptoms have completely abated, simple foods should be introduced gradually, and if these are retained, the diet may be increased.

Supportive Nursing Care

The nursing care of patients with food poisoning is largely one of making the patient comfortable. The patient is quite exhausted as the result of vomiting and diarrhea and wants to be disturbed as little as possible. He should be kept comfortably warm.

Bacterial Toxins—Botulism

GENERAL DESCRIPTION

Botulism is a type of food poisoning caused by the toxin of *Clostridium botulinum* and characterized by nervous symptoms resembling encephalitis.

The Causative Agent

The etiologic agent is a gram-positive, slightly motile, spore-bearing bacillus which grows best under anaerobic conditions. It is commonly found in the upper layers of the soil, thus gaining access to vegetables, fruits, straw, and hay. Occasionally, *Clostridium botulinum* is found in the feces of horses and cattle but rarely in human feces. The organism itself is not pathogenic for man or animals. However, it produces a powerful toxin which is highly poisonous.

Five types of *Clostridium botulinum* are known. These are designated as Types A, B, C, D, and E. The only two types commonly found in human outbreaks are A and B, but Type E has also been reported. Type C has been found in epidemics in fowl and Types C and D in cattle, horses, and sheep.

Clostridium botulinum multiplies in food, especially under anaerobic conditions, and produces a toxin which is one of the most powerful known. A teaspoonful of canned material containing botulinus toxin is sufficient to kill an adult. The toxin is not destroyed by gastric juice but is readily destroyed by heat.

The Host

Symptoms

The incubation period of botulism varies from 1 to 3 or 4 days. Occasionally, mild gastro-intestinal symptoms may occur a few hours after eating the offending food.

The earliest symptoms are a feeling of tiredness, followed by dizziness and headache. Nausea, vomiting, diarrhea, and abdominal pain sometimes are present at onset. The characteristic symptoms are those of the nervous system, chiefly disturbances of vision. There may be strabismus, double vision, loss of accommodation, and drooping of the lids. The patient gets weaker, finds it difficult to talk and to swallow, and may show dyspnea and cyanosis. The temperature is only slightly elevated, but prostration may be extreme. Death results from respiratory failure in about $1/2$ to 1 week after the toxic food was eaten. If the patient survives to the second week, he will probably recover.

Diagnosis

For a laboratory diagnosis of botulism, a small amount of the filtered material, prior and subsequent to boiling, is injected into mice. The mice receiving the unboiled material will be killed, and the others will survive. Mice are then protected with antitoxin A and others with antitoxin B. After 24 hours the filtered material is injected into the protected mice. If the material contains A toxin, the mice protected with antitoxin A will survive, and the others will die; if the material contains B toxin, the mice protected with antitoxin B will survive and the others die.

Immunity

There is no prophylactic toxoid available, since the disease is uncommon and active immunization is not worth while. Passive immunization is available to those exposed, as indicated under Treatment.

THE ENVIRONMENT

The organism does not grow in the animal body, so that contaminated vegetables, eaten raw, do not cause symptoms. The danger lies in canning contaminated foods, particularly vegetables, without treating the cans or jars with sufficient heat to destroy the spores. Under the anaerobic conditions of a sealed jar or can, the bacilli multiply and produce the toxin. Since the bacilli do not grow very readily in highly acid fruits and vegetables, these rarely cause symptoms even if insufficiently sterilized. Proper sterilization of canned food requires prolonged boiling, preferably under pressure. Directions for proper canning are available from the U.S. Department of Agriculture.

Control

The importance of proper sterilization of canned food is well known to the canning industry. So carefully is this controlled that nowadays cases of botulism are hardly ever reported as a result of commercially canned food. Most outbreaks result from food improperly canned in the home.

In contrast to the spores, which are not readily destroyed by heat, the toxin is easily destroyed by boiling for a few minutes. A safe precaution is to boil all home-canned foods in a saucepan for at least 10 minutes with constant stirring. If any toxin is present it will be destroyed. Since food containing the toxin does not necessarily taste bad, it should not be tasted before boiling.

MEDICAL CARE PLANS

Treatment

The best treatment is prevention. If symptoms develop, botulinus antitoxin should be used. Since too much time is necessary to determine the type of toxin ingested, an antitoxin of A and B types should be used and should be given in an initial dose of 5,000 to

10,000 units intravenously. Individuals known to have eaten the contaminated food, who have not yet developed symptoms, should be given antitoxin A and B prophylactically, in doses of 2,500 to 5,000 units intramuscularly.

The patient should be placed in an oxygen tent if he is cyanotic. When there is considerable accumulation of mucus in the pharynx, mechanical suction should be applied gently. Occasionally, breathing becomes so difficult that a tracheotomy has to be performed.

Diet

Patients who are very ill may be able to take liquids only. These should be given in small quantities. If there is great difficulty in swallowing, fluids may have to be given parenterally.

Supportive Nursing Care

The kind of nursing care that is needed varies with the severity of symptoms. Usually, the patient requires bed rest and limitation of physical activity. Unnecessary nursing procedures should, therefore, be dispensed with. The atmosphere in the room should be cheerful and quiet. Visiting should be limited to close relatives. A daily sponge bath may be given for general comfort, providing it does not tire the patient.

In communities where home canning is a common practice, the public health nurse should be familiar with agencies where demonstrations in home canning are available. She participates in the planned educational program for the prevention of botulism by instructing housewives in proper methods of canning, by providing current literature, and by encouraging attendance at demonstrations. The public health nurse should stress cleanliness in handling food and the adequate boiling of home-canned foods, the preparation of which is at all doubtful, before consumption.

Food Poisoning Caused by Bacteria—Salmonellosis

GENERAL DESCRIPTION

Salmonellosis is a generic term referring to a type of infection commonly present in food poisoning, which is characterized by nausea, vomiting, diarrhea, and cramps, and which is caused by one of a number of bacteria known as *Salmonella*.

THE CAUSATIVE AGENT

The salmonellae are gram-negative, motile, nonsporeforming bacilli which are pathogenic for man and animals, excepting

Salmonella typhi, Salmonella paratyphi A, and *Salmonella para-typhi* B, which are pathogenic for man only. There are many species of the genus, and they are distinguished from each other by their antigenic relationships. They grow readily in ordinary mediums and are easily destroyed by heat and disinfectants. In culturing stools, selective mediums are used to suppress the growth of *Bacillus coli*. Like typhoid, the other salmonellae have flagella, and two distinct antigens can be prepared, one from the flagella (H) and the other from the soma (O). By appropriate agglutination methods, the salmonellae can be separated into several groups. Each group has the same O antigen, but different members of the group differ in their H antigens.

THE HOST

Symptoms

The incubation period varies from 8 to 48 hours. The symptoms are chiefly nausea, vomiting, abdominal cramps, and diarrhea. Fever is usually present, and there is weakness, often with prostration. Symptoms may last 1 to several days, and recovery is the rule. Occasionally, the salmonellae enter the blood stream and cause an illness resembling typhoid.

Diagnosis

Confirmatory laboratory diagnosis is made by the recovery of the organisms from the stools of patients and from incriminated foods. The organisms should be typed by the antigenic schema of Kauffmann-White.

Immunity

No specific immunity is available.

THE ENVIRONMENT

The salmonellae are widely scattered in nature and affect most animals. Three of the salmonellae, *Salmonella typhi, Salmonella paratyphi* A, and *Salmonella paratyphi* B, do not occur naturally in the lower animals but usually cause severe infection in man. They are the only three in which the carrier state may be a prolonged one. The majority of the salmonellae are primarily pathogenic for animals but may also cause disease in man. These are the ones chiefly found in cases of food poisoning. The commonest ones found in this country are *Salmonella typhimurium, Salmonella choleraesuis, Salmonella enteritidis, Salmonella oranienburg, Salmonella montevideo, Salmonella newport, Salmonella anatum,*

Salmonella give, Salmonella panama, and *Salmonella derby.* They affect all types of animals including rodents and fowl. In the latter the organism may be found in the eggs and thus be transmitted to man. There is also a small group of salmonellae which infects animals but is rarely found in human infections.

Food is infected either by a food handler who is ill with salmonellosis or a carrier of salmonellae, or by contamination from infected rodents or dogs. The salmonellae may also be present in the raw meat of infected animals or in the eggs of fowl. If these are improperly cooked the salmonellae may survive and cause illness when eaten.

Control

The control of food poisoning depends on careful hygiene in the preparation of food, on the prevention of contamination, on thorough cooking, on good refrigeration, and on the careful selection of food handlers. Cleanliness is the first requirement and applies equally to the person who handles and prepares the food and to the place in which it is prepared. Adequate hand washing before handling foods should be stressed. Cooking utensils should be carefully washed with hot water and a detergent before they are put away. Roach powders and rat poisons are not needed in a kitchen which is clean. Utensils should not be lined with metals which are easily soluble and poisonous. Foods should be touched by hands as little as possible. Milk should be pasteurized.

Perishable foods should be refrigerated at a temperature of 50° F. or lower, both before preparation and after. There is a mistaken notion that once a food has been cooked it is safe. Cooked food as well as raw food can be infected, and this frequently occurs. It should not be permitted to remain in a warm kitchen for several hours while cooling. Custards and creamed fillings, for instance, are excellent culture mediums for staphylococci. After preparation they should be immediately cooled artificially and placed in a refrigerator. The rebaking of custard and cream-filled pastry has been recommended as one method of control.

Occasionally, foods are cooked in a central commissary and are then transmitted by wagon to distant places for sale or consump-. tion. Such foods should be refrigerated in transit and on arrival until shortly before use. Foods like hollandaise sauce, which presumably, lose their quality if refrigerated, should be prepared in small amounts which can be used up in a comparatively short span of time.

Individuals acting as cooks or bakers should be carefully screened for possible enteric, respiratory, or skin infections. They should not be permitted to work until clinically recovered and, in the case of specific enteric infections, until at least two stool specimens have been shown to be free of pathogenic organisms.

Inspections of food-handling establishments should be made. These should stress the need of adequate working room, regular inspection of foodhandlers, sanitary plumbing, adequate washing and toilet facilities, proper cleansing of cooking utensils, thorough cooking, rapid cooling of certain foods, and adequate refrigeration. Only by vigilant attention to details can outbreaks of food poisoning be prevented.

MEDICAL CARE PLANS

Treatment

There is no specific treatment. Therapy is symptomatic and has been described on page 343.

Diet

The patient may be given cracked ice or fluids that can be retained. Intravenous infusions of physiological saline and glucose may be given for dehydration.

Supportive Nursing Care

Nursing care plans are essentially directed toward making the patient comfortable. Home visits to reported cases of salmonellosis are made by public health nurses from or designated by the health department. The purpose of the visit is to give or demonstrate nursing care and isolation procedures to the attendant or family member giving care to the patient. The local regulations for disinfection of stools, immunization of contacts, and other precautionary measures should be explained.

Upon discharge from the hospital, home visits may be indicated to arrange for stool specimens and to counsel the family on other problems. If the laboratory report on the stool is positive, the patient may become a carrier and require periodic supervision by the health department. Prevention of salmonellosis includes teaching families proper refrigeration of foods, proper handling of fruits and vegetables, and thorough cooking of foods. Persons with boils or lesions should not be permitted to prepare food for consumption by others.

REFERENCES

1. Buchbinder, L.; Osler, A. G.; and Steffen, G. I.: "The Isolation of Entero-cocci from Foods Implicated in Several Outbreaks of Food Poisoning," *Pub. Health Rep.,* **63**:1, 1948.
2. Dack, G. M.: *Food Poisoning,* 2d ed., University of Chicago Press, Chicago, 1949.
3. Dickson, E. C.: *Botulism,* Monograph No. 8, Rockefeller Institute, New York, 1918.
4. Dolman, C. E.: "Bacterial Food Poisoning," *Canad. J. Pub. Health,* **34**:97, **34**:205, 1943.
5. Frant, S., and Kleeman, I.: "Cadmium 'Food Poisoning,'" *J.A.M.A.,* **117**:86, 1941.
6. Geiger, J. C.; Dickson, E. C.; and Meyer, K. F.: *The Epidemiology of Botu-lism,* Public Health Bull. No. 127, September, 1922.
7. Getting, V. A.; Wheeler, S. M.; and Foley, G. E.: "A Food-borne Strepto-coccus Outbreak," *Am. J. Pub. Health,* **33**:1217, 1943.
8. Greenberg, M.; Birnkrant, W. B.; and Schiftner, J. J.: "Outbreak of Sodium Nitrite Poisoning," *Am. J. Pub. Health,* **35**:1217, 1945.
9. Kauffmann, F.: *The Diagnosis of Salmonella Types,* Charles C Thomas, Publisher, Springfield, Ill., 1950.
10. Kleeman, I.; Frant, S.; and Abrahamson, A.: "Food Poisoning Outbreaks Involving Smoked Fish," *Am. J. Pub. Health,* **32**:151, 1942.
11. Mallam, P. C., and Alkadeff, R.: "Salmonella Infection in Man Conveyed by Duck Eggs," *Lancet,* **1**:887, 1946.
12. Rubenstein, A. D.; Feemster, R. F.; and Smith, H. M.: "Salmonellosis as a Public Health Problem in Wartime," *Am. J. Pub. Health,* **34**:841, 1944.
13. Trussel, R. E.; Stewart, C. B.; and Korns, R. S.: "Chemical Food Poisoning," *Am. J. Hyg.,* **51**:142, 1950.
14. Watt, J.: "An Outbreak of Salmonella Infection in Man from Infected Chicken Eggs," *Pub. Health Rep.,* **60**:835, 1945.
15. Wylder, M. K.: "Botulism in New Mexico," *Am. J. Dis. Child.,* **75**:203–205, 1948.

Chapter 39 HELMINTHIASIS (WORMS)

THE helminths include all worms. Some live as parasites in the intestinal tract of man. They are bisexual, multicellular animals. They are divided into two large groups, the roundworms and the flatworms. Some of those causing intestinal disease in man are discussed below.

Control of infestation with worms is a community problem. As such, it requires teamwork between the physician, parasitologist, sanitarian, health officer, public health nurse, and social worker. The International Health Division of the Rockefeller Foundation, in its campaign for the eradication of hookworm disease, concentrated on one procedure: the construction of sanitary privies in rural areas and the education of the public in their use. The program was highly successful and is equally so for the control of ascariasis. In the control of pinworm infection, emphasis must be shifted to personal hygiene. In trichinosis and the tapeworm diseases, emphasis must be laid on care in thorough cooking of meat and fish.

Obviously, the public health nurse assisting in such a program must be familiar with the life cycles of the different worms and understand where the chain can be broken. She should be familiar with general methods of therapy and with the precautionary hygienic measures to be taken to prevent infestation.

The nursing responsibilities for all helminthic infections consist of (1) proper management of ambulatory patients in hospital or health department clinics and (2) the preventive aspects which involve case finding and education of the patient and family.

In the clinic the nurse is responsible for the preparation of materials necessary for treatment, for arrangements to obtain proper specimens, for the interpretation of the medical findings, and for instruction of patients in proper hygienic and other protective measures.

Roundworms (Nematodes)

1. *Ancylostoma duodenale* and *Necator americanus,* the hookworms

2. *Ascaris lumbricoides,* the large intestinal roundworm
3. *Enterobius vermicularis,* the pinworm or threadworm
4. *Trichinella spiralis,* producing trichinosis

Ancylostomiasis (Hookworm Disease)

The Causative Agent

The causative agent is *Ancylostoma duodenale* or *Necator americanus.* Infection with the cat hookworm (*Ancylostoma braziliense*) and the dog hookworm (*Ancylostoma caninum*) causes a skin disease known as "creeping eruption." The adult worm is pink in color, cylindroid in shape, and somewhat curved. The male is about $\frac{1}{4}$ to $\frac{1}{2}$ inch in length, the female a little longer. Attachment is to the wall of the small intestine where copulation occurs and the female begins to lay eggs. An estimated total of 25,000 eggs is laid daily and discharged in the feces.

The discharged eggs must go through a developmental stage in moist, warm soil before they become infective. This takes about 5 days. The larvae enter the human body by piercing the skin. They reach the small veins, enter them, and are transported to the capillaries of the lungs. They break through into the air sacs, travel up the bronchioles to the trachea and pharynx, and are swallowed. They travel down the intestinal tract to the small intestine, attach themselves to the wall, and become sexually differentiated.

The Host

Symptoms

The incubation period, or the period between the piercing of the skin and the laying of eggs by the adult females, is about 5 weeks. The symptoms can be divided into those that affect the skin, lungs, and gastro-intestinal tract, and general systemic symptoms.

Skin Lesions. At the site where the worm enters the skin there are itching and burning, the area becomes red and swollen, and a papulovesicular rash may develop. This is often spoken of as "ground itch," and is more common in infection with the New World hookworm (*Necator americanus*) than with the Old World one.

Exposure to the larvae of canine or feline hookworm does not cause an intestinal infection, but causes a "creeping eruption" which is a serpiginous, erythematous, papulovesicular lesion caused by the migration of the larvae in the skin, which may continue for weeks or months until they die. The lesions itch, and as a result of scratching, eczema or infection may result.

Pulmonary Lesions. When the larvae break through the pulmonary capillaries into the air sacs there may be slight bleeding. Usually the symptoms are absent or minor.

Intestinal Symptoms. Most mild infections cause no symptoms. If infestation is heavy and repeated and if it has persisted for a long time, symptoms may result. These are poor appetite and mild digestive disturbances.

General Symptoms. When hookworm infestation is severe, these symptoms are the most prominent. Most notable is anemia, which is due to blood loss caused by the milking of intestinal capillaries by the worm. This is aggravated by poor nutrition, which is common in areas where hookworm infestation is marked. The results of malnutrition and anemia during a long period of time are evident not only in poor physical growth and development but in poor mental development.

Diagnosis

This is made by an examination of the stools, in which the characteristic eggs are found.

Immunity

No immunity results from infection. Reinfestation is the rule.

The Environment

The disease is present in many parts of the world, particularly in warm climates, where sanitary conditions are poor and privies are not used but excreta is deposited in the soil. If shoes were worn the opportunity for infection would be minimized. However, shoes are rarely worn in such climates by people who are poor and whose standards of personal hygiene are low. Persons from 5 to 19 years of age are most commonly infected.

Control

Isolation is not necessary, since the ova passed by patients are not infective until they have passed through a developmental stage in the soil.

The elimination of hookworm disease is largely an educational and economic problem. It involves the (1) education of the population in the danger of soil pollution, (2) construction of privies and their use, (3) raising the economic standards of people in hookworm areas so that they can obtain a good diet and may be able to afford shoes, and (4) mass treatment of infected individuals. Such a program appears simple. Its administration has been carried on by sanitarians all over the world with only partial success.

MEDICAL CARE PLANS

Treatment

The preferred drug is tetrachloroethylene. The adult dose is 3 cubic centimeters; for children, the dose depends on weight. A second choice of drug is hexylresorcinol crystoids in hard gelatin capsules (0.2 gram each). The adult dose is 1 gram; for children over 6 years the dose is 0.8 gram, and for children under 6 years, 0.6 gram. The capsules are given at one time before breakfast and are followed in 2 hours with a saline purge. No food is given for 5 hours. The capsules must not be chewed or the mucous membranes of the mouth will be irritated. Treatment may be repeated in three days. A blood transfusion may be necessary if the anemia is marked. If it is mild, iron may be given by mouth.

Diet

A well-balanced diet reinforced with essential nutrients and vitamins is prescribed.

Supportive Nursing Care

In severe infections the patient may be admitted to the hospital. Nursing care is essentially symptomatic.

In endemic areas the public health nurse plays an important role in a control program. She assists with case-finding surveys and mass therapy under the direction of a parasitologist. In such an educational program the nurse needs to be thoroughly familiar with the variety of symptoms that accompany hookworm infection, the ways in which it is acquired, and measures for prevention. Families and children should be indoctrinated in sound practices of personal hygiene and wearing of shoes. Unsanitary sewage-disposal facilities should be reported to the health officer. Instruction to the family should include nutrition and guidance with other health problems.

Ascariasis

THE CAUSATIVE AGENT

Ascaris lumbricoides is the commonest of all worms. It is elongated, the male measuring from 6 to 12 inches and the female a little more. The worms attach themselves to the small intestine and copulate, and the female lays her eggs, as many as 200,000 per day. The fertilized eggs require a period of incubation in the soil before they become infective for man. If the soil is moist and shady, the embryo develops into the larval stage, and the egg then becomes infective.

If embryonated eggs are swallowed, they pass down to the duodenum. Here the intestinal juices soften the shells of the eggs and the larvae tear through, penetrate the intestinal wall, and are carried by the veins or lymphatics to the lungs. They remain here a few days, then they break through the capillaries into the air sacs, pass up to the bronchi, trachea, and pharynx, and are then swallowed and pass down to the small intestine where they mature into adult males and females.

The Host

Symptoms

The incubation period, or the time between the swallowing of the eggs and the first laying of eggs by the mature female, is about 60 to 75 days. The time required for the egg to develop in the soil before it becomes infective is about 2 to 6 weeks.

As a rule, the presence of *Ascaris* in the intestines causes no symptoms. It has been stated that heavily infected children are less developed physically and mentally than uninfected ones. Occasionally, there is complaint of vague abdominal pain. Rarely, the worms may cause symptoms by blockage as of the lumen of the appendix.

Since the larvae migrate through the lungs before they come to their permanent resting place in the intestine, they occasionally cause symptoms there. These may consist of fever and other signs of pneumonitis as a result of the plugging of bronchioles.

Diagnosis

This is made by the finding of the characteristic eggs in an examination of the stool.

Immunity

An infestation does not confer immunity. Reinfection is the rule.

The Environment

The disease is found all over the world. It flourishes best in warm, moist climates, particularly where the sanitary conditions are poor and excreta are deposited in the soil. Since the eggs are not infective unless they have gone through a developmental stage in the soil, ascariasis can be eliminated by the use of toilets or privies. Children are most frequently infected, since they are more apt to play in the soil and put contaminated fingers into their mouths. Furthermore, where the level of sanitation is low, they are more apt to spread their excreta in the soil in which they play.

Where human excreta is used as fertilizer of crops, raw vegetables may become contaminated and cause infestation when eaten. Where the soil is polluted, the eggs may develop and be carried by the wind in dust and then be inhaled and swallowed.

Control

The most important item in the control of ascariasis is the provision of proper facilities for the disposal of excreta. People, especially those living in rural communities, should be impressed with the importance of using privies or other toilets. The importance of hand washing after going to stool and before eating should be stressed, especially to children.

The patient need not be isolated, since any eggs that he may pass are not infective until they have developed in soil. However, all members of the family, especially children, should have their stools examined and all positive cases should be adequately treated.

MEDICAL CARE PLANS

Treatment

Hexylresorcinol is the preferred drug. It is administered in gelatin capsules or crystoids of 0.1 or 0.2 gram each. The dose is 1 gram for adults, 0.8 gram for children above 6 years, and 0.6 gram for children below that age. It is given on an empty stomach in the morning; a saline purge is given 24 hours later. No food is given for 5 hours. The capsules must be swallowed whole, because if they are chewed the drug will irritate the mucous membranes. The treatment may be repeated, if necessary, after 3 days.

Diet

Maintenance of good nutrition is important to counteract debilitation. Easily digested foods containing essential nutrients are fed to the patient.

Supportive Nursing Care

Children with severe infections may be admitted to the hospital for medical care. Nursing care is essentially symptomatic.

All nurses concerned with care of children should be able to recognize symptoms of ascariasis and to make proper referral to a medical clinic or parasitologist for treatment. A history of residing in a tropical country may strongly suggest an infection with ascariasis. In her teaching of families, the public health nurse should emphasize cleanliness of the hands and fingernails, and washing the hands before eating and after use of the toilet.

Enterobiasis (Pinworm or Threadworm Infection)

The Causative Agent

Enterobius vermicularis (Oxyuris vermicularis) is a small round-worm which inhabits the cecum and adjacent colon and ileum. It is a tiny worm which looks like a thread. The male measures between $\frac{1}{8}$ and $\frac{1}{4}$ inch, and the female is slightly longer. A pregnant female is loaded with eggs, as a result of which she releases her attachment to the gut and migrates in the lumen, passing down the colon and out of the anus, and crawling on the perineal skin. As she does so, she deposits eggs and then dies. The eggs are fully embryonated and require no further development to become infective.

Eggs, when swallowed, reach the duodenum and hatch. The larvae pass down the bowel, become attached, and develop into adult worms. The life cycle takes about 2 months.

The Host

Symptoms

The incubation period, from the time the eggs are swallowed until they mature into adult worms, is 2 to 3 weeks. There are few symptoms resulting from infestation with *Enterobius* except pruritis of the anal region and vulva. This is caused by the migrating females and induces scratching. As a result, there may develop a dermatitis or eczema.

Diagnosis

The diagnosis is made by the recovery of the typical ova or worms from perianal swabs. Eggs are not commonly found in the feces. The NIH swab (National Institute of Health) is commonly used. This consists of a piece of Cellophane wound around the end of a glass rod. The rod is held in a test tube by means of a per-forated rubber stopper through which the upper part of the rod passes. Another method is to use Scotch tape at the end of a tongue depressor, adhesive side out. This is pressed against the perianal region early in the morning, the tape is removed and stuck to a glass slide, adhesive side down, and examined under the microscope. Occasionally, the tiny worms are seen crawling on the skin in the anal region. They should be placed in alcohol and brought to the doctor for examination.

Immunity

There is no immunity from infection. Reinfection is common.

THE ENVIRONMENT

Enterobiasis has a world-wide distribution. It is commoner in warm climates because standards of hygiene and sanitation are not as good as in temperate climates. It is seen at all seasons of the year. Children are more commonly infected than adults, but it is much more a group infection than are other helminthic infections. The presence of infestation in one member of the family requires the examination of all.

Since the eggs need not go through a developmental phase to become infective, reinfection is common. Children scratch the anal region, get the ova on their fingers or under the fingernails, and carry them promptly to their mouths to be swallowed. Uninfected children, sleeping in the same beds or playing on the floor, are infected from eggs which are freely scattered on the sheets or the floor. Treatment should therefore be directed to the entire family or group.

Control

Control is essentially a question of personal hygiene. The hands should be washed after using the toilet and before eating. The infected person should be promptly treated and should sleep alone until cured. All other members of the family should be examined, and treated, if infected. The bed linen and underclothes should be changed daily and boiled after use. Infected children should have their fingernails cut short and should be bathed regularly. Floors should be scrubbed after completion of treatment. The discovery of a case in a home or an institution requires the examination of all members of the group and the treatment of the infected ones.

MEDICAL CARE PLANS

Treatment

The same treatment may be employed as for ascariasis, fortified by a warm-water enema the night after treatment with 0.1 per cent solution of hexylresorcinol. However, the more reliable treatment is the oral administration of tablets of gentian violet before meals. The dose for adults is 1 grain (60 milligrams) three times a day for a week. For children the dose is $\frac{1}{20}$ grain (3 milligrams) per year of apparent age three times a day for 1 week. The treatment may be repeated after a week's rest. Tablets come in sizes of $\frac{3}{20}$ and $\frac{1}{2}$ grains (10 and 30 milligrams).

The wide-spectrum antibiotics have been shown to be effective in treatment and are preferable to gentian violet on account of ease of administration. Terramycin is given in a daily amount of about 25 milligrams, per kilogram of body weight, divided into four doses, for a period of 2 to 3 days. The daily dose can then be halved for another 2 to 3 days and then further reduced but maintained for about 2 weeks.

Diet

A full diet including basic nutritives is given to maintain general health.

Supportive Nursing Care

Since enterobiasis is fairly common, all nurses concerned with care of children should learn to recognize symptoms and refer individuals in need of treatment for medical care. If pinworms are discovered, all family members should be referred for examination and treatment at the same time. In her teaching of families, the public health nurse should place particular emphasis on hand washing for all members, care of fingernails, and good practices in personal hygiene. She should demonstrate proper hand washing to the patient or family and give reasons for keeping fingernails short and clean. Instruction in environmental hygiene should include washing the floors with hot water and detergent and boiling all bed linen and personal underclothing to prevent reinfection. Demonstration in the method of obtaining parasites from the perianal region for microscopical examination should be given to an adult family member.

Trichinosis

GENERAL DESCRIPTION

Trichinosis is a disease caused by a roundworm, *Trichinella spiralis,* and characterized by fever, gastrointestinal symptoms, facial edema, and muscle pains. The disease results from eating raw or insufficiently cooked infected pork products.

THE CAUSATIVE AGENT

Trichinella spiralis is a roundworm which can be seen by hand lens or under the microscope. The parasite enters the human body as an encysted larva in infected pork. The capsule of the larva is digested in the stomach by the acid juice, and the larva penetrates the mucous membrane of the duodenum or jejunum. The worms mature in a few days and mate, and the female then discharges larvae for a period of about 6 weeks. These penetrate the lymphatics or veins and are distributed through the circulation, penetrating striated muscle where they rest and become encysted. They may remain viable for many years, and the cyst becomes calcified. A similar process occurs in hogs that eat infected scraps. These hogs are then the source of infection in humans.

The Host

Symptoms

The symptoms are variable, depending on the number of larvae ingested and the tissues invaded. Gastro-intestinal disturbances may be present during the period of invasion—about 1 week following the eating of the pork. This stage may be entirely absent. During the second week, with the migration of larvae, serious symptoms arise; they consist of severe muscle pains resulting from the inflammation caused by the larvae. The muscles most commonly involved are the diaphragm, intercostals, and muscles of the extremities, mouth, and larynx. As a result, walking, masticating, and talking are very painful. Fever is usually very high, and edema around the eyes is very common. During the next stage, when the larvae become encysted, the patient feels very sick, looks toxic, and may be dehydrated. The pulse may be very rapid, and cyanosis may be marked. Death may occur, or the crisis may pass and gradual recovery ensue. The symptoms vary from the severe form described in fairly heavy infestation to comparatively mild symptoms in light infestations.

Diagnosis

An eosinophilia is almost always present. In the acute stage worms are occasionally found in the fecal discharges and in the cerebro-spinal fluid, but this is not usual. Biopsy of muscle is of greatest value after encystation has taken place. However, a negative result is not conclusive. The skin test, using 0.1 cubic centimeter, of a 1:10,000 dilution of trichina antigen intradermally is of value for confirmation, but it may be negative early in the disease. The precipitin test performed with the patient's serum is usually positive. However, it is not specific, since a number of other conditions give a positive reaction. The complement-fixation and flocculation tests are much more specific.

Immunity

Reinfections are not common but have been described. There is no active or passive immunizing agent.

THE ENVIRONMENT

Trichinosis is quite prevalent in the United States. Because of light infestation or errors in diagnosis, many cases are not recognized during life. Various estimates of the incidence have been made, a common figure being about 20 per cent. The infection in hogs is very wide spread due to the custom of feeding them meat scraps which are often infected trichinous meat. Rats may also become infected by eating infected scraps of hog meat or infected dead rats.

Control

In humans the infection occurs only as a result of eating infested pork. To prevent infection in man, a break in the chain of transmission from hog to man must be made. This can be accomplished in one of the following ways:

(1) All pork and pork products should be thoroughly cooked before eating.
(2) Hogs should be fed grain only.
(3) Hogs should be fed garbage only if it is thoroughly cooked before feeding.
(4) All raw pork should be frozen at a temperature of 5° F. for 20 days or 10° below zero for 10 days or 20° below zero for 6 days. These temperatures will kill the trichinae.
(5) Microscopic inspection of all pork should be made before it is allowed to be sold.

There are difficulties in the way of enforcement of all of these methods. The first depends chiefly on the householder. Unfortunately, many people are careless about or unaware of the dangers of raw or incompletely cooked pork. Smoking, pickling, and dry salting will destroy trichinae if properly done. Outbreaks caused by improperly smoked pork products have been reported. The feeding of cooked garbage is feasible, but many farmers will not do it, and since the raising of hogs is done by many small farmers, enforcement is difficult. Microscopic examination of pork is too time-consuming. Freezing is the most practical method for large-scale control. However, there is not enough storage space available, it would require holding meat for a considerable length of time, and would involve considerable expense to the industry. For the present, the avoidance of trichinosis is up to the individual and depends on his refusal to eat any pork which is not thoroughly cooked.

MEDICAL CARE PLANS

Treatment

There is no specific medication. Treatment is symptomatic. Mild cases are usually ambulatory and have few complaints besides general discomfort. They need no medication and require no nursing care. Severe cases are often quite sick.

Diet

A liquid diet is given during the early stage and is gradually liberalized with improvement in the general condition.

Supportive Nursing Care

Nursing care depends largely upon the degree and severity of the infection. If severe, bed rest is essential. Alcohol sponges may be given if there is an unusual rise in temperature. Cold or hot boric acid compresses may be applied to the eyes if edema is present.

Medication for muscular pain and sedation for discomfort from restlessness may be prescribed by the physician.

In the course of home visiting, the public health nurse should teach housewives the importance of slow, long cooking of pork and pork products as a safeguard against trichinosis. This includes hamburgers which are sold as beef and contain pork. The nutritive values and palatability of pork are not destroyed by long thorough cooking. The meat should be cooked until it appears white. This educational program may be carried out in conjunction with problems on nutrition, or by means of pamphlets, talks to special groups, or by films or other visual aids.

Flatworms (Platyhelminthes)

1. Flukes (trematodes)
     Schistosomiasis
2. Tapeworms (cestodes)
     a. *Taenia solium,* or pork tapeworm
     b. *Taenia saginata,* or beef tapeworm
     c. *Diphyllobothrium latum,* or fish tapeworm
     d. *Echinococcus granulosus,* or hydatid worm

Flatworms—Flukes

Schistosomiasis

General Description

Schistosomiasis is a disease caused by a blood fluke and character-ized by bloody urine or stools and enlargement of the spleen and liver.

The Causative Agent

There are two types of schistosomiasis: (1) the urinary form, some-times called bilharziasis, caused by the vesical blood fluke, *Schisto-soma haematobium;* (2) the intestinal form, caused by *Schistosoma mansoni* or by the oriental form, *Schistosoma japonicum.* There are minor differences in morphology of the three worms, but their essen-tial structures are alike. The sexes are separate, the female being longer and thinner than the male and measuring about 20 milli-meters.

Eggs are discharged into streams, pools, or canals by the urine or feces of infected individuals. The eggs hatch and become free-swim-ming forms (miracidia). They come in contact with an appropriate species of snail and infect it. Development goes on in the snail for 4 to 8 weeks, and finally fork-shaped larvae (cercariae) break out of the snail. The cercariae swim about in the water, and if they come in contact with human skin they pierce it, gain access to the small veins, and are transported to the right heart, from which they pass into the pulmonary capillaries. Over a period of about 3 days they squeeze their way through the capillaries into the pulmonary veins and they are then carried to the left heart and the systemic circula-tion. They pass to the abdominal aorta and through the mesenteric artery to the portal circulation. In the portal circulation of the liver, they feed and grow, become sexually mature, and move out after about 20 days from the time they penetrated the skin, against the blood current, to the mesenteric vein and the hemorrhoidal and vesical plexuses.

In the case of *Schistosoma haematobium,* the eggs pass to the small veins of the bladder, break through and are passed in the urine. In *Schistosoma mansoni* and *Schistosoma japonicum,* the eggs pass to the venules of the intestine and escape into the lumen of the bowel to be passed in the feces. Some of the eggs are deposited in the liver.

The Host

Symptoms

Incubation period. This is a period of about 10 to 12 weeks between the time the cercaria enters through the skin and the eggs are laid. At the point of entry there is an irritation, and in a few hours petechiae are visible at the sites of invasion of blood vessels. There may be fever, headache, backache, chills, and sweats. The abdomen is large and tender, and the liver and spleen are enlarged.

Period of deposition and extrusion of eggs. In *Schistosoma haematobium,* several months pass between the deposition of eggs and their appearance in the urine. There may be no subjective symptoms for a long time, but usually there are burning on micturition, urgency, and frequency, with bloody urine. There may also be dull pains in the lower back. In *Schistosoma mansoni* and *Schistosoma japonicum,* the extrusion of eggs is accompanied by bleeding from the bowels. The individual goes on to emaciation, anemia, and development of cirrhosis of the liver, and marked malnutrition.

Diagnosis

The most important laboratory finding is the characteristic egg in the urine or feces. During the incubation period a leukocytosis with eosinophilia is common. The complement-fixation test, with infected molluscan tissue as antigen, or a skin test assists in the diagnosis in late cases when eggs are not being discharged.

Immunity

No immunity is conferred. Reinfection appears to be the rule. There is no means of active or passive immunization.

The Environment

Schistosoma haematobium is endemic in Africa. *Schistosoma mansoni* is found in Africa, in Yemen (Asia), and in South America in northeastern Brazil, Venezuela, and Dutch Guinea. It is also found in the Lesser Antilles, Puerto Rico, and Santo Domingo. *Schistosoma japonicum* is confined to the Far East, particularly Japan, China, and the Philippines. In endemic focuses almost the entire population may be affected. This is due to the pollution of streams, canals, and pools and to the use of these waters by farmers, by children who swim in them, and by women who wash their clothes there. The practice of urinating in the streams and defecating on soil which is washed into them keeps them continuously infected. In the Far East the use of night soil for fertilizer adds an additional hazard.

There are no animal reservoirs of *Schistosoma haematobium* and *Schistosoma mansoni*, although monkeys have been found naturally infected with the latter. In Japan, domestic animals and field mice, and in China, dogs, cattle, and water buffaloes have been found to be reservoirs of *Schistosoma japonicum*.

Control

Schistosomiasis affects a large part of the world's population. Proper sanitary disposition of human fecal discharges could break the chain of infection from man through the snail and back to man. The educating of poor and backward populations in the use of properly constructed privies can be done, as was demonstrated by Heiser in Java, but it requires a forward-looking government with energy and money. The education must be carried further so that people will understand the dangers of polluting streams with urine or feces and of bathing or washing in such polluted waters.

MEDICAL CARE PLANS

Treatment

Specific treatment with antimony compounds is effective. Tartar emetic intravenously, Stibophen (Fuadin) or Anthiomaline intramuscularly may be used.

Flatworms—Tapeworms

Adult tapeworms are long, flat worms which are composed of a head, or scolax, which anchors the worm to the intestinal wall, and segments which develop from the distal end of the scolex. Tapeworms have no digestive system but absorb food from the medium in which they live. Their genital organs are well developed. Each segment contains both male and female genitalia. The eggs are fertilized in the segment and stored in a uterus, from which they are discharged into the host's intestines.

Taenia Solium (Pork Tapeworm)

THE CAUSATIVE AGENT

The adult pork tapeworm lives in the small intestine, attached to the wall by its head, or scolex, which is provided with cup-shaped suckers and hooklets. It attains a length of 6 to 20 feet. When the eggs escape from the segments and pass through the intestines, they may remain viable for several weeks if deposited in the soil. If ingested by hogs, they pass into the small intestine, the shell disintegrates, and the embryo penetrates the venules and is carried in the hog's blood stream, filtering out between the muscles and becoming encysted there. If man swallows the eggs as a result of contamination of food or water, the same process goes on in his body. If man eats infested pork raw or inadequately cooked, the larva is digested out of the pork meat in his stomach, travels down to his intestines, becomes attached to the intestinal wall, and develops into an adult worm in 5 to 12 weeks.

THE HOST

Symptoms

There are few symptoms resulting from the presence of the adult worm. Occasionally, there are complaints of vague abdominal pains or loss of appetite.

Diagnosis

This is made by finding the eggs or segments in the stools of man. However, the eggs cannot be differentiated from those of the beef tapeworm. The accurate diagnosis depends on examination of segments, if passed in the stool, or of the scolex, after treatment.

THE ENVIRONMENT

The worm is an important parasite wherever man eats pork. The pig is the only source of infection for man. Knowledge of the tapeworm goes back to ancient times, although it was confused with the beef tapeworm.

Control

Isolation of the patient is unnecessary. To prevent a patient's infection with the eggs of the tapeworm which he harbors, careful attention should be given to personal hygiene, stressing the washing of hands before mealtime. Infected individuals should sleep alone. To prevent infection from infested pigs, it is necessary to see that pork is well cooked before it is eaten. Federal inspection of pork assists in control, since infested meat looks "measly" and can be readily picked out.

MEDICAL CARE PLANS

Treatment

This is similar to that discussed under Fish Tapeworm, page 370.

Taenia Saginata (Beef Tapeworm)

THE CAUSATIVE AGENT

The worm lives in the intestine with its head embedded in the small bowel. Unlike the scolex of the pork tapeworm, this one has no hooks. The worm is larger than the pork tapeworm, attaining a size of 30 to 40 feet and sometimes as much as 75 feet. The usual-sized worm may have 1,000 or 2,000 segments. Man becomes infected by eating raw or underdone infected beef. The incubation period is about 10 to 12 weeks.

THE HOST

Symptoms

Few symptoms result from infection. Sometimes abdominal pain or diarrhea occurs.

Diagnosis

Since the eggs do not differ in appearance from those of the pork tapeworm, diagnosis can be made only by examining segments of the worm if they are passed in the stool.

THE ENVIRONMENT

The distribution of the worm is world wide. Cattle become infected by grazing on ground polluted by human excreta.

Control

The chief control for man is to see that all beef that is eaten is well cooked. Another method of control is to forbid the pollution of pasture land with human excreta. Federal inspection of beef helps in control, since infected beef looks "measly" and can be recognized with the naked eye.

MEDICAL CARE PLANS

Treatment

This is similar to that discussed under fish tapeworm, page 370.

Diphyllobothrium Latum (Fish Tapeworm)

THE CAUSATIVE AGENT

The adult worm measures from 10 to 30 feet and contains as many as 3,000 segments. A million eggs may be discharged daily by one worm. If the eggs get into a water medium after discharge from man's intestines, they mature in about 15 days and swim about as embryos in the water. Within 12 hours they must be ingested by a copepod in order to continue their development. If the infected copepod is ingested by a fresh-water fish, the development is further continued into the larval stage. If man consumes such infected fish raw or insufficiently cooked, he becomes infected, the larva attaches to the intestinal wall, develops into an adult worm, and begins to lay eggs in 5 to 6 weeks.

THE HOST

Symptoms

Symptoms are usually minimal with single infections. Multiple infections may cause abdominal pain and general discomfort and possibly anemia.

Diagnosis

Parts of the worm are occasionally passed. Usually, the condition is diagnosed by an examination of the stool and the finding of characteristic eggs.

Immunity

As in all helminthic infections, immunity does not develop.

THE ENVIRONMENT

The fish tapeworm is common in many European countries and in North America. It is also found in Siberia, Manchuria, and Japan. Although other mammals may become infected, such as the dog and cat, man is nevertheless responsible for continuing propagation.

Control

The patient need not be isolated, since the eggs which he sheds must undergo development in the copepod and fish before they become infective. The disease can easily be prevented by avoiding the use of raw or insufficiently cooked fish. The use of toilets or privies which prevent access of eggs to fresh water, and proper treatment of patients, adds to control of cutting off the supply of ova.

MEDICAL CARE PLANS

Treatment

Oleoresin of aspidium is the drug of choice. For 24 to 48 hours the patient is starved, only liquids being given. On the afternoon of each of these days, a saline cathartic is administered. On the morning of the third day oleoresin of aspidium in gelatin capsules, 1 minim per year of age, is given, the total dose being divided in three and one part administered at 8, 8:30, and 9 A.M. The maximum dose is 4 cubic centimeters. At 10:30 A.M. another purge is given. Food is allowed after the bowels have moved. All bowel movements for the next 48 hours are saved, strained, and examined for the head. If the head has not been passed, treatment may be repeated after a week.

Diet

No special diet is required.

Supportive Nursing Care

The average patient is ambulatory, and the general effect upon health is dependent upon the number and size of tapeworms and the intestinal irritation produced by the infection. Usually, there is much anxiety about the condition, especially when the patient discovers segments of tapeworms in his stools.

The essential responsibilities of the public health nurse working in the community are recognition of symptoms in individuals, referring them for medical treatment, and participation in educational programs. She should stress proper methods of cooking beef, pork, and fish, and reinforce her instruction with pamphlets or other illustrative materials.

Echinococcosis (Hydatid Disease)

THE CAUSATIVE AGENT

The tapeworm causing hydatid disease is *Echinococcus granulosus.* The adult worm lives in the small intestines of the dog, attached to the wall. It is a small worm, ⅛ to ¼ inch in length and discharges only a few eggs. Sheep are the usual intermediate hosts, but man becomes the intermediate host if he swallows the eggs, comparable to the pig and cow in pork-tapeworm and beef-tapeworm infections. The eggs hatch in the duodenum, and the larvae penetrate the intestinal wall, enter the small veins, and are carried to various organs. The liver is the most common site, accounting for about three quarters of human infection. The lungs and brain are also occasional sites of lodgment. Some of the embryos are killed by the white cells. Those that survive develop a cystic cavity. The cyst may attain a fairly large size. Usually, there develops around it a tough, fibrous capsule. From the inner layer of the cyst, smaller cysts may bud and remain attached or break off and float free in the cystic cavity.

The Host

Symptoms

The cyst itself causes no symptoms as a rule, except by its size or location. Infected individuals may live normal lives for many years until the cyst attains a size which causes pressure or dysfunction.

Diagnosis

The diagnosis is not easy. It must always be considered whenever a large liver mass is felt. In the lungs or bones, the X ray may be of assistance. In the liver, the X ray may disclose calcification. A blood count will often disclose an eosinophilia, as in other tapeworm infections. The intradermal test with hydatid fluid is usually positive, and the complement-fixation test with hydatid fluid as antigen is also of assistance.

The Environment

Many animals, in addition to man, are secondary hosts. Sheep, cattle, and pigs are common reservoirs, but many other animals may become infected. If the viscera of such animals are ingested by dogs, they become definitive hosts and the adult worm lodges in their intestines. Man becomes infected by eating contaminated food or drink or using contaminated utensils. Children playing with infected dogs or on infected soil may swallow the eggs and develop the disease.

Endemic regions are found in sheep-raising countries like Iceland, Australia, New Zealand, Argentina, Uruguay, and Chile. It is also found in the north and south of Africa and in many parts of Europe and Asia. It is uncommon in North America.

Control

Strict personal hygiene, with emphasis on hand washing before meals, should be enforced. In endemic areas dogs should be kept from eating the offal or viscera of sheep, cattle, or hogs.

Isolation is unnecessary, since the disease cannot be communicated from person to person.

Medical Care Plans

Treatment

The only effective treatment is surgery, provided the cyst is amenable to surgical removal.

REFERENCES

General

1. Craig, C. F., and Faust, E. C.: *Clinical Parasitology*, 4th ed., Lea & Febiger, Philadelphia, 1945.
2. Faust, E. C.: *Human Helminthology*, 3d ed., Lea & Febiger, Philadelphia, 1949.
3. Most, H.: "Protozoan and Helminthic Infections," *Bull. New York Acad. Med.*, 25:717, 1949.
4. Shookhoff, H. R.: "Common Intestinal Parasites," *Pub. Health Nursing*, 48:383, 1948.
5. Strong, R.: *Stitt's Diagnosis, Prevention and Treatment of Tropical Diseases*, 6th ed., The Blakiston Company, Philadelphia, 1943.

Ancylostomiasis

1. Bestowich, J. M.; Murphy, M.; and Reed, E.: "Hookworms and the Public Health Nurse," *Pub. Health Nursing*, 42:344, 1950.
2. Jacobs, L.: "Hookworm Disease," *Pub. Health Nursing*, 40:1191, 1940.
3. Rogers, H. L.: "Nursing Care in Hookworm Diseases," *Pub. Health Nursing*, 40:1197, 1940.

Ascariasis

1. Faust, E. C.: *Human Helminthology*, 3d ed., Lea & Febiger, Philadelphia, pp. 471–478, 1949.

Enterobiasis

1. Most, Harry: "Protozoan and Helminthic Infections," *Bull. New York Acad. Med.*, 25:717–739, 1949.
2. Shookhoff, Howard B.: "Common Intestinal Parasites," *Pub. Health Nursing*, 48:383–387, 1948.

Trichinosis

1. Massachusetts Department of Public Health: "Trichinosis in Massachusetts," *New England J. Med.*, 238:201, 1948.
2. Gould, S. E.: *Trichinosis*, Charles C Thomas, Publisher, Springfield, Ill., 1945.
3. Roueche, B. J.: "A Pig from Jersey," *The New Yorker Magazine*, Nov. 18, 1950.
4. Shookhoff, H. B.; Birnkrant, W. B.; and Greenberg, M.: "An Outbreak of Trichinosis in New York City," *Am. J. Pub. Health*, 36:1403, 1946.

Chapter 40 LEPTOSPIROSIS (WEIL'S DISEASE)

GENERAL DESCRIPTION

WEIL'S disease is an infectious disease characterized by fever and jaundice and by involvement of the kidneys and spleen.

THE CAUSATIVE AGENT

The causative organism is *Leptospira icterohaemorrhagiae*. It was isolated in 1915. It is a spirochete with many fine, short spirals and is actively motile. It can be seen on dark-field illumination. *Leptospira* survives in water for as long as 3 weeks. It can be grown on culture and may be stained with Wright or Giemsa stains. It passes through Berkefeld filters. It has been isolated from human beings, mice, rats, and dogs.

THE HOST

Symptoms

Leptospira icterohaemorrhagiae and a related spirochete causing the same disease, *Leptospira canicola*, have a wide distribution in dogs. Mice and rats are easily infected. In man, the infection has all degrees of severity. In mild cases, after an incubation period of 1 to 2 weeks, there occurs a mild, irregular febrile illness with conjunctival infection. In 2 to 3 days jaundice appears. Fever subsides after 3 days to 1 week.

In the more severe cases the onset is often sudden, with a chill, followed by fever of 104° to 106° F. Severe headache and muscle pains are common. There are loss of appetite, nausea, and vomiting, and, frequently, abdominal pain. Cough is a common symptom. The patient is flushed and appears prostrated. Often, there are conjunctivitis and petechial hemorrhages in the skin.

After about 5 days there come a fall in temperature and the appearance of jaundice, which increases in intensity in the next few days. Kidney involvement is manifest by oliguria, albumin, red cells, and casts in the urine and tenderness in the kidney region. If the renal involvement is severe, symptoms of uremia may develop. The patient is drowsy or stuporous and may lapse into coma. The liver is enlarged and palpable, but the spleen is usually not felt.

If the patient survives, there are gradual fall in temperature, diminution in the jaundice, increase in urine output, and fading of the skin hemorrhages. The patient looks better and improves gradually. Convalescence is prolonged. The mortality is from 5 to 10 per cent. At autopsy, hemorrhages are found in the kidney, liver, skin, muscles, and central nervous system.

Diagnosis

Leptospira may be found in the blood early in the disease by dark-field examination or by Giemsa stain. They can also be obtained by blood culture and by guinea-pig inoculation. In the guinea pig the organisms are found in the peritoneal cavity in a few days. After death of the animal, the organisms are seen in many of the organs.

Leptospira appear in the urine in the second week of illness, and can be demonstrated by dark-field examination or animal inoculation. Antibodies appear after the first week of illness. The agglutinins rise slowly to reach a peak in 6 to 8 weeks, when a titer of 1:30,000 or higher is reached.

Immunity

Recovery from the disease appears to confer a permanent immunity. Active immunization with a vaccine of killed or attenuated leptospira has been tried with questionable results. This also is true of passive immunization with hyperimmune horse serum.

The Environment

Rats are vectors of *Leptospira icterohaemorrhagiae,* the organisms being found in their urine and feces. The proportion of infected rats varies greatly in different communities; in this country it is between 10 and 40 per cent. Human infection usually results from contact with water contaminated by rat urine or feces, either by drinking or bathing in such water. The organism can enter through breaks in the skin or through mucous membranes. Sewer workers, butchers, fishmongers, miners, and farmers are the ones who most commonly come in contact with water or food polluted by rats. Dogs may serve as reservoirs and may transmit either *Leptospira icterohaemorrhagiae* or *Leptospira canicola.* Humans infected by contact with dogs are usually infected with *Leptospira canicola.*

The disease is world wide in distribution but is more common in warm climates. It occurs in all seasons but oftener in the summer and spring. Essentially, it is a disease of those who come in contact with rats or mice. It is, therefore, largely an occupational disease and is most common in males. For the same reason it is commoner in the young adult and early middle ages than in other age groups.

The disease is essentially a rat infestation. Man is infected accidentally if he drinks water or eats food contaminated by infected excreta, if he bathes or works in polluted water, or if he is bitten by an infected rat. The disease is transmitted from rat to rat in the same way.

Control

This depends largely on efforts to eliminate rats. The necessary measures will be discussed under Plague and Murine Typhus, pages 498 and 509. Those who work in polluted waters should wear proper clothing and shoes. All who come in close contact with rats should make sure that their food is protected from rodent excreta. Swimming in waters frequented by rats should be prohibited. Individuals handling mice or rats should wear rubber gloves.

MEDICAL CARE PLANS

Treatment

Specific treatment has been tried with hyperimmune horse serum. Reports of the results obtained are conflicting, some investigators finding the treatment of great benefit and others believing that it is not of great value. Both penicillin and Aureomycin appear to be effective in animals infected experimentally. There has not been enough experience with these or other antibiotics in humans.

Diet

The diet should be high in calories, carbohydrates, and proteins. Fat tolerance is low, and fat should be omitted from the diet. Fluids should be given in liberal amounts. If the fluid intake is inadequate, the patient should receive an intravenous infusion of 5 per cent glucose in physiological saline.

Supportive Nursing Care

The comfort of the patient is of prime importance in nursing care. Sponge baths may be given for high elevations in temperature. If there is headache or restlessness, an ice cap may be applied to the head. Occasionally, patients are delirious and should be watched in order to prevent accidents. Sedatives may be given for pain and restlessness.

The patient's urine may be emptied into a flush toilet. Otherwise, the urine should be mixed in its receptacle with 5 per cent chloride of lime or other antiseptic and held for 1 hour before its disposal.

The public health nurse should be familiar with preventive measures. These include veterinary care of sick cats and dogs, wearing of gloves when individuals are handling rat traps in heavily infested areas, to avoid contamination by urinary and excretal discharges of rats and mice, and the importance of wearing boots by individuals in damp areas where there is a possibility of being exposed to the infection.

REFERENCES

1. Ashe, W. F.; Pratt-Thomas, H. R.; and Kumpe, C. W.: "Weil's Disease," *Medicine,* 20:145, 1941.
2. Bertucci, E. A.: "Leptospirosis," *Am. J. M. Sc.,* 209:86, 1945.
3. Blake, F. G.: "Weil's Disease in the United States," *New England J. Med.,* 223:561, 1940.
4. Chirino, F.: "Leptospirosis," in *Pullen's Communicable Diseases,* Lea & Febiger, Philadelphia, 1950.
5. Heilman, F. R.: "Aureomycin in the Treatment of Experimental Relapsing Fever and Leptospirosis Icterohemorrhagiae," *Proc. Staff Meet., Mayo Clin.,* 23:569, 1948.
6. Larson, C. L., and Griffitts, J. J.: "Comparison of Effect of Penicillin and Immune Serum in Treatment of Leptospirosis in Young White Mice and Hamsters," *Pub. Health Rep.,* 60:317, 1945.
7. Raven, C.: "Canine Leptospirosis in Pennsylvania," *J. Infect. Dis.,* 69:131, 1941.
8. Strong, R. P.: *Stitt's Diagnosis, Prevention and Treatment of Tropical Diseases,* The Blakiston Company, Philadelphia, 1943.
9. Walch-Sorgdrager, B.: "Leptospirosis," *Bull. Health Organ., League of Nations,* 8:143, 1939.

Chapter 41 TYPHOID FEVER

GENERAL DESCRIPTION

TYPHOID fever is an acute infectious disease caused by the typhoid bacillus and characterized by fever and prostration.

THE CAUSATIVE AGENT

The typhoid bacillus is a gram-negative, motile bacillus with flagella. It grows readily on culture mediums, but its colonies cannot be distinguished from those of colon bacilli except by the use of special selective mediums. The typhoid bacillus is placed among the salmonellae by the Kauffmann-White classification and is called *Salmonella typhi*. It is also occasionally referred to by its previous classification as *Eberthella typhosa*. The salmonellae are a large group and contain, in addition to the typhoid bacillus, the bacilli of paratyphoid fever and the organisms frequently responsible for food poisoning. The salmonellae infect man and the lower animals, but typhoid and paratyphoid A and B are unique in that animals are not affected by them.

Salmonella typhi is readily destroyed by heat and disinfectants but may persist in the frozen state for a long time. In water and soil the organism will survive for weeks. Salmonella resists the action of certain dyes which inhibit the growth of the colon bacillus. On the other hand, certain salts favor the growth of salmonella over the colon bacillus. Advantage is taken of these differences in the preparation of selective mediums to isolate salmonella. The various types of salmonella are differentiated by agglutination reactions with specific immune serums.

THE HOST

Symptoms

The incubation period of typhoid fever is usually 7 to 14 days but may be as long as 1 month. The onset of the disease is insidious and the diagnosis is rarely made in the first few days unless the disease is suspected in the presence of an outbreak. The patient complains of malaise, headache, backache, and anorexia. Epistaxis and bronchitis may occur. Fever is present, but it is not high. The patient may be ambulant, but intensification of symptoms compels him to go to bed. The fever gradually increases until it reaches 103° to 104° F. at the end of the week. The patient is now bedridden, lethargic, somnolent, and disinterested. His tongue is coated, his lips are dry, and his teeth are covered with sordes. His pulse is slow and dicrotic, and he feels generally miserable. Occasionally, there are signs and symptoms of bronchitis. The spleen may now be felt, slightly enlarged and soft. The abdomen is tympanitic. The stools may be loose and frequent, or there may be constipation. A rash may appear for a few days, as discrete, rose-colored spots. The fever remains at a plateau for 1 or 2 weeks, during which time the symptoms are aggravated. Feeding becomes a real problem, and a nurse must exercise all her ingenuity to keep up the patient's nutrition and make him comfortable. He may develop tremors or become irrational or delirious. Gradually, defervescence occurs, and the temperature may reach normal within 1 week or 10 days. There is a regression of symptoms, the patient gradually recovers, and a long convalescence follows. Relapses, however, are not uncommon.

Complications

The mortality in typhoid fever is about 10 per cent, most of the deaths being due to complications. Of these, the commonest are hemorrhage and perforation. Hemorrhage results from rupture of a blood vessel in the necrotic lymphoid tissue of the intestine. There may be a considerable loss of blood. It does not usually occur until the second or third week of the disease. Hemorrhage is manifested clinically by pallor, a sudden increase in the pulse rate, and, usually, a lowering of the fever. Blood does not appear in the stool until several hours later, since the bleeding is high in the intestines.

Perforation results from the rupture of the intestine, usually at the site of one of the necrotic Peyer's patches. The chief manifestations are sudden acute pain and symptoms of shock. The patient is apprehensive, he may vomit, his temperature drops, and his pulse increases. The abdominal wall becomes rigid.

Phlebitis of the leg veins is also a late complication. The leg becomes painful, swollen, and edematous. The affected vein is thickened and tender.

Cholecystitis and cholelithiasis may not develop until after recovery. They are not uncommon complications, particularly in patients who become chronic carriers.

Osteomyelitis is another complication that develops late in the disease and may not be noted for many years. An abscess, which has the characteristics of a "cold abscess," develops in the bone. It lacks the acute symptoms of fever and localized pain. Many typhoid bone abscesses are discovered accidentally years later as a result of X ray examination and surgical exploration.

Carriers

From 3 to 5 per cent of persons recovering from typhoid fever become chronic carriers. Typhoid patients should therefore be followed for some time after recovery. In New York City a case of typhoid fever is not discharged until 1 year after recovery and until four sets of specimens of stools, taken 3 months apart, have been reported as negative for typhoid bacilli. Chronic typhoid carriers may excrete typhoid bacilli for the rest of their lives. They should therefore be under supervision and not permitted to engage in occupations requiring the handling of food, the nursing of the sick, or the care of children.

There is no treatment for chronic typhoid carriers. In about 85 per cent of chronic carriers, the focus of infection is in the gallbladder. If a specimen of bile is obtained, the typhoid bacillus can be cultured from it. Under those circumstances a cholecystectomy is advised. In a very large percentage of cases the carriers state will disappear after the gallbladder is removed. The remainder continue as carriers.

Carriers may be continuous or intermittent excreters of typhoid bacilli. Some may cease to be carriers after a number of years, apparently because the focus has disappeared. In New York City a carrier who has had a cholecystectomy or has gone with negative stools for 5 years is eligible for discharge from observation, if he submits a number of authentic stools and bile specimens and these are found negative for typhoid bacilli.

Diagnosis

A number of laboratory aids can be used to assist the physician in arriving at a diagnosis. Early in the disease the typhoid bacillus can be recovered from a blood culture—during the first week of illness, in as high as 80 to 90 per cent of cases. The organisms are shed in the stools, and positive cultures can be obtained from the stools in a very high percentage of cases. The organism may also be cultured from the urine in about 25 per cent of cases. Beginning with the second week of the disease, agglutinins in the blood of patients can be demonstrated by the Widal test. Tests are carried out for both the somatic or O agglutinins and the flagellar of H agglutinins. Both are usually present in cases of typhoid fever in increasing titers. In an individual with suspicious symptoms, a Widal test showing a titer of 1:80, or higher, with O and H antigens is considered significant.

A nonspecific laboratory aid is a low total blood count with a relative lymphocytosis.

Immunity

An attack of typhoid fever usually confers lifelong immunity; second attacks have, however, been reported. Prophylactic immunization with a vaccine of killed typhoid bacilli was begun in the United States Army in 1913 and resulted in a marked decrease of typhoid fever in Army personnel. The vaccine used today consists of a saline solution of killed typhoid bacilli, 1 billion per cubic centimeter. It is given subcutaneously in three doses of 0.5 cubic centimeter each, at weekly intervals. The immunity lasts for about 2 to 3 years, at which time a booster dose of the same vaccine, either 0.1 cubic centimeter intradermally or 0.5 cubic centimeter subcutaneously, should be given.

THE ENVIRONMENT

Typhoid fever is a widespread disease and occurs in all countries and climates. The condition of a country's sanitation is a more important determining factor than its climate or geography. Similarly, although the fall is generally considered to be the season of greatest prevalence, this does not hold true of all communities. The disease is more common in young and middle adult life than in infancy or old age. In the case of infants this is probably because they are more carefully protected from contaminated foods than are older individuals. Old people living in countries where typhoid is prevalent have probably developed some immunity as a result of contact with the disease. There is little difference in attack rates between the sexes and among whites and nonwhites.

Occupation is not an important factor in susceptibility to typhoid, although the disease is commoner among nurses and attendants treating typhoid patients and among sewer workers than in other occupations. The risk among soldiers, who drank unprotected and untreated water in the field, used to be very great. In the Spanish-American War, for instance, a mortality of 1,500 per 100,000 was reported. Compulsory immunization of all recruits and chlorination of water supplies in the field have reduced the incidence, so that in World War II the mortality in American troops was only 5 per 100,000.

The reservoir of typhoid bacilli is the human case or carrier, since animals are not susceptible to this infection. The infection is spread by the contamination of water or food supplies. In the past, epidemics occurred because lakes, ponds, or rivers that were sources of supply of drinking water were permitted to be polluted by sewage.

Contamination of a water supply may also result from cross connections between water and sewage pipes or from contamination of wells by seepage of surface water. A breakdown in the water-purification system may allow untreated water to pass to the consumer. Outbreaks may also be caused by a contaminated, nonpasteurized milk supply, or by the contamination of salads or other foods by a carrier who has not carefully scrubbed his hands. Outbreaks of typhoid have been reported that were traced to certain types of cheese which were not pasteurized or sufficiently aged. Several outbreaks have been traced to oysters grown in polluted waters. Single cases of typhoid fever are traced, in most instances, to a hitherto unknown carrier in the family. Although flies have been incriminated in some outbreaks of typhoid fever, they usually act only as mechanical transmitters from infected feces to food.

There has been a great decline in the cases and death from typhoid fever in the United States. In 1900 350,000 cases were reported, and the disease ranked fourth in causes of death. In the 5 years from 1945 to 1949, the median number of cases reported per year was 3,500, with 320 deaths. If the decline in cases continues, it will soon be a rare disease in this country. There is little reason to doubt that most of this progress has been a result of the improvement in environmental sanitation. The protection of our water supplies, the pasteurization of milk, the supervision over shellfish and other foods, and the proper disposal of sewage have been the most potent factors in the control of the disease. The supervision of chronic carriers is an important additional measure which communities should take.

Routine immunization against typhoid fever is hardly necessary in this country. It should be given, however, to all persons exposed to its hazards, such as those traveling to foreign countries, those in contact with cases and carriers, those working with polluted waters, or in instances where an entire community has been exposed as a result of a breakdown in the water supply.

Epidemics of Typhoid Fever. Numerous epidemics of typhoid fever have been described in the literature, the major ones being caused by the admixture of sewage with a drinking supply. In all instances where the community took measures to keep sewage out of the water supply or to purify its water supply, the epidemic was stopped. Most of the outbreaks reported in recent years have been caused by food contaminated by typhoid carriers. An unusual outbreak of this type occurred in New York City a few years ago:

A report was received of three cases of typhoid fever in a hospital, all living within a block or two of each other. Within another 5 days fifteen more cases were reported, all living in a radius of twenty-five adjacent city blocks. The normal expectancy would be less than one case per year in that area. Investigation of the water, milk, ice and ice cream ruled all of them out as causes of the outbreak. Food stores in the vicinity were canvassed, and stool cultures were obtained from employees. All, however, were negative for typhoid bacilli. There were twelve chronic carriers living in the neighborhood. None had worked in the neighborhood, nor had any engaged in food handling. It was noted that a vegetable store had been patronized by a number of the patients and was across the street from the block where seven cases had occurred. An alert clerk checked with the Bureau of House Numbering and discovered that although the vegetable store and the carrier had different street addresses they were both in the same building, the store being situated on the avenue side and the carrier on the street side.

A sanitary investigation disclosed that a blockage of the waste pipe had occurred several times about 3 to 4 weeks preceding the outbreak. This waste pipe drained the sewage from the carrier's apartment which was on the top floor over the vegetable store. About a month prior to the outbreak there had been a stoppage in the waste line, and sewage had backed up out of the toilet bowl in the apartment immediately over the store and had flooded the floor and adjacent foyer. It had dripped down through the floor to the store below and had contaminated the vegetables and fruits in the rear of the store. The storekeeper stated that he had discarded the vegetables that were grossly polluted but had cleaned off the others and sold them. The back of the store was roped off, and all food there was embargoed. Repairs were made to the plumbing, the store was cleaned, and fresh supplies of fruits and vegetables were obtained. No further cases occurred.

Control

The control of typhoid fever lies primarily in careful environmental sanitation—a clean water supply, pasteurization of milk, proper sewage disposal, and supervision over foods and shellfish. The disease may, however, also be transmitted by the patient directly and by carriers. For the elimination of these hazards, certain regulations should be enforced.

Typhoid fever patients should be isolated, and their rooms should be screened in the summer. The nurse caring for the patient should be immunized against the disease. The stools may be emptied from the bedpan into the toilet if the latter is water-flushed and connected with a sewer or a septic tank. If not, a cup of freshly made 5 per cent solution of slaked lime or other approved disinfectant should be poured over the stool in the bedpan and the stool should be broken up with a wooden spatula. It should be kept covered in the bedpan for 1 hour before disposal. Bedpans should be sterilized after use. Nurses should wash their hands thoroughly with soap and water after handling the patient and the bedpan.

Household contacts to cases should be immunized with typhoid vaccine. Food-handler contacts to a case should not be permitted to continue at work unless they move from the house or the patient is moved elsewhere, and until after two stool specimens taken at least 24 hours apart are reported as negative. Children who are contacts may continue at school.

The patient is kept isolated until after he has recovered clinically and is not discharged until two specimens of his stool, taken not less than 24 hours apart, have been examined and reported as negative for typhoid bacilli. He may then be discharged and resume his usual work, but a follow-up should be continued for 1 year, during which time he should be required to submit four stool specimens, at intervals of 3 months, to the laboratory for culture.

Typhoid carriers should not be permitted to be employed in any occupation where they handle food for others, exclusive of their own families. This includes nurses caring for patients, housemaids who serve or help to prepare meals, and baby nurses who feed infants. Carriers should remain under the supervision of the local health department as long as their carrier state continues, and they should notify the department when they move or change their occupations. Contacts to a carrier, who are food handlers, may be permitted to continue at their occupation if their stool specimens are negative for typhoid bacilli.

MEDICAL CARE PLANS

Treatment

Until recent years the treatment of typhoid fever was symptomatic. Chief reliance was placed on good nursing care, relief of the patient's discomfort, and keeping up his nutrition.

The specific treatment of typhoid fever is of recent origin. The drug of choice is the antibiotic chloramphenicol. A priming dose of 3 grams is given in the first few hours, and the drug is then continued in a daily amount of 100 milligrams per kilogram, divided into four equal doses. Temperature usually subsides in a few days after treatment is started. The administration of the drug should be continued for 2 weeks, or a relapse may occur. The dosage may, however, be reduced to 25 milligrams per kilogram after the fever has subsided. Although the antibiotic acts specifically in curing the patient, it does not prevent the occurrence of chronic carriers. Needless to say, it has no influence on the cure of carriers. Although a carrier may not excrete bacilli while taking the drug, the bacilli are again excreted soon after the cessation of its administration. Since chloramphenicol may cause hemolytic reactions, the patient's blood count should be checked frequently.

The patient may have discomfort from diarrhea, constipation, flatulence, or abdominal distention. Preparations of bismuth sulfate and small amounts of morphine may be necessary. A low enema is given if constipation is present. Enemas should be given slowly to avoid hemorrhage and distention of the colon. Flatulence is usually treated by attention to the diet. If there is diarrhea, the quantity of fruit intake should be limited.

Hemorrhage is treated by keeping the patient quiet, allaying his anxiety, and giving him a transfusion. Perforation requires immediate surgical intervention. Phlebitis is treated by keeping the leg elevated. Heparin or dicumarol may be employed as in phlebitis from other causes. Sedation may be necessary for restlessness.

Diet

The patient should receive a high-calory diet with vitamins added. Since the appetite is poor and distention not uncommon, feedings should be small and frequent, high in protein value, and readily digestible. Fluids are given freely.

Supportive Nursing Care

The most important factor in nursing care is general comfort of the patient. The room should be cheerful and well ventilated, and windows should be screened against flies.

Bed rest is essential. During the onset and prodromal period, the patient may be listless and drowsy. Tepid sponge baths should be given to relieve discomfort from high elevations in temperature.

As the circulation of skin is often impaired, the patient's position should be changed frequently. Rubbing sensitive skin areas with alcohol helps to harden the skin, stimulates circulation, and aids in preventing decubital ulcers. Rubber rings or cotton doughnuts should be used when there is evidence of pressure. Consideration should also be given to good body alignment. Ulceration and inflammatory conditions of the mouth may occur when mouth care is neglected. An alkaline mouthwash used before and after meals aids digestion and prevents accumulation of sordes. To prevent dryness, the mouth should be kept lubricated with a mixture of glycerin and lemon juice. Cold cream or camphor menthol should be applied to the lips. The patient's hands should be washed before meals and after using the bedpan. The fingernails should be kept clean and trimmed.

Home visits are made by public health nurses to patients ill with typhoid fever. The purpose of the visit is to give nursing care to the patient, under the physician's direction, or to demonstrate nursing care and isolation procedures to the attendant or member of the family caring for the patient. The nurse should explain to the family the importance of immunization of all contacts, and should refer them to the private physician. Home visits are made as often as necessary, depending on the condition of the patient and the home situation. If the patient has been removed to a hospital, a home visit is made to explain prophylactic and preventive measures and to render assistance with other familial problems.

Home visits are also made to chronic carriers to explain their condition to them, to suggest an interview with the health officer regarding the possibility of cure by means of cholecystectomy, to teach proper hygienic measures, to avoid transmission of the disease to others, and to interpret the regulations of the health department and explain why their enforcement is necessary. Contacts to carriers in the household are urged to be immunized, and they are referred to their physicians for this procedure.

REFERENCES

1. Bercovitz, Z. T.: *Clinical Tropical Medicine*, Paul B. Hoeber, Inc., New York, 1944.
2. Dubos, R. J.: *Bacterial and Mycotic Infections of Man*, J. B. Lippincott Company, Philadelphia, 1948.
3. New York City Department of Health: *Nursing Procedures Relating to Acute Communicable Diseases*, 1949.
4. Pullen, R. L.: *Communicable Diseases*, Lea & Febiger, Philadelphia, 1950.
5. Siler, J. F.: *Immunization to Typhoid Fever*, Johns Hopkins Press, Baltimore, 1941.
6. Woodward, T. E.; Smadel, J. E.; Ley, H. L., Jr.; Green, R.; and Mankikar, D. S.: "Chloromycetin in Treatment of Typhoid Fever," *Ann. Int. Med.*, 29:131, 1948.

Chapter 42 CONTACT DISEASES

GENERAL CHARACTERISTICS

CONTACT diseases may be caused by noninfectious materials such as chemicals and allergens or by microorganisms. An example of chemicals is beryllium, which causes granulomas if rubbed into cracks in the skin, and an example of allergens is poison ivy, which causes an itchy skin eruption. Microorganisms causing skin affections may be viruses, bacteria, fungi, or metazoa. Examples are trachoma, erysipelas, ringworm, and hookworm.

Manifestations

The symptoms of contact diseases usually manifest themselves locally in the skin, hair, or mucous membranes where the agent enters. These may be minor but may be followed by serious systemic disease.

Transmission

This may be direct contact from person to person, as in the venereal diseases or impetigo, or from animal to man, as in animal ringworm. Transmission may also occur indirectly as a result of contact with contaminated substances. Epidermophytosis may be spread by moist bath mats; oil dermatitis may be caused by oil-soaked clothes; and granulomas may result from the escape of beryllium into the air from broken fluorescent bulbs.

THE CAUSATIVE AGENT

Incubation Period

This varies with the agent. In general, inorganic substances have the shortest incubation period, and organic allergens have a somewhat longer one. The microorganisms have varying incubation periods, from 1 or 2 days in impetigo to 1 month in syphilis.

Viability of the Agent

Some organisms, like the gonococcus, are readily destroyed outside the body; others, such as ringworm, may survive on fomites for long periods of time. They vary also in their resistance to destructive agents. The gonococcus is readily destroyed by the antibiotics, while *Treponema pallidum* is much more resistant. Ringworm of the scalp requires prolonged treatment with physical and chemical agents.

Prevalence of the Agent

The prevalence of the causative agent varies widely. Syphilis is fairly widespread over the globe, but yaws is rare in North America. Poison ivy occurs in summer only, and chiefly in rural areas. Contactants are found in industry chiefly, and the presence of specific ones depends on the industry.

Reservoir

The reservoir of infection of most of the contact diseases is in humans. This is true of all the virus and bacterial diseases. Ringworm may occur in cats and dogs, and hookworm is found in the soil. The allergens are chiefly in plants, and the chemicals have their reservoir in inorganic bodies such as machinery.

Pathogenicity

Many of the agents of contact diseases cause illnesses which are uncomfortable and disagreeable; for instance, ringworm or dermatitis. Others are somewhat more deleterious to health; for example, chancroid or gonorrhea. Only a few are sufficiently serious to be reflected in mortality tables. The most important of these is syphilis.

THE HOST

Customs and Habits

The customs and habits of people influence the spread of contact diseases to a considerable extent. This holds true especially of personal hygiene, including sex hygiene, which plays a large part in the spread of venereal disease as well as diseases like impetigo and trachoma. Handshaking and kissing transmit very few diseases, although syphilis may be transmitted that way. The method of excreta disposal plays a large part in the transmission of diseases such as hookworm; these diseases cannot take hold in a community that uses privies or flush toilets. In communities where the soil is infected, the chain of infection could readily be broken if shoes were worn. Household pets may determine the presence or absence of ringworm, and the type of recreation enjoyed may contribute to the spread of diseases like athlete's foot or poison ivy dermatitis.

Defense Mechanism

The constitutional factors of race, sex, and age play a role in contact diseases as in other types of disease. Ringworm of the scalp is rare after puberty; it is more common in boys than in girls. Puerperal sepsis occurs, of course, only in parturient women. Lymphogranuloma venereum is more common in Negroes than in whites, but it is doubtful if this is a racial characteristic; it is more probably due to greater crowding and poorer economic conditions.

The local factors of resistance are an intact skin and mucous membrane which offer resistance to the entrance of microorganisms but which can nevertheless be penetrated by the hookworm, secretions like those of the eyes which wash out foreign substances, and oil and sweat which dilute the action of alkalies and acids.

The last line of defense in these as in other diseases is the immune process that is set up in the blood, and that includes phagocytosis. It must be stated, however, that there is a high susceptibility of man to the contact diseases and very little active immunity even following an attack of one of the diseases.

THE ENVIRONMENT

Physical Environment

The climate and season play a role in determining the presence and spread of contact diseases. The survival of hookworm in the soil is favored by a warm climate, and the growth of poison ivy or sumac is dependent on warm weather and rain. Also, during the warm weather, people spend more time out of doors, go out to the country more, and wear fewer clothes.

Social and Economic Environment

This is a very important factor in the spread of venereal diseases. There is no question that men whose economic status is low and who have poor housing facilities seek their pleasures elsewhere. Their ethical and hygienic standards are lower, and they are more apt to enter into relationships with women of low standards. Crowding influences the amount of contact and consequently the spread of diseases like pediculosis, scabies, and ringworm. Occupations determine the substances one comes in contact with, and thus the opportunities for close contact. As in the other diseases discussed, the wealth of a community determines the amount of general education that can be spread, the amount of intensive health education, the number of treatment centers, the opportunities for environmental sanitation, and the social and ethical awareness of the people.

Medical Aseptic Techniques

Gowns, Caps, and Masks

The aseptic techniques used to prevent spread are predicated on the biological survival of infectious agents outside the host environment. Meticulous care in hand washing is of primary importance in all contact diseases. This should be done with soap or other detergent and warm water.

Caps and masks are not required during care of diseases spread by contact. A gown should be worn during nursing care of the infectious periods in most of these diseases. Rabies and tetanus may be listed as exceptions.

Gloves

Rubber gloves should be worn when changing dressings of discharging lesions, when applying medication locally, and when in contact with infectious material.

Concurrent Disinfection

Contaminated dressings from discharging lesions should be handled with forceps and placed in a paper bag, wrapped securely, and disposed of by incineration. Personal and bed linen should be handled with care and placed in a separate canvas bag, properly tagged. Linen may then be sent to the laundry without previous disinfection, since ordinary handling in mechanical laundries is safe and disinfects the materials. Dishes do not require separate handling. They should be washed with a detergent and warm water and rinsed with boiling water after use. Ambulatory patients should receive instructions in hand washing, the use of separate towels, washcloths, and other toilet articles, and should be cautioned to sleep alone.

Terminal Disinfection

After the discharge of the patient, the unit is aired and cleaned thoroughly with warm water and soap. All equipment used by the patient is cleaned with soap and water and boiled for 5 minutes or autoclaved. Heavy equipment should be thoroughly scrubbed with soap and warm water. It is doubtful whether the use of disinfectant solutions is of any value.

REFERENCES

1. Berens, C.: *The Eye and Its Diseases,* 2d ed., W. B. Saunders Company, Philadelphia, 1949.
2. Conn, H. T.: *Current Therapy,* W. B. Saunders Company, Philadelphia, 1951.
3. Dubos, R. J.: *Bacterial and Mycotic Infections of Man,* J. B. Lippincott Company, Philadelphia, 1948.
4. Ormsby, O. S., and Montgomery, H.: *Diseases of the Skin,* 7th ed., Lea & Febiger, Philadelphia, 1948.
5. Rivers, T. M.: *Viral and Rickettsial Infections of Man,* J. B. Lippincott Company, Philadelphia, 1948.
6. Van Rooyen, C. E., and Rhodes, A. J.: *Virus Diseases of Man,* Thomas Nelson & Sons, New York, 1948.

Chapter 43 ANTHRAX

GENERAL DESCRIPTION

ANTHRAX is a disease caused by *Bacillus anthracis* and characterized by the formation of a malignant pustule in the skin which progresses often to a septicemia. Occasionally, the disease occurs as a pulmonary or intestinal infection.

THE CAUSATIVE AGENT

The causative agent of anthrax is a fairly large, nonmotile, gram-positive rod which occurs singly or in chains and which forms spores. Smears from tissues frequently show encapsulated forms. The organism grows well on ordinary mediums in the presence of oxygen. The spores are resistant to heat and disinfectants. They are destroyed by boiling for 5 minutes, by oxidizing agents such as potassium permanganate 4 per cent solution in 15 minutes, and by hydrogen peroxide in 1 hour. Iodine and chlorine destroy the spores as well as the vegetative forms, but the mercurials, phenols, and detergents are not very effective. The spores resist desiccation and freezing for years.

THE HOST

Symptoms

The incubation period is from 1 to 3 days, rarely up to 7 days. The most common form is cutaneous anthrax, which occurs in 95 per cent of cases. It is known as malignant pustule. A papule forms at the point of inoculation of the skin. It has a reddened base. The papule changes into a vesicle, which dries with a hard, black crust. There are pain and itching. There is considerable edema around the lesion, and reddened lymphatics may be observed, spreading to the regional lymph nodes, which become enlarged and tender. Many small vesicles may occur in the tissues surrounding the eschar.

With the development of the local lesion, general symptoms occur. These consist of fever, headache, and general malaise. The temperature may not be elevated very much. The white blood cells are variable in number, occasionally there is a slight leukocytosis, and at other times a mild leukopenia. The seriousness of the disease depends on the invasion of the blood stream by the organism. When this occurs, the patient may become quite ill, with marked malaise, disturbance in circulation, cyanosis, and collapse. Death may occur in a few days. However, septicemia does not necessarily mean a fatal termination.

In 5 per cent of anthrax infections the presenting symptoms are pulmonary or gastro-intestinal. Pulmonary symptoms result from inhalation of the organism. Onset is sudden, with chills and fever. Respirations are increased. There may be cough, pain in the chest, and dyspnea, and the sputum is occasionally blood-tinged. Symptoms increase in severity, and death may occur in 24 to 48 hours.

The gastro-intestinal type of anthrax is rare. It is caused by the ingestion of infected food. Local symptoms consist of vomiting and abdominal pain. General symptoms consist of fever and restlessness. If peritonitis occurs, there are abdominal rigidity and tenderness.

The case fatality from anthrax in the United States varies but is about 20 per cent. Cases that recover usually get well in a period of 3 to 6 weeks.

Diagnosis

The laboratory diagnosis of cutaneous anthrax is readily made by a film of fluid from a vesicle or serum under the eschar, stained by the Wright or Giemsa method. A culture should be made at the same time. The diagnosis is presumptive. To distinguish the bacillus from the nonpathogenic ones resembling it, mice or guinea pigs should be inoculated with infected material or with blood. The organism may be recovered from the blood stream, if septicemia has occurred. In pulmonary anthrax the sputum should be examined for the bacilli. If filtered extracts of boiled, infected tissue are layered over immune serum, a ring of precipitate will show. This is the Ascoli test.

Immunity

An attack of the disease does not confer permanent immunity. Second attacks have occurred with an interval of less than 1 year. There is no vaccine available for immunization of humans, although vaccination of livestock with a spore vaccine, Carbozoo, is effective.

THE ENVIRONMENT

Anthrax is predominantly a disease of animals and has been known since antiquity. However, proof that *Bacillus anthracis* is the etiologic agent was first offered in 1877 by Robert Koch. The disease has world-wide distribution. It is commonest in cattle, sheep, horses, and swine and occurs in them in the form of a septicemia as a result of infection following the eating of contaminated pasture or artificial food. It is rarely spread from animal to animal. In the United States anthrax is commonest in the southeastern part of South Dakota, the northeastern part of Nebraska, and along the Texas Gulf Coast and the Mississippi Delta.

In man, anthrax occurs as a result of contact with infected animals or their products. It is, therefore, largely an occupational disease, affecting farmers, butchers, veterinarians, and others who come in contact with ill animals, longshoremen, tanners, and other workers who handle infected hides or skins, and woolsorters or other workers who handle infected wool, hair, and bristles. Occasional disease in man occurs from the use of unsterilized shaving brushes.

The incidence of the disease in the United States is low, about 85 cases a year. Secondary cases in man do not occur. It is commonest in adult males because of occupational exposure.

Control

This depends on control of the source. Animals that have anthrax should be killed and incinerated. Vaccination of livestock should be carried out. Disinfection of hair, wool, hides, and skins from suspected areas should be compulsory. Workers in tanneries and wool mills should be protected from dust by proper ventilation and by education in methods of personal hygiene. The sale of unsterilized shaving brushes should not be permitted.

Patients with anthrax should be isolated until their lesions have healed. Quarantine of contacts is not necessary. Contaminated dressings from wounds should be placed in a paper bag and burned. Gloves should be worn when dressing lesions. Linen contaminated with discharges should be autoclaved or boiled for not less than 5 minutes. Upon recovery or death of the patient, the room and bedstead should receive a thorough cleaning.

MEDICAL CARE PLANS

Treatment

The use of penicillin has been shown to be effective in treatment. Large doses should be used, in the range of 300,000 units a day, until bacteria cannot be cultured from the wound and clinical symptoms indicate recovery. Specific antianthrax serum may be administered intravenously in a dose of 300 to 600 cubic centimeters diluted in 5 to 10 per cent glucose solution. It may be repeated, if necessary.

Diet

Dietary adjustments are made during the acute febrile period. Following decline in temperature, a well-balanced diet is served.

Supportive Nursing Care

Since the majority of patients admitted to hospitals have a cutaneous type of anthrax, nursing care is symptomatic. The discomfort generally arises from edema of the lesion and its location. When lesions are situated on face, neck, or shoulders, the nurse should observe the patient for signs and symptoms of meningitis.

Occasionally, patients remain at home, and the public health nurse may be called to give or supervise nursing care. The family member giving care should be instructed in proper disposal of dressings. Since anthrax is an occupational disease, a nurse giving service in industry should instruct workers to report skin abrasions promptly.

REFERENCES

1. Gold, H.: "Anthrax," *Arch. Int. Med.*, **70**:785, 1942.
2. La Boccetta, A. C.: "Anthrax: 36 Human Cases of External Type Treated Successfully with Penicillin," *Am. J. M. Sc.*, **216**:407, 1948.
3. Medwid, I., and Jakszta, W.: "Nursing Care in Anthrax," *Am. J. Nursing*, **48**:761, 1948.
4. Simpson, R. C.: "Anthrax," *Am. J. Nursing*, **48**:759, 1948.

Chapter 44 IMPETIGO CONTAGIOSA

General Description

IMPETIGO contagiosa is an acute communicable disease characterized by the formation of vesicles and crusts in the superficial layers of the skin.

The Causative Agent

The agents commonly found in the lesions of impetigo are staphylococci and streptococci, but there is no experimental evidence to indicate that such organisms cause the lesions if injected into the skin.

The Host

Symptoms

The incubation period is about 2 days. The lesion appears as macules, which rapidly become vesicular. The fluid in the vesicle becomes cloudy, and the vesicle then dries and becomes crusted. The crust is usually golden yellow in color and is superficial, as if it were stuck on. In children, it is most commonly seen on the face. In newborn infants the vesicles usually burst or dry without leaving a crust, or they leave only a very thin crust. At this age the lesions are commonest on the lower abdomen, although they appear on any part of the body. In newborn infants the disease is spoken of as *pemphigus neonatorum* or *impetigo contagiosa neonatorum*. There are no constitutional symptoms, and recovery is the rule.

Diagnosis

No laboratory tests are of aid in the diagnosis. In children the disease may sometimes be confused with chickenpox.

Immunity

An attack does not confer immunity. There are no known active or passive immune procedures.

The Environment

The disease is not dependent on climate or season for spread. It is seen in men and women of all races and colors and in children and adults. It is more common in children than in grown-ups. It is spread chiefly by person-to-person contact but also by indirect contact with articles soiled with the discharges of impetigo. It is seen chiefly where there are crowding and poor personal hygiene.

In nurseries for newborn infants, impetigo spreads rapidly once it occurs. It is a constant dread to the administrators as well as to doctors and nurses, since the spread cannot often be stopped without quarantining the nursery. Various methods of control have been tried, from daily baths or daily inunctions with various types of antiseptic ointments to routine injections of penicillin. It is certain that the less crowded the nursery and the more rigid the aseptic technique of the nurses, the less frequently does impetigo occur. The use of the dry technique of handling infants in nurseries has become more and more popular and appears to cut down the incidence of impetigo. Where this method is used, the infant's face is cleaned of blood and vernix in the delivery room, and it is then sent down to the nursery. No bath or oil rub of any kind is given to the infant until its discharge. Usually, in about a week's time the dried vernix and superficial layer of skin peel off, leaving the skin beneath pink and supple. The infrequent handling gives less opportunity to injure the baby's delicate skin and to transmit superficial infections.

Children suffering from eczema, scabies, and other itchy rashes frequently scratch and thus infect themselves and develop impetiginous lesions. These have to be treated like other lesions of impetigo. After they are cured, the underlying condition should be treated.

Control

Children with impetigo should be kept out of school and away from other children until cured. Contacts may continue at school. Meticulous care should be taken in the personal hygiene of the patients and siblings. Cases of scabies, eczema, and other itchy rashes should be treated promptly. Nursing care in nurseries for newborns should follow aseptic procedures, and infants should be handled as little as possible. Bathing and oiling should be discontinued. Temperatures should not be taken regularly, and certainly not more than once a day. Infants should not be weighed routinely more often than twice a week.

The nurse should wash her hands with soap and water after caring for an infant. Physicians should examine infants as infrequently as possible and should wash their hands with soap and water and put on a clean gown before entering the nursery.

If an infant develops impetigo in a nursery, the child should be immediately isolated. If several infants develop impetigo, they should be isolated, and the nursery should be quarantined until no further cases arise.

MEDICAL CARE PLANS

Treatment

A number of measures have been used. The most common is ammoniated mercury ointment, 2 to 5 per cent, applied to the lesions after the scabs have been softened with water and removed. Sulfadiazine and penicillin ointments have also been used. Some investigators have reported favorable results from the use of sulfadiazine by mouth and penicillin by injection. As a matter of fact, the lesions will heal without medication if kept clean and dry.

Diet

No dietary adjustments are necessary.

Supportive Nursing Care

The nurse in the hospital clinic, school, or community agency should instruct the patient or family in proper care of lesions. The patient should have his own towels and washcloths. If at all possible, he should sleep alone. The fingernails should be kept clean and short, and patients should be instructed not to touch lesions with their hands. All materials and dressings used in cleansing, removing crusts, or in applying medication should be placed in a paper bag or newspaper and burned.

REFERENCES

1. Fox, E. C., and Shields, T. L.: "Résumé of Skin Diseases Most Commonly Seen in General Practice," *J.A.M.A.*, 140:763, 1949.
2. Pillsbury, M.: "The Management of Bacterial Infections of the Skin," *J.A.M.A.*, 132:12, 1946.
3. Tobias, N.: *Essentials of Dermatology*, 3d ed., J. B. Lippincott Company, Philadelphia, 1948.

Chapter 45 KERATOCONJUNCTIVITIS

KERATOCONJUNCTIVITIS is an acute inflammatory condition of the conjuctiva characterized by edema, lymphoid hyperplasia, and corneal infiltrations, and often occurring in epidemic form.

THE CAUSATIVE AGENT

The causative agent is said to be a virus. Sanders isolated such a virus by inoculating conjunctival scrapings into tissue culture and then injecting the tissue culture into the brains of mice. According to Sanders, patients recovering from the disease develop neutralizing antibodies to the virus.

THE HOST

Symptoms

The incubation period is about 1 week. The earliest symptoms are those of itching or burning of the eye and the feeling that there is a foreign body in it. Edema of the eyelid occurs and soon becomes marked; there is a profuse serous discharge from the eye. The lid is often so swollen that the eye cannot be opened. There may be mild constitutional symptoms, such as headache, malaise, and low-grade fever. These may, however, be absent. In about 48 hours after onset, the follicles in the palpebral conjunctiva appear enlarged, and the areas between them are red and swollen. The preauricular lymph node is enlarged and slightly tender. The submaxillary glands may also become enlarged. There is considerable chemosis of the bulbar conjunctiva, and there may be ecchymosis. Often a thin, delicate membrane is present on the palpebral conjunctiva. After about 1 week there is regression in the swelling of the lid, the discharge diminishes, the conjunctival surface shows a decrease in the size of the follicles and the subjective symptoms diminish. The lymphadenopathy may also disappear, or it may persist for some time longer.

Corneal infiltrations are now visible. They are seen both in the

399

periphery and in the pupillary center. They are subepithelial, gray in color, and minute in size. They give the appearance of ulcers, although the tissue over them is intact, and they do not stain with fluorescein. The opacities may cause blurring of vision and photophobia. They gradually clear, but it may take months before they are completely gone. The lesions may occur in only one eye or in both.

Diagnosis

Diagnosis is made by the clinical findings, which are characteristic. Also, the disease occurs most commonly in epidemic form. Neutralizing antibodies are said to be present in the serum following recovery.

Immunity

No active or passive immunizing procedures are available. It is not known whether an infected individual develops immunity or for how long it lasts.

The Environment

The disease was first described in 1889 in Vienna. Later, epidemics were reported in India, China, and Malaya. In the United States Hobson reported some cases in California in 1938. In 1942, Holmes reported an epidemic of several thousand cases in Hawaii, and in the same year Hogan and Crawford studied an outbreak in San Francisco and gave the disease its present name. Since then, outbreaks have occurred in various parts of the country. Most of the outbreaks occurred in industrial plants.

Although the disease may occur in any age group and in both sexes, most of the cases have been reported in male adults, since they made up the largest percentage of industrial workers. However, small outbreaks have occurred in homes and in doctors' offices and these have involved both men and women. Because of its occurrence in outbreaks in shipyard workers, it was referred to as shipyard conjunctivitis. However, the disease has no relation to occupation. Spread appears to occur as a result of person-to-person transmission, either directly or by means of infected instruments or objects.

Control

The patient should be isolated during the acute stage of the disease. Rigid personal hygiene should be enforced in the use of personal towels and washcloths. The patient should be taught to wash his hands with soap and water after touching his eyes directly or with tissues. The use of paper tissues as eye wipes should be insisted upon. All eye syringes, pus basins, and other equipment used by the patient should be kept apart and sterilized before use by others. The patient should be impressed with the manner of spread and the need for careful personal hygiene.

MEDICAL CARE PLANS

Treatment

No specific treatment is available. Sulfonamides and the antibiotics have been used locally as well as by mouth and parenterally without apparent benefit. Convalescent serum has been employed by some with questionable benefit.

Nonspecific treatment consists in keeping the eyes clean with warm water and the use of mild anesthetic solutions to relieve pain. Wet compresses applied to the lids often give comfort. Since the disease is highly contagious, it is important that patients use disposable paper tissues and that instruments and other objects coming in contact with discharges from the infected eyes be thoroughly cleaned and sterilized after use.

Supportive Nursing Care

Inasmuch as patients are seen by nurses in hospital clinics, in industry, and in school medical offices, education of the patient in personal hygiene, careful disposal of paper tissues, separate towels, and correct instillation of eyedrops are very important to control spread of the disease.

REFERENCES

1. Braley, A. E.: "Epidemic Keratoconjunctivitis," *Med. Clinics N. Amer.,* 27:1641, 1943.
2. Hobson, L. C.: "Acute Epidemic Superficial Punctate Keratitis," *Am. J. Ophth.,* 21:1153, 1938.
3. Hogan, M. J., and Crawford, J. W.: "Epidemic Keratoconjunctivitis with Review of Literature and Report of 125 Cases," *Am. J. Ophth.,* 25:1059, 1942.
4. Pellitteri, O. J., and Fried, J. J.: "Epidemic Keratoconjunctivitis, Report of a Small Office Outbreak," *Am. J. Ophth.,* 33:1596, 1950.
5. Perkin, J. E.; Korns, R. F.; and Westphal, R. S.: "Epidemiology of Epidemic Keratoconjunctivitis," *Am. J. Pub. Health,* 33:1187, 1943.
6. Sanders, M.: "Epidemic Keratoconjunctivitis. I. Isolation of a Virus," *Arch. Ophth.,* 28:581, 1942.

Chapter 46 LEPROSY (HANSEN'S DISEASE)

GENERAL DESCRIPTION

LEPROSY is a chronic infectious disease caused by *Mycobacterium leprae* and characterized by lesions in the skin and peripheral nervous system.

THE CAUSATIVE AGENT

The causative agent of leprosy is believed to be *Mycobacterium leprae,* although the disease has never been transmitted to animal or man with cultures or tissues of lesions of the disease. The organism grows with great difficulty in artificial culture mediums and has not been propagated in chick embryos. The organism is found quite regularly in certain types of leprous lesions.

Mycobacterium leprae is acid-fast and resembles *Mycobacterium tuberculosis.* In tissues the bacilli appear in round masses, known as globi. Differentiation from the tubercle bacillus is made by this characteristic but must be corroborated by injection into guinea pigs which can be infected with tuberculosis but not with leprosy.

THE HOST

Symptoms

The incubation period is very long. It varies from a few to 20 or more years, the average being 5 to 10 years. The onset is extremely insidious, so that many individuals may not come to the attention of a physician until the process is well advanced. They usually seek attention for a skin lesion which fails to heal, or a chronic nasal discharge with nasal bleeding and obstruction, or on account of burns of the skin, which, to their surprise, are found by the physician to be anesthetic.

The lesions of leprosy occur in two forms, the lepromatous (nodular, cutaneous) and the tuberculoid (macular, maculo-anesthetic, neural).

Lepromatous Lesions. These appear as raised areas of the skin, either diffuse or as nodules or both. They are seen chiefly in exposed areas. On the face, the occurrence of the nodules, the thickened skin, and prominent, nodular ears give the well-known leonine facies. Nodules also appear on the extremities; however, they are not seen in the folds, on the palms and soles, or on the scalp.

The mucous membranes of the nose and mouth are frequently involved. In the nose, ulceration occurs, and the septum may become perforated. The nasal cartilages are involved, and as they become destroyed a saddleback nose may result. In the larynx, infiltration and swelling of the mucosa occur, and frequently ulceration. Huskiness of the voice and cough are common. If the process goes on to scarring, laryngeal stenosis occurs, with difficulty in breathing.

Conjunctivitis, keratitis, and iridocyclitis are seen in about 10 per cent of patients. Corneal opacities result, leading to partial or complete blindness.

Spread of the leprous process to lymph glands and visceral organs is the rule. There are few organs that escape its ravages.

Tuberculoid Lesions. In the tuberculoid form the skin lesions are macular in type, atrophic and depigmented, with sharply defined borders. The lesions are irregular in distribution, the patches being small or extensive and occurring chiefly on the covered parts of skin, as the trunk, back, buttocks, and thighs. They spread more rapidly than lepromas. They may involve the peripheral nerves and spread to the nerve trunks, which become enlarged, infiltrated, and indurated. The nerve trunk can frequently be palpated; a common site is above the elbow, where the ulnar nerve is fairly superficial. While the leprous process is going on in the nerve, there may be neuralgic pains along its distribution. When the nerve is destroyed, anesthesia results in the parts of the skin served by it, with muscular atrophy and trophic changes. Contractures of fingers and toes may result. In the upper extremities these result in the so-called "claw hand." Resorption of bone is not uncommon in the small bones of the hands and feet. Fingers and toes may be partially or completely resorbed. The nails remain attached to the tips, since they ascend with the retracting skin and bones. Both feet and hands become distorted and shortened.

Other trophic disturbances are malformed and brittle nails, loss of sweating, and ulcers of the skin. As a result of loss of sensation, burns from a lighted match or from leaning against a hot stove or implement occur, and heal very slowly. Ulcerations on the soles of the feet add to the discomfort of walking.

Mixed lepromatous and tuberculoid lesions are the rule in advanced cases.

Constitutional symptoms are not usually present at onset, or if they are, they are not severe enough to make the patient complain of them. In the course of the disease, febrile episodes may occur and are usually referred to as "lepra reactions." They consist of fever, chills, general discomfort, and various acute skin eruptions, such as erythema nodosum, erythema multiforme, and erysipeloid. These episodes usually last a few weeks.

Diagnosis

The diagnosis is not too difficult when lesions are far advanced. Because of its comparative rarity in temperate climates, the disease is frequently confused with a number of other conditions, particularly syphilis, tuberculosis, eczema, and the mycoses. What adds to the confusion is that a positive Wassermann or other serologic test for syphilis is obtained frequently in leprosy.

In lepromatous leprosy a positive bacteriologic test can be obtained by superficial incision of the lesion with a sharp razor blade and smearing the tissue juice on a slide. After fixation in heat, a Ziehl-Neelsen stain is made. A positive result is almost always obtained. The bacteria are usually not found in the skin scrapings of the tuberculoid lesions. If there is involvement of the nasal mucosa, a smear will often be positive for *Mycobacterium leprae*. Nasal smears and skin scrapings should be made in all cases.

The lepromin test is used by some investigators but is not uniformly considered of value. It is a skin test made with an extract of leprous tissue containing *Mycobacterium leprae*. It is usually positive in the tuberculoid, but not in the lepromatous type of leprosy.

Immunity

There is no serologic test of any value in the diagnosis of leprosy. No active or passive immunization procedures against the disease are available.

THE ENVIRONMENT

Leprosy is probably one of the oldest of known diseases. It originated in Africa or Asia and spread to Europe during the Middle Ages, when it occurred in epidemic form. It spread to America during the early colonization of this country and by the slave trade. In Europe the disease is seen only in a few focuses in some countries in the south and those bordering on the Baltic Sea. In America, focuses are found in Louisiana, Texas, Florida, and Southern California. Of 770 native patients admitted to the national leprosarium in Carville, La., from 1921 to 1950, 635 were natives of these four states, and an additional 77 were residents of them. It is still prevalent in South America, the Caribbean area, and Mexico. It is estimated that of the approximately 3 million lepers in the world, 30,000 are in the Americas, 750 of them in the United States.

Leprosy is found chiefly in tropical and semitropical countries, but whether this is the effect of climate or poor personal hygiene is not certain. It must be remembered that at one time it was quite prevalent in the Temperate Zone of Europe. In New York City, although lepers are not isolated and many of them have married and brought up families, no new case has ever arisen. All cases followed by the Department of Health got their leprosy elsewhere. It appears to affect men more than women, and children are more susceptible than adults. Crowding and poor personal hygiene are important predisposing factors. All races and colors may get the disease. In countries where leprosy is endemic, it is wise to separate young children from adult lepers.

The method of transmission of leprosy has not been definitely established. Two methods appear probable—contact with discharging ulcers or inhalation of bacilli from nasal and mouth discharges. However, the lack of an animal that can be infected with the disease and the long incubation period make it difficult to determine which of the two factors is responsible. Prolonged and intimate contact appears to be necessary.

Control

The isolation of lepers in colonies has been practiced since Biblical days. Yet it seems that in the United States, except in limited communities where the disease is endemic, such a procedure is hardly justified. The disease is only slightly contagious, particularly in the Temperate Zone, and can be treated on an ambulant basis. Many lepers can continue to do their usual work for a great many years, since the progress of the disease is slow. The newer drugs offer some hope of arrest. There is, therefore, no good reason for shutting lepers out from society for the rest of their lives. If they are permitted to partake of the life of the community under a hygienic environment and with careful attention to personal hygiene, the risk of transmission is negligible. Unfortunately, the word leper has carried with it a connotation of uncleanliness and horror since Biblical days, and most individuals shrink from the word. Teaching the public the significance of the disease is worthwhile public health education.

MEDICAL CARE PLANS

Treatment

No specific treatment is available for the disease. Chaulmoogra oil by mouth and by injection has been used for many years, but its value is doubtful. Since the introduction of the sulfonamides, sulfones have been used with encouraging results in a number of clinics. The compounds most intensively investigated have been Promin, Diasone, Sulphetrone, and Promacetin. Promin is given intravenously in a daily dose of 1 to 5 grams. The others are given by mouth, Diasone in a tablet (0.3 gram) three times a day; Sulphetrone in a total daily dose of 3 to 6 grams (tablets of 0.5 gram); Promacetin in a dose of 2 to 3 grams a day. Treatment must be continued for a long time.

The nonspecific treatment of leprosy is purely symptomatic. Conditions are treated as they arise. Anemia responds to iron medication. Ulcerations and necrosis of the bone are treated surgically. Tracheotomy is occasionally necessary on account of laryngeal stenosis. Analgesics, sedatives, and hypnotics may be required on account of pain, nervousness, and sleeplessness.

Diet

A well-balanced diet supplemented with vitamins is given.

Supportive Nursing Care

Most patients are ambulatory and are permitted outdoor activity. The nursing care is essentially directed toward mental hygiene, alleviation of pain and discomfort, and cleanliness and care of lesions. Patients usually develop severe anxieties and hostility as a result of enforced isolation in a leprosarium. Separation from family, friends, and community accentuate feelings of rejection, and the patient needs constant encouragement and suitable diversional activity. Occupational therapy is an essential part of treatment.

Patients should be instructed in personal hygiene and care of secretions from discharging lesions. In the Temperate Zone the danger of spread as a result of casual contact is minimal, so that a nurse need not take unusual precautions. Good medical aseptic technique, including careful hand washing, is a sufficient protection against spread.

In a community where there are a number of lepers either in the arrested or in a mildly progressive stage, home visits should be part of a generalized public health nursing service to the family. The contacts should be supervised and referred for periodic examination. The public health nurse should assist both the leper and his family in making a satisfactory adjustment to the disease and should point out its hopeful aspects. She should enlist the aid of other agencies, if necessary, to obtain employment for the patient or to make other social and economic provisions.

REFERENCES

1. Carroll, L. D.: "The Role of the Local Public Health Nurse in Hansen's Disease Control," *CDC Bulletin*, **10**:8, 1951.
2. Cochrance, R. G., "A Critical Review of the Present Position of Sulfone Therapy in Leprosy," *Tr. Roy. Soc. Trop. Med. & Hyg.*, **44**:259, 1950.
3. Faget, G. H., and Pogge, R. C.: "Treatment of Leprosy with Diasone," *New Orleans M. & S. J.*, **98**:145, 1945.
4. Gillen, M. E.: "Leprosy—The Larger View," *Am. J. Nursing*, **47**:86, 1947.
5. Godbout, R. A.: "Public Health Nurse and Leprosy," *Pub. Health Nursing*, **41**:30, 1949.
6. Johanson, F., and Erickson, P.: "Leprosy. Current Status of Therapy," *J.A.M.A.*, **144**:12, 1950.
7. McCoy, G. W.: "Leprosy: Factors in Public Health Management," *Pub. Health Rep.*, **65**:1522, 1948.
8. McCoy, G. W.: "Modern Public Health Measures against Leprosy," *Pub. Health Nursing*, **41**:28, 1949.
9. Senior, M. O.: "The Call Slip Read Leprosy," *Am. J. Nursing*, **47**:83, 1947.

Chapter 47 THE MYCOSES—RINGWORM

THESE are diseases caused by fungi, which are a large group of plants characterized by lack of chlorophyll. They live on decayed organic matter. Fungi are composed structurally of vegetative and reproductive portions. The vegetative part is made up of branching filaments called *hyphae,* which intertwine into a dense mass known as the *mycelium.* The reproductive portion is made up of *spores,* which are individual cells or groups of cells that separate from the mycelium and carry on an independent existence.

There are several ways in which fungi may be classified. One of these divides the pathogenic fungi into (1) yeasts or yeastlike fungi, (2) ringworm fungi, and (3) imperfect fungi. The yeasts and yeast-like fungi are characterized by their method of reproduction which is by budding. The true yeasts are composed of single cells only which multiply by budding; the yeastlike fungi have hyphae in addition to the budding cells. Among the diseases caused by this group of fungi are torulosis or cryptococcosis, which may occur as a localized skin infection or as a generalized infection with invasion of the central nervous system and the production of a form of meningitis; and moniliasis, a group of disorders caused by the genus *Candida,* which may affect the skin, nails, or lungs.

The ringworm fungi or *dermatophytes* are a closely related group which invade the superficial layers of the skin, hairs, and nails of man or animals but do not cause systemic infections. They appear as mycelial fragments and reproduce by a variety of spore forms which characterize them. The three genuses which commonly cause disease in man are the *Microscorum, Trichophyton,* and *Epidermophyton.* The common diseases are tinea capitis or ringworm of the scalp, tinea corporis, or ringworm of the skin, and tinea pedis (epidermophytosis), or athlete's foot.

The most important members of the pathogenic imperfect fungi are the *Actinomyces, Blastomyces dermatitidis, Coccidioides immitis,* and *Histoplasma capsulatum.* Actinomycosis is the disease caused by several species of the genus *Actinomyces.* It is a disease characterized by the formation of deep abscesses. About half the cases have involvement of the jaw and neck, and infection is believed to occur through the mucous membranes of the mouth. The infection may spread to the bones of the jaw and even to the skull. It may also involve the lungs and the chest wall. Actinomycosis sometimes involves the abdominal organs.

The disease caused by *Blastomyces dermatitidis* is known as "blastomycosis" and is most commonly seen as a lung infection. It resembles tuberculosis, histoplasmosis, and coccidioidomycosis in its clinical aspects and must be differentiated from them. The fungus can usually be cultured from the sputum. Blastomycosis can also occur as a skin disease. It begins as a reddish papule which increases in size and then becomes warty in appearance. Small abscesses develop and are followed by ulceration.

Coccidioides immitis and *Histoplasma capsulatum* are important causes of pulmonary disease in some sections of the country. They are discussed on pages 156 and 189.

Tinea Capitis (Ringworm of the Scalp)

GENERAL DESCRIPTION

Ringworm of the scalp is a superficial disease of the scalp and hair follicles caused by varied species of *Microsporum* or *Trichophyton* and characterized by brittleness and loss of the affected hairs.

THE CAUSATIVE AGENT

The chief causative agents are *Microsporum canis (lanosum)* and *Microsporum audouini*. Other causative fungi are *Trichophyton violaceum* and *Trichophyton gypseum*. The first two are the more important causative agents, and of the two, *Microsporum audouini* is the more persistent and difficult to cure. *Microsporum canis* is an infection of animals and may be transmitted to humans who come in close contact with infected dogs and cats. *Microsporum audouini* infects only humans and is spread from person to person. Differentiation between the two types is made by culture of infected hairs and examination by a trained mycologist.

THE HOST

Symptoms

The incubation period is undetermined. There are usually no subjective symptoms. Ringworm caused by *Microsporum audouini* appears as grayish patches of varying sizes, round or oval, which are covered by scales and in which the hairs are broken off close to the scalp. No inflammation is apparent. There may be only a single patch or several, or the scalp may be entirely covered with them. They vary in size from an area no larger than a dime to one the size of a silver dollar. In ringworm caused by *Microsporum canis,* the area of involved scalp usually shows evidence of inflammation. The hair is broken close to the scalp or may be lost in the center of the lesion and appears broken at the periphery only. The edges of the lesion are frequently raised and may appear more inflamed than the center. There may be tiny vesicles in the lesion or there may be scaling or crust formation.

Diagnosis

When the lesions have progressed to the condition described above, they are readily recognized by the naked eye. However, at this stage, the infection has already lasted for some time. In the early stages the infection can be recognized only by the use of a Wood light, which is a filtered ultraviolet light. In a dark room the infected hairs stand out under the light as greenish, fluorescent particles. Under the light it is possible to pick out single or multiple infected hairs, which appear perfectly normal to the naked eye. The Wood light does not distinguish between the different kinds of fungi. This can only be done by culturing the hair in Sabouraud's or other medium, or by direct examination under the microscope by an experienced mycologist.

Immunity

No immunity results from an infection. Reinfections are common. There is no known immunizing agent against the disease.

The Environment

Ringworm of the scalp has been recognized for many years in both epidemic and endemic form. It occurs in all climates and at all seasons of the year. It is essentially a disease of children and disappears after puberty even if untreated. It is much more common in boys than in girls, the ratio being 9 to 1. Negro boys have a higher rate in infectivity than white boys, possibly because their hair is shorter. The extent of infection is usually not known unless surveys are made by means of the Wood light. Since 1943 extensive epidemics have been described along the eastern coast of the United States. There is reason to believe, however, that these epidemics were discovered as a result of new interest in the disease and extensive surveys made.

In New York City, surveys of school children were made in the academic years 1943–1944 and 1944–1945. All cases discovered were referred for treatment and not readmitted until cured. In the 1943–1944 survey about 198,000 children were examined and the over-all incidence was found to be 1.08 per cent. It varied from no cases in some schools to a high of 8 per cent in others. The higher percentages were in schools where the children were almost all colored. In the 1944–1945 survey, some 430,000 children were examined, and an incidence of 0.4 per cent was found. The highest percentage (2.0) was in a school in a Negro district. The ratio of boys to girls was about 3 to 1, a lower ratio than commonly found.

From the results of these surveys, it appears evident that removal of cases from school and treatment of the cases has a definite influence on reducing the incidence the following year. Experience during these surveys also indicated a considerable number of familial infections. Although some investigators have found infected hairs in barbers' clippers and on the backs of seats in theaters, the experience in New York City, where surveys were made in theaters and barbershops, did not corroborate the findings. It appears that ringworm of the scalp is most commonly transmitted in the home, particularly in homes where there is crowding. Transmission may possibly occur in schools, also, but the importance of this is doubtful.

Control

Children with ringworm of the scalp should be kept out of school if not treated. If there are a considerable number of cases in a school, a special class may be arranged for them and they should be given treatment in the class. If special classes are not available, they should be permitted to attend school, provided they remain under treatment. All household contacts should be examined under the Wood lamp. If affected, they should be treated similarly. If unaffected, they should be permitted full activity. The use of individual combs and other toilet articles should be stressed.

MEDICAL CARE PLANS

Treatment

Infections with *Microsporum canis* are more easily cured than those with *Microsporum audouini*. A number of ointments have been introduced for treatment. Among the most effective are those containing undecylenic or propionic acids. The hair should be clipped short and the ointment applied to the scalp. Frequent examination should be made under the Wood light, and dead hairs should be removed with tweezers. Most cases of infection with *Microsporum canis* will be cured by this method. Infections with *Microsporum andouini* are more resistant, and only 50 to 60 per cent of cures are obtained by topical application. A much larger percentage of cures results from epilation by means of X ray, and the application of salves thereafter. X ray epilation should be done only by competent and experienced workers with this medium. An insufficient dosage does not cause the hair to fall out. An overdose may cause permanent baldness. In the hands of competent doctors there is little risk. Since 1943, cases found in surveys in New York City have been referred to proper agencies without the occurrence of a single mishap.

Supportive Nursing Care

Plans for nursing care are essentially educational and preventive. The public health nurse assists in ringworm control by working co-operatively with the health officer, school physician, family physician, teachers, and treatment agencies. Under the direction of the health officer, she plans for Wood light surveys in areas where the infection is prevalent and refers children with positive findings to a proper treatment agency. When surveys with Wood light are planned, the nurse should instruct children and parents to shampoo the hair the night before and should stress the avoidance of hair tonics or other hair dressings. In giving instruction to families, she should emphasize use of separate combs, brushes, and towels. Written instructions regarding hygienic measures to be observed are helpful to the family. If the child is excluded from school, the parent should be interviewed and the necessary treatment explained or demonstrated.

Continued supervision of the infected child is necessary, since the long duration of treatment often brings about negligence by the parents. As a result, treatment is not continued, the child becomes a truant, misses schooling, and becomes a psychologic and social problem.

Tinea Corporis (Ringworm of the Skin)

GENERAL DESCRIPTION

This is a disease of the glabrous skin and may be caused, like ringworm of the scalp, by any species of *Microsporum* or *Trichophyton*.

THE CAUSATIVE AGENT

The agent is a fungus of any species of *Microsporum* or *Trichophyton*. Differentiation is made by culture of scrapings and examination under the microscope.

The Host

Symptoms

The incubation period is undetermined. The lesions of ringworm of the skin vary in appearance. They usually start as small, raised lesions with a reddened base, covered by numerous tiny vesicles. The lesion advances peripherally by the formation of new vesicles at the edges. Coincident with the advance, the center clears, giving the appearance of a ring. If several adjacent lesions coalesce, intricate patterns may form. Sometimes the central part does not clear but remains scaly and eczematoid in appearance. Various modifications of the two types may occur.

Diagnosis

The disease must be distinguished from other inflammatory conditions not of fungous origin, such as eczema and psoriasis. Scrapings of the edges examined under the microscope will usually demonstrate fungous filaments. Culture of the scrapings will confirm the diagnosis.

Immunity

There is no immunity. Reinfections are not infrequent.

The Environment

Ringworm of the skin has a wide distribution in all climates. It affects white and colored, young and old, male and female. However, it is more commonly seen in children than in adults. The dermatophytes that cause ringworm include a number of species that infect animals primarily and infect humans only incidentally, as a result of contact with animals. The disease never causes deaths and hardly ever causes disability. Symptoms are negligible except for the rash. The main disturbance is the cosmetic one.

Control

Children with ringworm of the skin should be excluded from school until cured. Household contacts should be examined and, if they are free of the disease, should not be placed under restrictions.

Medical Care Plans

Treatment

Treatment is usually simple and effective. Isolated lesions can usually be cured by painting with tincture of iodine 4 per cent solution in alcohol twice daily for a few days. If the lesions are widely spread the use of an ointment is advisable. A variety of drugs has been recommended. Among them is Whitfield's ointment, half strength, a salve containing undecylenic acid—undecylenate mixture in petrolatum and an ointment containing 2 per cent salicylic acid and 3 per cent sulfur.

Tinea Pedis (Epidermophytosis: Athlete's Foot)

General Description

This is an infection of the upper layers of the skin caused by an invasion of the cornified epithelium by some species of *Trichophytons* and *Epidermophytons*.

The Causative Agent

Several species of *Trichophyton* and *Epidermophyton* may be causative agents. All cause similar clinical symptoms and can be differentiated by cultural examination.

The Host

Symptoms

The incubation period has not been definitely determined. In the acute cases the initial lesion is a deep-seated vesicle or a group of vesicles. These are most commonly seen on the soles of the feet or the palms of the hands. The fluid may be absorbed, leaving a brown, stained area. The vesicle may rupture and discharge its gelatinous fluid. Scaling will follow.

The intertriginous type is more commonly seen. In its mildest form it occurs as a maceration of the skin between the toes or as a dry scaling with fissures. As the macerated skin desquamates a red base with a scaly border is seen. Secondary infection may supervene.

A third type is the chronic, thickened form, which is dry and occurs on the heels, soles, and sides of the feet. Symptoms are minimal in contrast to the other two types, which may cause itching or pain.

All three types of lesions, which commonly occur on the feet, may also occur on the hands.

Diagnosis

The diagnosis of athlete's foot is usually made without much difficulty. For confirmation, scrapings of the edges of the lesion should be cultured and examined under the microscope.

Immunity

No immunity appears to develop. Indeed, many individuals have recurrent exacerbations and recurrences if careful hygienic measures are not followed.

THE ENVIRONMENT

The disease is widespread and is seen in all climates. It is seen more commonly, however, in the summer, when sweating occurs. Males appear to be somewhat more susceptible than females, but this may be due to their habits and occupations. It is said to be frequently contracted in gymnasiums and locker rooms where many individuals walk barefoot, and particularly if they use common mats.

Preventive measures are largely hygienic measures. Cleanliness of the body and underclothing, and careful drying between the toes are essential. Lesions should be treated early. A wise protection against contamination is the use of sandals in shower or dressing rooms that are used by many people.

Control

Ringworm of the feet is so prevalent among older children, particularly in hot weather, that it is impractical to isolate them or exclude them from school. Furthermore, the wearing of shoes is a protection against spread. The nurse in school and in industry has an opportunity to stress the preventive measures outlined to students and employees.

MEDICAL CARE PLANS

Treatment

Treatment differs, depending on the clinical appearance of the disease. In the acute types, where there are considerable inflammation and swelling, patients must be kept off their feet and wet dressings should be applied. After the subsidence of acute symptoms the application of ointments, such as half-strength Whitfield's ointment, is recommended. White cotton socks should be worn and laundered after use. Individuals susceptible to ringworm of the feet should bathe their feet regularly, dry them well, especially between the toes, and dust ordinary talcum powder lightly between the toes.

REFERENCES

1. Carrick, L.: "Methods of Local Therapy for Tinea Capitis Due to Microsporon Audouini," *J.A.M.A.*, **131**:1189, 1946.

2. Culbert, R. W.; Robinson, A. E. R.; and Reiner, M. N.: "Study in the Reduction of Absence from School of Children with Tinea Capitis," *Am. J. Pub. Health,* **40:**1089, 1949.

3. Mitchell, H. H.; Story, S. S.; and Macdonald, J. C.: "An Epidemic of Ringworm of the Scalp," *Pub. Health Nursing,* **35:**1564, 1943.

4. Moorehead, M. A.: "Epidemic Ringworm of the Scalp," *Pub. Health Nursing,* **40:**86, 190, 1948.

5. Moorehead, M. A.: "Control of Epidemic Ringworm of the Scalp," *M. Woman's J.,* **56:**11, 1949.

6. Rothman, S.; Smiljanic, A.; Shapiro, A. L.; and Weitkamp, A. W.: "The Spontaneous Cure of Tinea Capitis in Puberty," *J. Invest. Dermat.,* **8:**81, 1947.

7. Schwartz, L.; Peck, S. M.; Botwinick, I.; Leibovitz, A. L.; and Frasier, E. S.: "Control of Ringworm of the Scalp among School Children in Hagerstown, Md.," *J.A.M.A.,* **132:**58, 1946.

8. Swartz, Jacob H.: *Elements of Medical Mycology,* 2d ed., Grune and Stratton, New York, 1949.

Chapter 48 OPHTHALMIA NEONATORUM

GENERAL DESCRIPTION

OPHTHALMIA neonatorum is an acute conjunctivitis which occurs in newborn infants. It may be caused by a variety of organisms, among the most common of which are the virus of inclusion conjunctivitis, which is discussed elsewhere, and a number of bacteria, among which are the gonococcus, meningococcus, pneumococcus, and staphylococcus. The latter are discussed here.

THE CAUSATIVE AGENT

Any one of a number of organisms may be responsible for the infection. At one time the gonococcus was the most common and the most virulent. At present the gonococcus is surpassed in frequency by other organisms.

THE HOST

Symptoms

The disease is limited to newborn infants. A similar conjunctivitis may occur in adults, but since the epidemiology is different, it is not considered in this discussion.

The incubation period is usually 2 to 3 days after birth. There are swelling of the lids, redness of the conjunctivae, and a thin discharge. The swelling increases, and the discharge becomes purulent. The swelling may be so great that the infant is unable to open its eyes. Before the introduction of antibiotics, the condition lasted for several weeks, and complications were not unknown. Occasionally, the infection is limited to one eye.

Diagnosis

A diagnosis can be made by examining a smear and a culture from the purulent material. One must exclude chemical conjunctivitis which results from the installation of silver nitrate and which clears up fairly rapidly. The diagnosis of inclusion conjunctivitis or blennorrhea is discussed under that disease.

417

Immunity

All newborn infants are susceptible.

THE ENVIRONMENT

The condition is limited to newborn infants. It usually results from contact with an infected birth canal during passage at birth. Occasionally, the infection may be transmitted by a mother or nurse who has conjunctivitis, by direct contact or by contact with articles freshly soiled. Gonorrheal ophthalmia used to be a frequent condition in newborn infants as a result of gonorrhea in the mother. With the requirement by law of the use of the Credé method, the incidence decreased. The method consists in the introduction of a drop or two of 1 per cent silver nitrate in the infant's eyes at birth. The use of penicillin in the treatment of gonorrhea has greatly lessened the incidence of gonorrheal ophthalmia, since a pregnant woman with the disease can be cured in 1 or 2 days.

Control

The infected infant should be isolated until cured, and great care should be taken in its handling and in the disposition of soiled articles. The nursery need not be quarantined.

All newborn infants should have silver nitrate or a similar effective agent instilled in the eyes at birth. All pregnant women who have a gonorrheal infection should be treated with penicillin. Great care in personal hygiene should be exercised in the handling of infants at and after birth.

MEDICAL CARE PLANS

Treatment

The disease responds promptly to the use of sulfadiazine by mouth or penicillin by injection. The former is used in a dose of 1 to $\frac{1}{2}$ grains per pound of body weight per day and the latter in a dose of 100,000 units a day. Treatment is usually not required for more than 2 or 3 days.

REFERENCES

1. Berens, C.: *The Eye and Its Diseases*, W. B. Saunders Company, Philadelphia, 1949.
2. McKee, S. H.: "Ophthalmia Neonatorum," *Am. J. Ophth.*, **25**:52, 1942.
3. Sievers, J. J.; Knott, L. W.; and Soloway, H. M.: "Penicillin in Treatment of Ophthalmia," *J.A.M.A.*, **125**:690, 1944.

Chapter 49 RABIES (HYDROPHOBIA)

GENERAL DESCRIPTION

R A B I E S is an acute disease of the central nervous system, caused by a virus to which all warm-blooded animals are susceptible. Dogs are most commonly affected, but it is often present in other canines, such as foxes, wolves, jackals, and hyenas. Man is accidentally infected when bitten by a rabid animal.

THE CAUSATIVE AGENT

The rabies virus is a large one and is not readily filterable. Infected nervous or salivary-gland tissue can be stored in neutral glycerin for several weeks at room temperature and for months in the refrigerator. The virus is best preserved by drying in the frozen state and keeping it refrigerated. If a 10 per cent suspension of such tissue is centrifuged, the virus will be found in the supernatant. Aqueous suspensions are readily destroyed by heat, sunlight, and chemicals.

The potency of a virus to immunize against rabies is tested by its action in protected and unprotected mice.

Pasteur was the first to experiment extensively in order to produce a vaccine. By serial injections into the brains of rabbits, the virus became modified so that the disease had a fixed, short, incubation period. This was called *fixed virus* to distinguish it from the virus occurring naturally in animals, which was called *street virus*. After many passages in rabbits, fixed virus became so attenuated that it had little power to infect dogs but preserved its antigenic powers. Pasteur exposed the spinal cords of rabbits injected with fixed virus to drying, so as to attenuate the virus further. He injected first the virus that had been dried for the longest number of days, and was therefore noninfective, and followed this with daily injections of infected rabbit cord that had been dried for fewer and fewer days. In this way dogs became more and more resistant and were able to tolerate infective doses. The success of this led Pasteur to try it in humans, with good results. There was always danger, however, that the living virus might harm rather than protect. Experiments in the early twentieth century indicated that if tissue suspensions of fixed virus were treated with chemical agents, the virus was killed but its antigenicity remained. Semple introduced a phenol-killed vaccine which is widely in use today.

The disadvantage of vaccine made from nerve tissue is that certain individuals injected with it develop postvaccinal paralysis. Johnson, in 1939, recovered from a fatal case rabies virus which he was able to grow serially in brains of day-old chicks until it became fixed for the chicks. This virus, known as the Flury strain, has been grown in chick embryos, and a dried vaccine has been obtained for use. It has been tried in dogs with good results and no resulting cases of encephalitis. Its use in humans has not been sanctioned as yet.

The Host

Symptoms

The incubation period of rabies is from 2 to 6 weeks but may be as long as 6 months. The onset is gradual with headache, fever, malaise, nausea, and sore throat. There are increasing irritability and anxiety. The patient complains of pain in the region of the bite. He becomes more and more anxious, his muscles are tense, his pupils dilate, and there is increase in sweating and salivation. As his nervousness increases, there occurs difficulty in swallowing, not only of solid food but of liquids. This is due to a spasm of the muscles of deglutition. It progresses to a point where the mere sight of water precipitates a spasm of the throat muscles. This symptom has given the disease the name of hydrophobia. As a result of the inability to swallow, dehydration results, with dry skin, mouth, and tongue, unless parenteral fluids are given. Convulsions with opisthotonos may occur. The patient becomes delirious, lapses into coma, and dies within a few days after onset. Occasionally, a patient survives the acute stage of excitement and goes on to the stage of apathy and paralysis. Weakness is followed by paralysis of the flaccid type, and death does not supervene until 1 week to 10 days after onset. The white blood count is usually increased. The spinal fluid is normal. Rabies is a fatal disease. No recoveries are known.

At autopsy no characteristic changes are found except in the central nervous system. The pathognomonic lesion is the Negri body. This is an inclusion body found in the cytoplasm of nerve cells, particularly in Ammon's horn of the hippocampus. It is a spherical or oval eosinophilic body with basophilic granules and is sharply outlined. There may be several inclusion bodies in one neuron.

Diagnosis

Diagnosis of rabies is made by the history of a bite, typical clinical symptoms, and the fatal outcome. The finding of Negri bodies in the brain is conclusive. When Negri bodies are not found, portions of the brain are inoculated into mice, and these are observed for a period of 1 to 3 weeks. If virus is present they usually die in a week with flaccid paralysis. Negri bodies can then be demonstrated in their brains.

Immunity

An attack of rabies is fatal in 100 per cent of cases. Humans and animals can be immunized with antirabies vaccine, after which they develop neutralizing and complement-fixing antibodies, the former of which persist for some time, but the latter of which disappear in a few months. A number of vaccines are available for prophylactic treatment. The first to be used was the Pasteur vaccine, which was an active, rabbit-fixed virus. Infected rabbit spinal cords were dried in a jar with potassium hydroxide for a varying number of days. Injections were begun with the cords that had been dried for the longest period and continued with cords dried for shorter and shorter periods. The Harris vaccine is also a living attenuated virus dried from the frozen state. The Semple virus is the one most widely in use in this country. It is a virus which has been inactivated by treatment with phenol. The final product contains 0.25 per cent phenol. Recently, a new vaccine has been introduced. This is from virus obtained from a fatal case which has been passed in day-old chicks, and then maintained in chick embryos. It has the advantage of being free of brain tissue and is said to cause a longer lasting immunity than other vaccines. It has been used in dogs only.

The effectiveness of vaccines in preventing rabies has not been definitely determined, although the prevailing opinion is that it is effective. Statistics are not readily obtainable, since the incidence of infection in individuals bitten by rabid animals varies according to the severity of the bite, its location, the amount of protective clothing, the amount of virus in the saliva, and other factors. In general, from 10 to 15 per cent of persons bitten by rabid animals develop rabies, whereas only a small percentage will develop it after treatment. If we exclude those that develop rabies within 2 weeks of the bite and who have, therefore, not received the full benefit of the vaccine, the fatality rate is less than 0.5 per cent of those treated.

One disadvantage of vaccine made from mammalian nerve tissue is that a certain percentage of individuals treated with it develop postvaccinal encephalitis. The incidence varies. In New York City it averages 1 case in about 2,000 persons treated. One must therefore weigh the advantages of the vaccine against the risk of encephalitis.

Passive immunization by the use of immune serum has been used to a limited extent. The combined use of immune serum and vaccine has also been tried and is said to be somewhat more effective than vaccine alone. Its value remains to be determined.

The Environment

Rabies has been known since antiquity and was described by Greek writers as long ago as 500 B.C. It occurred at first chiefly in wild animals but was known to attack domestic animals occasionally. The experimental proof that rabies could be transferred from wild animals to domestic dogs by the inoculation of saliva was given early in the nineteenth century. The Scandinavian countries acted on this information by quarantining domestic dogs and destroying all strays and thus eliminating rabies in their countries. Where the disease is prevalent in wild animals, reinfection of domestic animals may occur.

The extent of rabies in humans depends on its extent in domestic animals, and this, in turn, depends on its prevalence in wild canines which infect domestic dogs. In the beginning of the nineteenth century, rabies in dogs was quite prevalent in Europe as a result of extensive epizootics in wolves and foxes. Men became infected by the bites of dogs, and as many as 250 cases a year occurred in Prussia for a considerable period of time. At present, rabies is prevalent in most of Europe. Rigid quarantine of dogs has kept it out of England, Switzerland, and Scandinavia.

In Asia and Africa the principal wild animal propagating the disease is the jackal, although the mongoose is also involved. As elsewhere, the domestic dog becomes infected when bitten by the wild animal and keeps the disease alive by biting other dogs and occasionally man.

In North America rabies was apparently introduced by imported dogs in the beginning of the nineteenth century. Its presence was first noted along the eastern shore, but by the end of the century it had spread west to the Mississippi. Its presence in California may be explained by its spread eastward from Mexico where it is present in coyotes. The chief wild animals that are hosts of the disease in the United States are the coyote, skunk, and fox. Epizootics of rabies in foxes are quite prevalent at present in the Eastern and Southeastern states. In recent years about 9,000 cases of rabies a year in animals and 35 cases in man have been reported in the United States.

There is little rabies in Canada, except what is imported from the United States, but it is quite prevalent in dogs in Mexico,

Central America, and South America. An unusual discovery in these countries was that there exists a carrier of rabies. Most animals, including man, invariably die when they develop rabies. However, the vampire bat may become infected and recover and then act as a carrier of the disease. The discovery of the part played by the vampire bat in rabies transmission is quite dramatic. For many years a paralytic disease in cattle, called *malde caderas,* was known in Brazil. A similar disease was known in other countries of South America and Mexico and went by the name of *derriengue.* It was only after considerable study that both diseases were proved to be rabies and were shown to be transmitted by vampire bats. These animals subsist on blood only, which they suck from animals after biting them. When other animals are scarce, they attack man. In 1925, a similar paralytic disease in cattle appeared in Trinidad, and thousands of animals died as a result. Its nature was not recognized at first but was later shown to be rabies which was spread by vampire bats that had migrated from South America.

In Hawaii and Australia rabies does not occur, chiefly because of the rigid quarantine maintained in those countries.

The disease can be said to be world wide in distribution, in all climates and all seasons. It attacks males and females equally and children as well as adults.

Control

No isolation of the patient is necessary, since the disease is spread by bite. For the same reason, quarantine of contacts is unnecessary.

In the control of rabies it is important to have a carefully planned program, well integrated. This should include the following:

1. Leashing of all dogs at large, and the picking up of those found unleashed and their destruction or quarantine
2. Annual immunizaton of dogs with a potent antirabic vaccine, the procedure to be tied in, preferably, with licensure
3. Compulsory reporting of all dogbites, the immediate examination of biting dogs by a veterinarian, and their surveillance for 1 week
4. Maintenance of antirabic clinics for the vaccination of persons bitten by rabid, suspiciously rabid, or stray dogs.

It is possible to keep rabies out of a country by maintaining strict quarantine against dogs coming from elsewhere. This has been accomplished by England and Australia, for instance. In the United States, where rabies is well established among wild and domestic animals and where there are no sharp physical lines of demarcation between states, quarantine alone would hardly be effective. Where rabies has become epizootic among wild animals, there must be added to the program outlined the capture and destruction of the infected wild animals and the immunization of livestock with a potent antirabic vaccine.

Medical Care Plans

Treatment

There is no specific treatment for the disease once it has set in. Death results in all cases. Treatment is directed toward the patient's comfort. Sedatives are employed to control anxiety, and to prevent convulsions, and parenteral fluids are given for dehydration.

The prophylactic treatment of rabies is extremely important. The wound caused by the bite should be washed thoroughly with a 20 per cent soft-soap solution. The former method of cauterization with fuming nitric acid seems to have no greater value, is more painful, and may cause scarring.

Vaccine treatment should be begun immediately. The Semple vaccine (phenol killed) is administered subcutaneously in fourteen daily injections. Slight local reactions may occur. It is wise to use a different site each day. Of considerable concern is the fact that a certain percentage of those injected develop postvaccinal encephalitis. In the experience of the New York City Department of Health, the ratio is about 1 to 2,000 injected persons. Most persons developing this complication recover completely. However, an occasional death does result, and of those surviving some may have nervous sequelae. It is, therefore, good medical practice not to recommend immunization unless the danger from rabies is greater than the risk of encephalitis. In New York City it is recommended only if the individual has been bitten by (1) a rabid dog, (2) a dog suspected of being rabid, or (3) a stray dog whose condition is not known. If the dog is known, he is kept under observation for 1 week. If symptoms of rabies do not develop in him in a week, observation is discontinued. If symptoms suspicious of rabies develop, antirabic vaccination is offered to the person bitten.

Diet

Laryngeal spasms make it difficult for the patient to swallow food. Soft, easily digested foods may be given if tolerated.

Supportive Nursing Care

Nursing care plans include measures which contribute to the comfort of the patient. Since the patient is emotionally upset and has fears related to water, bathing should be omitted. Hand washing should not be done within the room.

The patient is usually restless, excitable, and very apprehensive. These symptoms increase with progression of the disease.

The public health nurse plays an integral role in a rabies control program. She stresses the need of reporting all dog bites and of getting first-aid treatment, followed by antirabic inoculations in specified circumstances. The name and address of the owner of the biting animal should be obtained and the information given to the rabies control officer at the time of report, so that the animal may be kept under observation.

REFERENCES

1. Casals, J.: "A Current View of the Rabies Problem," *Ann. Int. Med.,* **23**:74, 1945.
2. McKendrick, A. G.: "A Ninth Analytical Review of Reports from Pasteur Institutes on the Results of Anti Rabies Treatment," *Bull. Health Organ., League of Nations,* **9**:31, 1940.
3. Pawan, J. L.: "Transmission of Paralytic Rabies in Trinidad by Vampire Bat," *Ann. Trop. Med.,* **30**:101, 1936.
4. Rabies. *CDC Bulletin,* **9**:1, 1950.
5. Steele, J. H., and Tierkel, E. S.: "Rabies Problems and Controls," *Pub. Health Rep.,* **64**:785, 1949.
6. Webster, L. T.: *Rabies,* The Macmillan Company, New York, 1942.

Chapter 50 TETANUS (LOCKJAW)

TETANUS is an acute infectious disease caused by the toxin of *Clostridium tetani* and characterized by convulsive contractions of the muscles.

THE CAUSATIVE AGENT

The causative agent is *Clostridium tetani,* a gram-positive, non-motile, sporeforming bacillus, which grows best under anaerobic conditions. Its natural habitat is the soil and the intestinal tract of higher animals. *Clostridium tetani* produces a powerful exotoxin which causes the symptoms of tetanus in man. It is readily destroyed by heat and by acids and alkalies.

THE HOST

Symptoms

The incubation period is generally from 5 to 10 days, but may be as long as several weeks. The onset is usually manifested by a stiffness of the muscles of the arms, legs, neck, and jaw. There is usually an accompanying fever, along with restlessness and irritability. As the disease progresses the rigidity of the neck and the stiffness of the jaws become prominent features. The latter may be so marked that the patient is unable to open his mouth. This is known as *trismus.* Other muscles of the body also become stiff and rigid. Convulsions frequently occur. These may be precipitated by minor stimuli and are painful because of the rigidity of the muscles. Difficulty in swallowing usually occurs, and cyanosis may result from spasms of respiratory muscles. Death occurs in about 50 per cent of all cases.

Diagnosis

The diagnosis is not difficult in a fully developed case. The stiffness of the neck and pain in the back may suggest meningitis, but the spinal tap shows a normal fluid. Peritonsillar abscess may cause trismus, but this is easily ruled out by proper examination. A history of injury helps in the diagnosis. There are no laboratory procedures of value in the early diagnosis. If the wound is still open, it should be cultured for *Clostridium tetani*.

Immunity

There is no quick test for immunity to tetanus. Laboratory and field investigations indicate that the preferred method of active immunization is to inject alum-precipitated tetanus toxoid in two doses of 1 cubic centimeter each, 1 month or more part. Tetanus toxoid may be combined with diphtheria toxoid or pertussis vaccine or with both for active immunization. This is discussed under Whooping Cough, page 304. A booster dose of 1 cubic centimeter fluid tetanus toxoid should be given at the end of 1 year and also whenever an injury with a lacerated wound occurs. Individuals who have not been actively immunized against tetanus should receive a prophylactic injection of 1,500 units of tetanus antitoxin if they are accidentally injured and suffer a laceration or burn.

THE ENVIRONMENT

The disease has been recognized since ancient times, but its cause and transmission were not known until the nineteenth century. In 1890 von Behring and Kitasato demonstrated that cultures of the organism contain an exotoxin and that its injection into animals results in the development of an antitoxin. Tetanus is widely distributed and occurs wherever wounds are contaminated with soil or other material in which the organism grows. Persons of all ages and colors and both sexes are susceptible. The disease is more common in males, due probably to their greater opportunity to be injured. The organism itself is not harmful and is frequently found in the intestinal tract of animals. In deep wounds the bacillus is able to grow under anaerobic conditions and thus produce the toxin, which is absorbed and causes injury to nerve tissue.

Tetanus is not a common disease in large urban centers. It is more common in rural areas, where there is a greater opportunity for wounds to be infected with contaminated soil. Its occurrence among the wounded in war used to be high. In World War I, tetanus antitoxin was introduced as a prophylactic measure in the British army in October, 1914. During August and September, no prophylaxis was used. There were 2,000 wounded in the home military hospitals during those 2 months, and 62 cases of tetanus occurred, a case rate of 32 per 1,000. During the rest of the war, among 2,000,000 wounded, 2,323 cases of tetanus occurred, a rate of 1.16 per 1,000.

In World War II, tetanus toxoid was used prophylactically for all troops. Only 12 cases of tetanus occurred among 2,734,819 wounded, a case rate of 0.0004 per 1,000. Furthermore, in only 1 of the cases was the wound caused in battle. On the other hand, in the Marshall Islands there occurred 12 cases among 266 Japanese wounded prisoners, and 14 cases among 284 wounded Japanese civilians, case rates of 45 and 49 per 1,000, respectively.

It is obvious that immunization with tetanus toxoid has practically eleminated tetanus in the armed forces.

Tetanus in the newborn still occurs in communities where midwives who have had no training in asepsis are permitted to deliver and care for babies. At one time, contamination of calf lymph smallpox vaccine with tetanus spores occurred now and then. The introduction of an aseptic technique in the preparation of the calves, the preservation of the lymph, and the careful bacteriological testing of the lymph have done away with this hazard.

Control

The case need not be isolated, since tetanus is not transmitted from man to man. Children should be actively immunized against tetanus with two doses of 1 cubic centimeter of alum toxoid 1 month apart. A booster dose of 1 cubic centimeter of the toxoid should be administered 1 year later, and again immediately following an injury. Individuals receiving an injury, who have not been previously immunized with toxoid, should be given tetanus antitoxin 1,500 units.

MEDICAL CARE PLANS

Treatment

Specific treatment should be given as early as possible, since it has no effect once the tetanus toxin has been fixed to the cells in the nervous system. A dose of 50,000 units of tetanus antitoxin diluted in 300 cubic centimeters of saline should be given intravenously as soon as possible after the diagnosis, to neutralize the free toxin in the body. Thereafter, smaller doses, of about 5,000 to 10,000 units should be given daily subcutaneously, to ensure the neutralization of any further toxin that may be elaborated. If the wound is not completely healed it should be opened wide to ensure exposure to air.

Although the antibiotics are of no value in counteracting the effects of tetanus toxin, they are nevertheless used for their possible effect on the tetanus bacillus and in the prevention of complications, such as pneumonia. Penicillin is the antibiotic of choice.

Continued sedation is often necessary to prevent the patient from going off into convulsive attacks. The drugs most commonly used are phenobarbital by mouth, Avertin by rectum, or Sodium Amytal intramuscularly or intravenously.

Diet

Feeding the patient is difficult because the neck muscles are rigid and the patient is unable to open his mouth. Between spasms, high-calory protein and carbohydrate fluids should be fed to the patient through a glass drinking tube with tip adequately protected by a small piece of rubber tubing. The fluid intake and output should be measured.

If the patient has difficulty in swallowing or is unconscious, oral feeding is discontinued. Fluids in the form of 5 per cent glucose are given intravenously. If the patient becomes very restless or the treatment induces spasms, it is discontinued.

As soon as convulsions diminish in severity and frequency, a high-calory soft diet is fed to the patient and is increased to a full diet when convalescence begins.

Supportive Nursing Care

Skilled nursing is essential in the management of patient care. As the patient is usually hypersensitive and reacts readily to any stimulus, noise and unnecessary movements by the nurse should be avoided. The room should be dimmed and have a minimum amount of furniture. The temperature of the room should be kept warm and constant. Bed covering should be light and easily adjustable. When convulsions occur, a padded tongue depressor should be placed between the teeth to prevent the patient from swallowing or biting his tongue. A suction apparatus should be available to remove secretions from the pharynx, and a tracheotomy tray should be available near by for an emergency. The patient should be carefully watched, and unusual symptoms, such as spasms, convulsions, cyanosis, and respiratory difficulty, should be noted by the nurse and reported immediately to the physician.

The position of the patient should be changed frequently to prevent pulmonary complications. The care of the mouth is important; it needs frequent cleansing with antiseptic mouthwash.

The public health nurse should be familiar with the prevention of tetanus. Children in rural areas and those going to camps should be protected against tetanus and should be referred to their physician for tetanus toxoid.

REFERENCES

1. Bruce, D.: "Analysis of 1,458 Cases which Occurred in Home Military Hospitals during the Years 1914–1918," *J. Hyg.*, **19**:1, 1920.

2. Caviness, V. S.: "Treatment of Tetanus," *North Carolina M. J.*, **4**:6, 1943.
3. Dietrich, H. F.: "Tetanus in Children," *Am. J. Dis. Child.*, **59**:693, 1940.
4. Firor, W. M.: "Treatment and Prevention of Tetanus," *Surg. Gynec. & Obst.*, **75**:185, 1942.
5. Harris, I., and Shapiro, S. K.: "Tetanus—A Challenge to Nursing," *Am. J. Nursing*, **50**:362, 1950.
6. Long, A. P.: "Tetanus Toxoid. Its Use in the U.S. Army," *Am. J. Pub. Health*, **33**:53, 1943.
7. Long, A. P., and Sartwell, P. E.: "Tetanus in U.S. Army in World War II," *Bull. U.S. Army M. Dept.*, **7**:371, 1947.

Chapter 51 TRACHOMA

GENERAL DESCRIPTION

TRACHOMA is an infectious eye disease caused by a virus of the psittacosis-lymphogranuloma group and characterized by a granular conjunctivitis and inflammation of the cornea, leading to scarring.

THE CAUSATIVE AGENT

The causative agent is a large virus of the psittacosis-lymphogranuloma venereum group which is found in the epithelium of the cornea and conjunctiva, and takes a basophilic stain. Inclusion bodies, consisting of groups of elementary bodies, are usually seen in cells, while elementary bodies can be seen free in the exudate. Both can be stained with Giemsa and are visible under a high-power microscope. The virus is readily destroyed by heat and drying but may be preserved in 50 per cent glycerin in a refrigerator. It cannot be cultivated in vitro, or in chick embryo, or in lower animals. Apes, baboons, and monkeys can be infected with the virus, causing a follicular conjunctivitis.

THE HOST

Symptoms

The incubation period is 5 to 12 days. The onset is acute, with inflammation of the conjuctiva, infiltration of the subepithelium, and papillary hypertrophy. The cornea becomes inflamed, the lids are swollen and the preauricular nodes become enlarged. There is a mucopurulent exudate from the eye. The acute stage lasts for several weeks and is followed by the subacute and chronic stages during which there is less discharge and the inflammatory symptoms gradually subside. The disease progresses slowly, with the formation of scars of the conjunctivae, pannus formation of the cornea, and deformity of the eyelids. Vision is reduced, often to a considerable extent. Bacterial infection may complicate the picture.

Diagnosis

The diagnosis is based on the clinical picture of follicles, pannus formation on cornea and cicatrices, and the finding of cytoplasmic inclusion bodies in scrapings from the conjunctiva and cytologic changes of the follicles, which show necrosis.

Immunity

Immunity to trachoma has not been shown. No methods are available for the active or passive immunization against the disease.

THE ENVIRONMENT

Trachoma is an old disease, having been recognized in ancient times. It is most prevalent in the Middle East, particularly in Egypt, where the majority of the population seems to be infected. It is widespread in the Orient but is also present in Europe and on the Western Continent. In this country it is most commonly found among the Indians and in some of the Middle Western and Southern states.

Its distribution is not dependent on climate or season but rather on poverty, crowding, and poor personal hygiene. All races and colors are susceptible. The acute stage is commonest in young children who obtain it from their mothers. Transmission is probably by means of fingers or fomites which are contaminated with secretions from the eyes or nasal discharge. The fly has been incriminated as an intermediate agent. The disease is usually not contagious in the chronic stage unless there is a lighting up with a recurrence of discharge.

Control

The basis of control of the disease is improvement in social conditions, better housing, less crowding, and careful personal hygiene. Cases should be discovered early and promptly treated. In endemic areas the regular examination of the eyes of school children should be made, and those infected should be isolated and treated. The use of common handkerchiefs and toilet articles should be prohibited. Patients should be instructed in the need of meticulous care in personal hygiene.

Children with trachoma in the acute stage should be excluded from school. Home visits by the public health nurse may be necessary to instruct the family in management of nursing care and in treatment.

The patient should be taught to wash his hands thoroughly each time there is contact with eye discharges. Paper tissues should be used and either disposed of in a flush toilet or collected in a paper bag for incineration.

Patients with trachoma should sleep alone. They should not use common towels or washcloths. Washbasins should be thoroughly cleaned after use.

MEDICAL CARE PLANS

Treatment

The sulfonamides are effective in the early treatment of trachoma. Cures have been reported in a few weeks. In the chronic stage when scars have formed and deformities of the lids are present, surgery has to be resorted to for relief.

Diet

A basic diet containing all nutrients is recommended.

Supportive Nursing Care

In endemic areas the nurse in the school program and the public health nurse in a community agency participate in eye surveys for case finding of trachoma. Home visits are made to instruct the family in nursing care procedures, measures for prevention of spread, and eye conservation. Family contacts to a case should be referred for examination and early treatment.

Inclusion Conjunctivitis

This disease, also known as inclusion blennorrhea and swimming-pool conjunctivitis, is a benign form of conjunctivitis often seen in newborn infants but also seen in adults, especially bathers in certain swimming pools. In the acute stage the disease resembles trachoma; however, pannus and cicatrization do not develop, and the disease does not go on to a chronic stage, although months may elapse before a complete cure results.

Scrapings of the cunjunctiva, when examined under the microscope, show inclusion bodies similar to those in trachoma. Expressed follicles have the same histologic picture as in trachoma but show no evidence of necrosis. Apes and baboons can be infected as in trachoma, and, as in that disease, they show a follicular conjunctivitis.

The infection also occurs in the genital tract of the female and in the male urethra. Infection in newborn infants is believed to occur during birth from contact with an infected vaginal tract. Adult infections of the eyes probably also result from accidental contact with genito-urinary discharge. Water in a swimming pool may act as the medium by which urethral or vaginal discharges reach the eyes. Proper chlorination of the water destroys the virus.

The virus of inclusion conjunctivitis does not differ in structure or cultural characteristics from that of trachoma. There is a theory that the two viruses were originally identical but that, as a result of prolonged infection of the genito-urinary tract, the former has changed its virulence. The diagnosis in newborns is easy, since trachoma does not occur at that early age. In older children and adults the diagnosis rests on the clinical picture, which is different in the two diseases, and on the cytologic difference of expressed follicles, which show no necrosis in inclusion conjunctivitis.

Control

The control of the disease consists of treating cases, as soon as discovered, with a sulfonamide. In newborn infants a 5 per cent sulfadiazine ointment is effective. Swimming pools should be properly chlorinated. Newborn infants with the disease should be isolated, and proper precautions should be taken by nurses to prevent transmission of the disease to others. The mothers of infected infants should be examined and, if virus is found, should be treated with sulfadiazine.

REFERENCES

1. Berens, C.: *The Eye and Its Diseases*, W. B. Saunders Company, Philadelphia, 1949.
2. Foote, F. N.: "Progress in Meeting the Eye Problems of Children," *Am. J. Pub. Health*, 40:313, 1950.
3. Forster, W. G., and Gibony, J. R.: "Trachoma," *Am. J. Ophth.*, 27:1107, 1944.
4. Howard, W. A.: "Inclusion Blennorrhea," *J. Pediat.*, 12:139, 1938.
5. Juliavelle, A.: *The Etiology of Trachoma*, Commonwealth Fund, Harvard University Press, Cambridge, Mass., 1938.
6. Siniscal, A.: "Trachoma—Blight on Mankind," *National Parent-Teacher*, 44:7, 1950.
7. Smith, J. E.; Julianette, L. A.; and Gamet, J. H.: "Sulfonamide Therapy of Trachoma," *Am. J. Ophth.*, 24:172, 1941.
8. Thygeson, P.: "Etiology of Inclusion Blennorrhea," *Am. J. Ophth.*, 17:1019, 1934.

Chapter 52 VENEREAL DISEASES

THE venereal diseases most commonly seen in this country are syphilis, gonorrhea, lymphogranuloma, granuloma inguinale, and chancroid. Although these diseases vary in their etiology and clinical manifestations, they are united by their manner of spread, which is chiefly through sexual contact. The procedures used in their control are, therefore, similar.

Syphilis is by far the most important of them because of its wide distribution, its chronicity, the seriousness of the lesions it causes, and the deaths and disabilities resulting from it. Organized efforts to control the venereal diseases suffered in the past on account of the social and moral stigmas attached to them and because of the reluctance of people to discuss them publicly or even to mention the terms in public print. Happily, the efforts of public health workers have convinced the public that effective control can be brought about only by frank discussion of the problem, by carrying on an educational program, especially among young people, by organizing facilities for diagnosis and treatment in order to lessen the rate of infection, and by an active case-finding program.

In past years, the program suffered from the fact that treatment was long drawn out, unpleasant, and expensive. Also, it was often an economic hardship because it took the patient away from his usual employment. As a result, lapses in treatment occurred, and late effects of some of the diseases were common. The introduction of penicillin has made a revolutionary change in the treatment of syphilis and of gonorrhea. The latter can now be cured with one or two treatments; the former, with treatment extending over a period of 2 weeks. The patient is ambulant and can continue at his usual work. The result is that many more infected individuals complete the treatment, and a considerable number of those who do not finish receive a sufficient amount of penicillin in the beginning to render them noninfectious. Syphilis has joined the other communicable diseases in the downward path of incidence and prevalence.

In the following pages the diseases are discussed individually. The program for control and for nurse participation is given in detail in the section on syphilis (pages 449–453) and applies equally to the other venereal diseases.

Chancroid

GENERAL DESCRIPTION

Chancroid is an acute disease of the external genital organs characterized by an ulcer commonly spoken of as a "soft chancre."

THE CAUSATIVE AGENT

The cause of the infection is the *Hemophilus ducreyi*. It is a small, gram-negative bacillus, which tends to grow in chains. It does not grow well on ordinary mediums but can be cultured on defibrinated rabbit's blood or on blood agar. It stains irregularly. It is best demonstrated by the Unna-Pappenheim stain.

THE HOST

Symptoms

The incubation period is 3 to 5 days. The lesion begins as a papule, which softens and becomes pustular. The pustule ruptures, and an ulcer forms; it is raggedy and the edges are soft, unlike the indurated edges of a syphilitic chancre. The regional glands are usually enlarged and may become purulent.

The lesion is usually present on the genitals. However, as a result of contact with such a lesion, chancroids may appear on other parts of the body. The ulcers are single as a rule, but they may be multiple and may be of various sizes and shapes. There is usually swelling of the adjacent tissues.

Diagnosis

Experienced clinicians usually make the diagnosis on clinical grounds. One should always rule out syphilis. Since the incubation period of the latter is longer, the patient should be kept under observation, and a Wassermann test should be taken immediately and after 3 months. Chancroid and syphilis may occur in the same individual as a result of one exposure. The syphilitic chancre may not appear until after the ulcer of chancroid has healed.

There are several laboratory aids in diagnosis:

Examination of smears. Smears from the ulcer should be examined for *Hemophilus ducreyi*.

Cultures from the ulcer. These are usually unsatisfactory, owing to overgrowth of contaminants. However, if pus can be aspirated from a regional gland, it is satisfactory for culture.

Skin test. The Ito-Reenstierna reaction or Ducrey skin test consists of the intradermal injection of 0.1 cubic centimeter of Ducrey

bacillus vaccine. It is read in 48 hours. A positive reaction is indicated if there are induration and redness in an area of at least 7
millimeters. The test is usually not positive until about 2 weeks
after the appearance of the lesion. The test continues positive after
healing of the lesion, so that positivity may be due to a previous
infection.

Auto-inoculation. This consists in rubbing some of the material
obtained from the lesion into a scarified area of the skin. In a few
days a chancroidal lesion will appear. Scrapings from this lesion
will usually give a positive smear.

Immunity

There is general susceptibility to the disease. One attack does not
confer immunity.

THE ENVIRONMENT

Chancroid was first recognized as a specific disease in 1889. However, it is frequently confused with some of the other venereal
diseases. It occurs in all climates and seasons, and among all races
and both sexes. It is a venereal disease predominantly, but is easily
transmitted by other than sexual contact. It is common in individuals who are sexually promiscuous and is therefore more frequent in
males than females. It is especially prevalent in such individuals if
their standards of personal hygiene are low. For this reason it is
more common in individuals of low-income groups.

Control

The prevention of this disease is part of the prevention of all
venereal diseases and includes rapid and adequate treatment,
epidemiological investigation of source cases and their treatment,
education of the public and repression of commercialized prostitu-
tion. Since the disease is largely one of uncleanliness, it is particularly important to teach adults the needs of personal hygiene.

MEDICAL CARE PLANS

Treatment

The treatment of choice is the use of sulfadiazine by mouth, 0.5
gram, four times a day for 10 days. Previous to the introduction of
this drug, treatment was a long-drawn-out affair, unpleasant both
for patient and doctor. The use of sulfonamides clears up most
infections in a few days. Aureomycin, Terramycin, and streptomycin
have been used in some cases, and reports indicate that these
drugs are as effective as sulfadiazine. Local treatment may help in

the patient's comfort. It consists of wet dressings for the inflamed and edematous tissues. If the inguinal glands have softened, they should be aspirated but not incised.

Gonorrhea

GENERAL DESCRIPTION

Gonorrhea is a venereal disease caused by the gonococcus and characterized by a purulent urethal discharge in the male and a mucopurulent cervical discharge in the female.

THE CAUSATIVE AGENT

The *Neisseria gonorrhoeae* is a gram-negative coccus which can be recovered from the exudate of gonorrheal infections. It appears as a bean-shaped diplococcus, the flattened sides approximating. It does not form spores or capsules and is not motile. It grows best on special mediums in an atmosphere of 8 to 10 per cent CO_2. It is destroyed by heat, drying, sunlight, ultraviolet light, and the usual disinfectants. It is readily destroyed by penicillin and is also susceptible to the sulfonamides and to streptomycin. Gonorrhea occurs in nature in humans only. Animals cannot be infected with the gonococcus.

THE HOST

Symptoms

The incubation period is 3 to 5 days. In men the onset is usually sudden, with an inflammation of the anterior urethra, which causes pain and burning on urination and a purulent discharge. The inflammation tends to progress backward, involving the posterior urethra, prostate, seminal vesicles, and epididymis. If untreated, it has a chronic course. In women, there is chiefly an involvement of the cervical canal of the uterus, causing a mucopurulent discharge. The infection may progress backward and involve the fallopian tubes, causing an abscess which may give pain, simulating appendicitis, and which may lead to sterility.

Occasionally, the gonococcus will gain entrance to the blood stream and be disseminated to other organs. It may cause valvular endocarditis or arthritis. In newborn infants an inflammation of the eyes, known as "ophthalmia neonatorum," may result from contact of the eyes with gonorrheal material either in passage through the birth canal or as a result of improper hygiene. If not treated, this may result in destruction of the eye structures and blindness.

In female children the inflammation of the urogenital tract is chiefly in the vulva and vagina, causing a vulvovaginitis with purulent discharge.

Diagnosis

The gonococcus is found without difficulty in the discharges of acute cases and is usually present in the pus cells. Although a nonspecific urethritis may occur in males, it is usually not so severe as gonorrhea, and the gonococcus cannot be recovered by smear or culture. The organism is not readily obtained by smear from subacute or chronic cases or from cervical smears. Better results are obtained from cultures of exudate.

Immunity

An attack of gonorrhea does not confer immunity. Antibodies in the blood are not found in significant titers. There is no method of active or passive immunization.

THE ENVIRONMENT

References to gonorrhea are found in ancient texts, but the term was used by Galen in A.D. 130. In the Middle Ages it was confused with syphilis. The organism was first identified by Neisser in 1879.

Gonorrhea has a world-wide distribution and occurs at all seasons of the year and in all climates. There is no racial immunity. Its spread depends on promiscuous sexual contact. Its incidence is greatest where economic conditions are poor, where crowding is marked, where ethical and educational standards are low, and where a community has a poor health program. All ages and colors and both sexes are susceptible to the disease, but, because of the nature of its spread, its greatest prevalence is in young adults. Spread by infected fomites may occur but is rare.

Control

The general principles that apply to the control of syphilis apply also to the control of gonorrhea and are discussed under Syphilis, page 449. Early treatment of cases of gonorrhea undoubtedly reduce the infective reservoir. Since syphilis and gonorrhea may be contracted at the same time, or shortly before or after each other, it is important for every physician who treats a case of gonorrhea to take a Wassermann test before beginning treatment and to repeat it once a month for 4 months.

In former years it was customary to take vaginal smears of all girls admitted to institutions or hospitals. This cluttered up the admitting wards and frequently caused delay in treatment of a sick child with a suspicious smear. The taking of such routine smears should be discouraged. If a child has a vaginal discharge, she should be admitted and isolated pending bacteriological examination of a smear. If this is negative, precautions should be removed. If it is positive, the child should be treated with penicillin.

Medical Care Plans

Treatment

Previous to the introduction of antibiotics the treatment of gonorrhea was a protracted and unpleasant experience, and chronicity was common. At present the treatment of choice is penicillin given in one injection of 300,000 units of procaine penicillin G in oil, with 2 per cent aluminum monostearate, which cures about 95 per cent of all cases. The rest require an additonal dose. The criteria for cure are a negative urethral smear and culture. If there is no discharge, the prostate is massaged, and a smear and culture for gonococci are made from the fluid expressed. In women, a smear and culture are made from the urethra and cervix. Complications are uncommon nowadays. Gonorrheal ophthalmia and vulvovaginitis, if they do occur, are also treated with penicillin. The broad-spectrum antibiotics may also be used in treatment.

Granuloma Inguinale

General Description

Granuloma inguinale is a venereal disease characterized by a chronic granulomatous infection of the skin.

The Causative Agent

The causative agent is said to be the Donovan body. This is an ovoid body consisting of one or two coccoid or bacillary forms surrounded by a capsule. Donovan bodies are found in smears from the granulating skin lesions both inside and outside of mononuclear cells. They are gram-negative and stain best with Wright or Romanowsky stains. They have not been cultured in ordinary culture mediums, nor has the disease been transmitted to animals. There are reports of their successful growth in the yolk sac of developing chick embryos and in artificial tissue culture. Donovan bodies are considered to be the etiologic agent of the disease because of ʾhe constant association of the two, but the nature of the bodies is still a matter of dispute.

The Host

Symptoms

The incubation period varies from a few days to several months. The disease begins as a papule or nodule which is soft and reddish in color. As a result of rubbing and maceration, it develops into a granulomatous lesion which is soft, bleeds easily, and ulcerates, and which spreads by contiguity. The disease tends to be chronic and, if untreated, may continue for months or years. Secondary infection may occur, and as a result ulceration and necrosis may cause extensive destruction of tissue.

Scarring frequently results, but islands of actively progressive disease may be present in the scars. The granulomatous lesions may be hypertrophic and resemble keloids. Enlargement of glands is characteristically absent and is one of the diagnostic differentiations from lymphogranuloma venereum.

Diagnosis

The diagnosis is made by the appearance of the lesion, the absence of lymphadenopathy, and the presence of Donovan bodies in scrapings from granulations.

Immunity

There is no method of active or passive immunization.

The Environment

The disease is prevalent in all parts of the world and attacks all races and ages and both sexes. It is particularly widespread in tropical and semitropical countries. It is seen most commonly in persons of young adult or middle age and in those who are sexually promiscuous and whose habits are not clean. In this country it is more common in Negroes than in whites and in men than in women.

Control

This is similar to that of the other venereal diseases and is discussed under Syphilis, page 449.

Medical Care Plans

Treatment

Treatment in former years consisted in the use of antimony compounds. With the introduction of the antibiotics, these have replaced other forms of therapy. Streptomycin has been the drug of choice. It is given in a daily amount of 4 grams in divided doses for a period of 5 to 10 days. Since the advent of the broad-spectrum antibiotics, they have been used either alone or in combination with streptomycin with favorable results. The largest experience has been with Aureomycin. Relapses with the use of antibiotics occur in about 10 per cent of cases. Most of these respond to a second course of treatment. Aureomycin, Terramycin, and chloramphenicol may be used instead of streptomycin, in the same dose as for lymphogranuloma venereum.

Lymphogranuloma Venereum (Lymphogranuloma Inguinale)

GENERAL DESCRIPTION

Lymphogranuloma venereum is an infectious venereal disease characterized by an initial lesion on the genitalia and inflammation of the regional lymph glands, usually resulting in suppuration.

THE CAUSATIVE AGENT

The disease is caused by a virus which can be isolated from the purulent lesions. It is closely related to the virus of psittacosis. Pus from the lesions contains inclusion bodies and elementary bodies similar to those of psittacosis. The disease can be transmitted experimentally to monkeys, guinea pigs, and mice. The virus can be propagated in the yolk sac of developing chick embryos. The virus remains active for a few days at 37° C. but loses its infectivity within 10 minutes at 56° C. It can be preserved for at least 1 year at a temperature of —70° C. The virus is destroyed by ultraviolet light within ½ hour and by Formalin within 24 to 48 hours.

THE HOST

Symptoms

The incubation period is 1 to 4 weeks. A primary lesion appears on the prepuce, glans, or shaft of the penis in the male and on the cervix, vaginal wall, or labia of the female. It may be a papule, vesicle, or small ulceration. The lesion is evanescent and frequently disappears without having been noticed. Soon the regional glands begin to enlarge. They are hard at first, and somewhat painful. There is considerable matting and adherence to the skin, which becomes red, edematous, and indurated. At this stage there often are constitutional symptoms of fever, malaise, and headache. Areas of softening appear in the mass. They rupture to the surface with discharge or seropurulent fluid. The discharge continues for weeks or months from sinuses that have formed and persist. When healing finally occurs, considerable scarring results.

In men the initial lesion usually drains into the inguinal glands. In some cases, and particularly in women, when the drainage of the infected area is to the perirectal glands, these become enlarged and purulent. As a result, proctitis and anal fistulas occur and, after healing, scarring and strictures of the rectum may result. Occasionally, the patient does not present himself until stricture has resulted, and a determination must then be made whether the stricture is due to lymphogranuloma venereum or to some other condition.

Diagnosis

A laboratory aid in diagnosis is the Frei test. This is a skin test originally performed with antigen obtained from pus of a case. The material is heated to destroy the virus and is properly standardized. It is injected intradermally in a dose of 0.1 cubic centimeter. In about 48 to 72 hours an indurated, red area, having a diameter of at least 0.5 centimeter with a small central necrotic zone, will be seen. This indicates infection but not necessarily recent infection.

The virus has been grown in mouse brain, and an antigen obtained from it has been used for the intradermal test. It is also possible to grow the virus in the developing chick embryo. An antigen obtained from such embryos, know as "Lygranum," may be used for the skin test. Lygranum may also be used as an antigen in the complement-fixation test with serum from the patient.

Immunity

Neutralizing and complement-fixing antibodies are present in the serum of patients with the disease and can be demonstrated by testing. There are no methods for active or passive immunization.

THE ENVIRONMENT

The disease is widespread throughout the world but is more common in the tropics. Males in young adult life are most often affected, probably because they are most active sexually. Like the other venereal diseases, it is most common among the poor, where there are crowding, lack of personal hygiene and education, and lack of stable home life. Since transmission is chiefly by sexual contact, the incidence is greatest in those areas where the incidence of syphilis is high. In the United States the Negro is more frequently infected than the white.

In men the commonest site of bubo formation is the inguinal region. This is due to the fact that lymphatic drainage of the glands and prepuce is by way of the inguinal glands. In females, only the anterior part of the vulva is drained by the inguinal glands. The posterior portion, much of the vagina, and the cervix drain into the perirectal and retroperitoneal glands. As a result, the anal and rectal lesions are commoner in women than in men.

As in syphilis, extragenital lesions may occur as a result of accidental inoculation or of irregular sexual practices. The progress of the lesions is the same as in cases where the infection is venereal, except that different glands are involved.

Control

The control of lymphogranuloma venereum is similar to that of syphilis and is discussed under that disease, page 449. In surveys, blood samples may be taken and tested for both syphilis and lymphogranuloma venereum by the complement-fixation method. The Frei test, which was discussed under Diagnosis, may be also used in surveys.

MEDICAL CARE PLANS

Treatment

No specific treatment was available prior to the introduction of the sulfonamides. Sulfadiazine in a dose of 4 grams a day appears to be effective in early cases if used for several weeks. Penicillin does not seem to affect the disease in any way. Since the introduction of Aureomycin, chloramphenicol, and Terramycin, these have supplanted the use of sulfadiazine. They give better results and in a shorter period of time. Aureomycin and Terramycin are given in a daily dose of 15 to 20 milligrams per kilogram of body weight, divided into four or six doses; chloramphenicol is given in a daily dose of 60 to 100 milligrams per kilogram, similarly divided, all for a period of about 2 weeks.

Nonspecific treatment consists of aspirating fluctuating buboes when they occur. Discharging sinuses and ulcerations should be cleaned, and a sterile dressing should be applied. If scarring has occurred and interferes with lymph circulation or if rectal strictures have resulted, surgery must follow.

Syphilis

GENERAL DESCRIPTION

Syphilis is a disease caused by the *Treponema pallidum* and characterized by the development of a chancre at the site of inoculation, followed by constitutional symptoms and skin lesions and by late manifestations of a variety of diseases, chief of which are those affecting the circulatory and nervous systems.

THE CAUSATIVE AGENT

Treponema is the generic term for one of a group of spiral organisms known as "Spirochaetaceae." The specific organism which is the cause of syphilis is *Treponema pallidum,* a motile, spiral organism with about 6 to 14 turns, which rotates on its long axis. It does not stain well with ordinary dyes but can be stained black in tissues with silver nitrate. In fresh specimens the *Treponema* is best seen by dark-field examination under the microscope.

The organism remains alive in vitro from a few hours to a day. It dies when dried. It may remain alive in blood stored in the refrigerator for 24 hours. It is readily destroyed by heat and the ordinary chemical disinfectants.

Treponema pallidum is not infectious in nature for any animal other than the human. It is prevalent in all parts of the globe. Infection may be induced artificially in the monkey and rabbit. Mice can be infected with the organism but show no symptoms of illness.

THE HOST

Syphilis is transmitted chiefly by sexual contact. In about 5 per cent of cases the infection is extragenital, being transmitted chiefly by contact with lesions in the mouth. Although the treponema can apparently penetrate mucous membranes, it does not penetrate intact skin.

Symptoms

The incubation period of syphilis is about 3 weeks. A hard, indurated papule, known as a "chancre," appears at the site of inoculation. This is usually some part of the external genitalia. However, extragenital chancres may occur on the lips, in the mouth, on fingers, breasts, or other parts of the body.

Often there is ulceration of the papule, so that on examination there appears to be an indolent ulcer covered with a membrane and exuding serum, the edges of which are firm and indurated. Sometimes the chancre begins as an erosion of the skin, which enlarges, exudes serum, and is indolent. Induration may not occur until a few days later. It is painless and causes no general symptoms. The regional lymph glands become enlarged and remain hard and discrete but not tender. This is known as the *primary* stage of syphilis. The chancre, whether treated or not, disappears ultimately, leaving a small scar.

After about 4 to 8 weeks from the appearance of the chancre, the *secondary* stage begins. This is manifested by constitutional symptoms of fever, headache, sore throat, loss of appetite, and a skin rash which is extremely varied in appearance. Occasionally, the symptoms of the secondary stage are so mild as to be overlooked. It is not possible, within the limits of this book, to describe the various skin manifestations. They may resemble almost any other skin disease. They are usually symmetrical and generalized, vary in color and configuration, and cause no subjective symptoms such as itching, burning, or pain. No part of the skin is immune to lesions. The lesions may be macular, papular, or pustular. They appear rapidly and usually attain their maximum development in about 2 weeks. If the patient is not treated, the rash lasts several weeks or months.

In areas of the body where two surfaces are apposed, the papules become flattened and moist. Such lesions occur often in the genital region, particularly near the anus, vulva, or scrotum. They are spoken of as "condylomas." In the perineal area they may become papillomatous or fungating growths, and their secretions are highly contagious. Similarly, in the mouth and on other mucous surfaces, the papules tend to become flattened and moist. They are pink or whitish and often covered with a film, and are known as "mucous patches."

During the secondary stage there is usually a generalized enlargement of the lymph glands. These do not attain a large size, but they are palpable and firm but not tender.

With the subsidence of the secondary stage the individual feels well and has no abnormal symptoms. The *tertiary* stage does not set in until several months or, more often, several years after this latent period. This stage consists in the development of glanulomatous lesions, known as "gummas," in different parts of the body. They are nodular, firm, circumscribed, and of varying sizes. They may break down and cause ulcerations, which heal slowly, causing considerable scarring. There are few parts of the body which may not be affected by the tertiary process. The commonest sites, or those most frequently called to the doctor's attention, are in the skin, bones, and circulatory and nervous systems.

In bones the tertiary lesions are chiefly periostitis or osteomyelitis. These may be symptomless or may cause pain and tenderness on pressure, or swelling. There is little fever, and there are few general symptoms. A joint lesion may occur, develop slowly, and end by causing considerable destruction. It is spoken of as the "Charcot joint."

The commonest lesion of the circulatory system is aortitis. This is an inflammation of the aorta, causing weakening of the walls of the vessel and often resulting in an aneurysm. When aortitis affects the first part of the aorta, it is frequently associated with a dilatation of the aortic ring, resulting in aortic regurgitation.

The nervous system is apparently invaded in most cases of early syphilis. However, late manifestations of neurosyphilis occur in only a fourth of all untreated cases. The lesions vary and give a variety of clinical symptoms, mimicking almost every kind of neurologic disease. Two that stand out especially are tabes dorsalis and paresis.

As already stated, tertiary lesions occur in other parts of the body, too. They cause symptoms similar to those produced by other granulomatous masses. It becomes imperative, therefore, to exclude syphilis when considering the diagnosis of almost any chronic disease.

Not all persons infected with syphilis develop tertiary lesions, although practically all have primary and secondary ones. About a quarter are cured spontaneously and another quarter do not show clinical symptoms, although they have a positive serology.

Congenital Syphilis. If a woman is infected with syphilis during or before pregnancy and is not treated, the child may be born dead or may be born alive but poorly developed, with evidence of skin lesions, snuffles, ulcerations of the lips, enlargement of the spleen and liver, and destruction of bone. The last of these can usually be demonstrated by X ray. Sometimes the child appears normal at birth but in a few weeks develops symptoms of rhinitis or snuffles, skin lesions, fissures at the angles of the mouth, enlarged spleen, and inflammation of the bones. If the child does not succumb, the lesions heal, as secondary lesions usually do, and the tertiary lesions may not occur until puberty. These resemble those in adults, but characteristic of the tertiary symptoms of congenital syphilis are (1) Hutchinson teeth, notched and peg-shaped upper incisors, (2) interstitial keratitis, a clouding of the cornea, (3) deafness, and (4) anterior bowing of the tibial bones.

Diagnosis

The diagnosis is made on the clinical examination. Confirmation by the laboratory in primary and in some secondary lesions consists in examining a drop of exudate obtained by scraping the lesions, under a dark-field microscope. The examiner should be acquainted with the structure of *Treponema pallidum* since other treponemas and spirochetes resemble it. The serologic diagnosis depends on the demonstration of antibodies in the blood by the complement-fixation or the flocculation tests.

The complement-fixation test for syphilis is known generally as the Wassermann test. Several modifications are also used. The test was originally made with syphilitic antigen and serum from the suspected individual. A positive test indicates the presence of syphilis. In actual practice, an extract of mammalian lipids is used as antigen. Why such an antigen should fix complement in syphilitic persons and not in normal ones is not quite clear. The fact, is, however, that it does.

The flocculation test is performed by mixing a similar antigen with the suspected serum in proper dilutions. If the serum comes from a syphilitic person, a precipitate or flocculate forms in the tube. Examples of flocculation tests for syphilis are the Kahn, Kline, Mazzini, V.D.R.L. (Venereal Disease Research Laboratory), and Hinton tests. The flocculation test takes much less time and trouble to perform than the complement-fixation test, but it is much more sensitive, and more false positives are obtained. In the New York City Department of Health a flocculation test is used as a screening test. All negative serums are so reported. Positive serums are confirmed by a Wassermann and a V.D.R.L. test.

There are several nonsyphilitic diseases which occasionally give a false positive flocculation or Wassermann test. Examples are malaria and leprosy. It is therefore necessary to correlate a positive result with the clinical findings. Several laboratories are co-operating in research to develop a serologic test which will be specific for syphilis.

Immunity

An infection with syphilis appears to confer immunity against further infection. However, if the infected individual is treated in the early stage and cured, reinfection may occur. There is evidence that the development of antibodies in the serum of the infected person plays a part in the resistance to further infection. There is no known method of immunizing any individual either actively or passively against the disease.

THE ENVIRONMENT

Syphilis appeared in Europe in epidemic form at the end of the fifteenth century. There is a great deal of discussion among medical historians as to whether the disease was imported into Europe from America by Columbus' returning sailors or whether it had existed there before the return of Columbus. In the early sixteenth century syphilis spread in Europe with great rapidity; many cases were apparently transmitted without sexual contact. The French called it the Neapolitan disease and the Italians called it the French disease. It was at first treated with the use of purgatives, but mercury soon became the drug of choice and was used widely.

For many years syphilis was confused with other venereal diseases, particularly gonorrhea. Discussions were widespread and heated on the unitary and dualist doctrines. Ricord (1800–1889) proved that pus from a case of gonorrhea could not cause syphilis and thus indicated the specific nature of the disease. He also divided its course into the three stages which are still applicable today. In 1905 Schaudinn discovered the *Treponema pallidum* and established the etiologic cause of syphilis.

The spread of syphilis does not depend on climate or season. It does occur more commonly in the poorer, more crowded, and less educated groups than in those more favored. Its extent is difficult to determine even in America, since it is still clouded in considerable secrecy, and reporting is inadequate. An opportunity presented itself to determine the prevalence of syphilis among young adults during the period of induction in World War II, when a Wassermann test was performed on each inductee. Of the first 2 million men between the ages of 21 and 35 tested, the over-all rate was 4.8 per cent. It was 2.4 per cent in whites and 27.2 per cent in Negroes. The rate varied tremendously in the different states, from a low of 0.7 per cent in New Hampshire to a high of 17.2 per cent in Mississippi. Syphilis is more common in men than in women owing to the more sheltered lives of the latter. Because it is transmitted chiefly by sexual contact, the incidence is highest in young adults. There is no race or color immune to the disease. Its higher prevalence in some racial groups is due chiefly to the lower economic and educational level of those groups.

The disease is most contagious in the primary and secondary stages. Untreated patients remain potentially infectious for several years after the initial lesion, but patients in the tertiary stage rarely transmit the disease.

Control

For many years the disease has been vigorously attacked in the United States by public health agencies. The control program varies in different communities. Essentially, however, the methods are similar. They consist of (1) case finding, (2) early recognition of cases, (3) treatment of cases, and (4) health education.

Case finding has many facets. First is the attempt to trace the source and contacts of every early case. This is a difficult procedure requiring adequate personnel to question the patient and to do field work. It also requires that the investigators have patience, sympathy, and sound common sense. Since the disease is one that has a good deal of social stigma attached to it, a great deal of secrecy prevails, and it is not easy to break this down.

Other methods of case finding are surveys, by means of the serologic test, of large groups in industry, particularly among young and middle aged adults. These may be part of a multiphasic screening for several other diseases. The requirement of a serologic test for syphilis of all couples contemplating marriage and of every pregnant woman is another one of the case-finding methods.

The early recognition of cases is largely a matter concerning the doctor. He must be trained not to overlook suspicious lesions, to avail himself of consultation, if necessary, and to take a blood specimen for serologic testing in all questionable cases.

Effective treatment is, obviously, an important part of control. In previous years, when treatment was uncomfortable and long drawn out, lapses were common. Modern therapy with penicillin has simplified procedures, shortened the time of treatment, and offered a way of rendering the patient noninfectious in a short period of time.

Health education is as important a measure of control in this as in other communicable diseases. The message must be brought to infected individuals that hiding symptoms will only make their condition worse. Stress should be laid on the fact that syphilis is an infection which can be cured and an effort should be made to remove the stigma of the disease. Emphasis should be laid on the importance of clean living and on the importance of family life, and opportunities should be provided to young adults to engage in social and athletic events which are wholesome.

The question of prophylaxis involves so many extraneous questions in the realm of sociology and religion that it is difficult to discuss in a medical textbook. In previous years such prophylaxis consisted in cleansing the genitalia and applying a mercury ointment. Recent experiments indicate that penicillin in a dose of about 1.5 million units is effective prophylactically. Experiments are being carried on with the oral use of the newer antibiotics in both the prophylaxis and the cure of syphilis.

MEDICAL CARE PLANS

Treatment

For centuries it has been known that mercury is curative in syphilis. The difficulty with the drug is that it is toxic to body tissue. After considerable experimentation Ehrlich developed salvarsan, an arsenic product, which was used for a great many years. Various modifications of this drug were introduced later, and bismuth was added to the armamentarium. Treatment with all of these drugs had to be prolonged over a considerable period of time, and the drugs were toxic. With the discovery of the antibiotics the entire picture was changed. Penicillin is now the drug of choice. It is not toxic and can be given in large doses. In a comparatively short period of time, penicillin administered in adequate doses will cure about 90 per cent of early cases of syphilis. Pregnant syphilitic women treated with penicillin almost never give birth to syphilitic infants, and congenitally syphilitic children born to mothers who have not been treated can be cured in most instances with adequate doses of the antibiotic.

There is no uniform method of dosage. For primary, secondary, and latent syphilis and for syphilis during pregnancy, many clinics begin treatment with a dose of 4 cubic centimeters of procaine penicillin in oil with 2 per cent aluminum monostearate (1.2 million international units) given intramuscularly, and continue daily treatment with 2 cubic centimeters (600,000 units) for a period of 15 days. Some clinics double the dose for the first day, so that if the patient does not finish the course there will still be a probability that he has been rendered noninfectious.

In cardiovascular syphilis and neurosyphilis the venereal disease clinics of the New York City Department of Health begin treatment with a weekly injection of 2 cubic centimeters bismuth salicylate in oil for 3 or more weeks prior to penicillin treatment. The latter is then given in an intramuscular injection of 2 cubic centimeters of procaine penicillin (600,000 units) every other day until 20 injections have been given.

In congenital syphilis an injection of 1 to 2 cubic centimeters (300,000 to 600,000 units) of procaine penicillin, depending on the baby's weight, is given daily, intramuscularly, for 15 days.

The dosage methods used render most cases of syphilis noninfectious and cure a large percentage of cases. Those not cured must be retreated. Investigations are in progress to determine the effectiveness of the newer antibiotics which can be administered orally.

Diet

There are no dietary restrictions.

Supportive Nursing Care

The simplicity of modern therapy for syphilis and the other venereal diseases has shortened the nurse-patient contact in the clinic and decreased the need for long-term follow-up of these patients in the home. However, the nursing responsibilities for case finding, education of the patient and family, and investigation of contacts are still basic concepts in a control program for venereal diseases and apply to all nurses whether in a hospital or in a public health agency.

The public health nurse in a generalized family program has an opportunity to discover undiagnosed cases, particularly in infants and expectant mothers, and to refer them for diagnosis. In instances where a case of syphilis has occurred in the family, she should instruct the family about the disease, allay their fears and worries as far as possible, and arrange for treatment. Frequently, there is need for giving assistance and guidance with other problems. The nurse should be especially concerned with recreational activities for the adolescent members of the family. She should be familiar with community facilities for recreation and utilize every opportunity to promote wholesome patterns of family living.

In industry the nurse may be helpful in interpreting to management the newer concepts in treatment and the importance of retaining the worker as long as treatment is continued.

The nurse in the school program should be alert in recognizing suspicious symptoms of congenital syphilis and arrange for follow-up conferences with a parent either in school or by visiting the home. In working with students in the older age group, she should be prepared to give counseling and guidance to those who request help with sex problems. This is important psychologically as well as in the prophylaxis of venereal diseases.

Case Finding. This is the most fundamental factor in venereal-disease control. The undiscovered case constitutes a constant source of infection in a community. The nurse needs to have an understanding of the prevalence and incidence of the disease as well as an understanding of people, their mores, and the community resources. Her approach, skill, and objectiveness in interviewing patients determine her effectiveness in finding infectious cases and in obtaining information about exposure and contacts.

Education of the Patient. The initial interview with a patient coming to the clinic for diagnosis and the conference following physical examination determine to a great extent the co-operation of the patient. The interpretive interview should be patient-centered and should be directed toward helping the patient to accept syphilis as an illness. It involves an explanation of the disease, treatment, and the importance of clinic attendance. The nurse should solicit the aid of the patient in controlling the spread of infection by explaining the precautions to be taken and obtaining accurate information about his contacts. The instructions given by the physician should be interpreted and supplemented by appropriate literature.

The nurse should stress the confidential nature of this interview and should encourage the patient to communicate his feelings freely. She should try to understand his social behavior, taking note of essential points which may need to be pursued by further questioning. Every effort should be made to have the patient assume responsibility for examination of contacts. The need for this procedure should be carefully explained and supported with valid reasons. The nurse should be prepared to give guidance as to the best approach and make the necessary arrangements for diagnostic screening. Since feelings of guilt are often increased when the family is involved, all barriers should be uncovered before giving specific instruction to the patient.

Investigation of Contacts. Home visits may be made by public health nurses or trained lay workers to persuade persons to report for a physical examination to their physician or to a treatment clinic. The nurse needs to be cautious and diplomatic in her approach if she is to succeed in finding the contact and in getting him under care. Ascertaining the identity of the contact is dependent upon the willingness of the patient to divulge accurate information concerning his contacts and on the methods that are employed in locating them.

Clinic Services. The quality of medical and nursing service influences the attitudes of patients regarding their disease and their regularity in keeping appointments. Operation and control on an appointment basis contribute to greater efficiency and aid in making provision for individual needs of patients.

The physical environment should be cheerful and friendly, and every courtesy should be accorded the patient on admission. For successful interviewing, separate rooms are essential for maintaining privacy and safeguarding the secrets of the patient. The waiting room should have current educational pamphlets and materials available for reading by patients.

Serological Tests. In some clinics nurses take blood specimens for serology. Sterile syringes, intravenous needles, and test tubes are required. The patient's arm is extended and is supported on a small table. The skin is cleansed with a cotton pledget saturated with alcohol 70 per cent. A rubber tourniquet is applied to the forearm, and the patient is instructed to clench his fist. The bracial vein is punctured with the needle and about 10 cubic centimeters of blood are withdrawn into the syringe. The tourniquet is then released, and an alcohol pledget is applied to the puncture with pressure as the needle is withdrawn. The patient is instructed to flex his arm. The blood is immediately transferred to the labeled sterile test tube and placed in a wire rack. The specimen is slightly slanted. It remains at room temperature for a brief period and is then transported to the laboratory.

When cisternal and lumbar punctures are employed, the nurse prepares the equipment and assists the physician. Rooms with cots

should be provided for the patient to rest on for at least 1 hour
before leaving the clinic.

REFERENCES

Chancroid

1. Greenwald, E.: "Chancroidal Infection," *J.A.M.A.*, **121**:9, 1943.
2. Kornblith, B. A.; Jacoby, A.; and Chargin, L.: "Chancroid," *J.A.M.A.*, **117**:2150, 1941.
3. Sullivan, M.: "Chancroid," *Am. J. Syph., Gonor. & Ven. Dis.*, **24**:482, 1940.

Gonorrhea

1. Heller, J. R., Jr.: "The Adequate Treatment of Gonorrhea," *J. Ven. Dis. Inform.*, **27**:225, 1946.
2. Jacoby, A., and Rosenthal, T.: "Revised Criteria of Cure in Gonorrhea," *Am. J. Syph., Gonor. & Ven. Dis.*, **34**:57, 1950.
3. Meads, M., and Finaldn, M.: "Penicillin in the Treatment of Gonorrheal Infections," *A. J. Syph., Gonor. & Ven. Dis.*, **30**:568, 1946.
4. Pelouze, P. S.: *Gonorrhea in the Male and Female*, 3d ed., W. B. Saunders Company, Philadelphia, 1944.

Granuloma Inguinale

1. Donovan, C.: "Ulcerating Granuloma of the Pudenda," *Indian M. Gaz.*, **40**:414, 1905.
2. Greenblatt, R. B.; Dienst, R. B.; Chen, C.; and West, R.: "Oral Aureomycin in the Therapy of Streptomycin-resistant Granuloma Inguinale," *South. M. J.*, **41**:1121, 1948.
3. Hill, L. M.; Wright, L. T.; Prigot, A.; and Logan, M. A.: "Aureomycin in Granuloma Inguinale," *J.A.M.A.*, **141**:1047, 1949.
4. Jacoby, A.; Rosenthal, T.; and Sobel, N.: "Ambulatory Treatment of Granuloma Inguinale with Streptomycin," *Am. J. Syph., Gonor. & Ven. Dis.*, **33**:76, 1949.
5. Thomas, W. L.: "A Clinical Study of Granuloma Inguinale with a Routine for the Diagnosis of Lesions of the Vulva," *Am. J. Obst. & Gynec.*, **61**:790, 1951.

Lymphogranuloma Venereum

1. Costello, M. J., and Cohen, J. A.: "Lymphogranuloma venereum," *Arch. Dermat. & Syph.*, **44**:391, 1941.
2. Coutts, W. E.: "Lymphogranuloma Venereum," *Bull. World Health Organization*, **2**:545, 1950.
3. Grace, A. W.: "Lymphogranuloma Venereum," *Bull. New York Acad. Med.*, **17**:627, 1941.
4. Grace, A. W.; Rake, G.; and Shaffer, M. F.: "New Material (Lygranum) for Performance of Frei Test for Lymphogranuloma Venereum," *Proc. Soc. Exper. Biol. & Med.*, **45**:259, 1940.
5. McKee, C. M.; Rake, G.; and Shaffer, M. F.: "Complement Fixation Test in Lymphogranuloma Venereum," *Proc. Soc. Exper. Biol. & Med.*, **44**:410, 1940.

Syphilis

1. Bauer, T. J., and Shortal, H.: "The Prevention of Congenital Syphilis," *Pub. Health Nursing,* **42**:81, 1950.
2. Bird, B.: "Social Hygiene—A Psychiatric Viewpoint," *J. Soc. Hyg.,* **35**:9, 1949.
3a. Morris, E. H.: *Public Health Nursing in Syphilis and Gonorrhea,* W. B. Saunders Company, Philadelphia, Chaps. 3, 4, 7, and 11, 1946.
3b. Nelson, Nels A.: "Modern Venereal Disease Control," *Am. J. Nursing,* **50**:75, 1950.
4. Rosenthal, T.: "The Modern Treatment of Venereal Disease," *Am. J. Nursing,* **49**:81, 1949.
5. Shortal, H.: "The Nurse and Family in Venereal Disease Control," *Pub. Health Nursing,* **38**:56, 1946.
6. Steiger, H. P., and Taylor, B. J.: "Venereal Disease Interviewing," *J. Ven. Dis. Inform.,* **28**:55, 1947.
7. Stokes, J. H.: "The Practitioner and the Antibiotic Age of Venereal Disease Control," *J. Ven. Dis. Inform.,* **31**:1, 1950.
8. Stokes, J. H., and Taylor, B. J.: *Dermatology and Venereology for Nurses,* 4th ed., W. B. Saunders Company, Philadelphia, 1948.
9. Thomas, E.: "Modern Treatment of Syphilis," *Bull. New York Acad. Med.,* **27**:175, 1951.

Chapter 53 YAWS (FRAMBESIA)

General Description

YAWS is a disease caused by *Treponema pertenue*, an organism closely resembling, if not identical with, *Treponema pallidum*, the cause of syphilis. The disease is common in tropical countries and chiefly affects children and young adults. It is not a venereal disease.

The Causative Agent

Although yaws has been recognized clinically for centuries, the organism responsible for the disease was first demonstrated by Castellani in 1905. It cannot be distinguished from *Treponema pallidum*. It is destroyed by drying, heat, and the common antiseptics. It has not been grown successfully in the test tube. Only man is infected in nature, but the organism can be passed in rabbits, producing characteristic lesions quite regularly.

The Host

Symptoms

The incubation period is not definitely known but is probably from about 3 weeks to 3 months. As in syphilis, there occurs a *primary* lesion. This consists of a papule, which soon changes into a vesicle and ruptures. Crusting results, and ulceration and secondary infection occur under the crust. The lesion enlarges and may reach a size of 1 to 2 inches in diameter. The lesion occurs most commonly on the lower extremities but may occur on any part of the skin. A previous break in the skin, such as an abrasion or burn, may determine the localization of the primary lesion. Unlike syphilis, it occurs only rarely on the genitalia. The regional lymph glands enlarge. The organisms causing the disease may be recovered from the edges of the primary lesion as well as from the lymph glands. They can be seen in a dark field, as in syphilis, or can be stained by the Fontana method, which is a silver-impregnation stain. After 3 to 4 weeks the Wassermann, as well as the various flocculation tests used in syphilis, becomes positive.

There are usually no constitutional symptoms. However, there may be a low-grade fever and joint pains, and the primary lesion itself may be painful. Untreated, the lesion may persist for weeks or even a few months and then subside, or it may subside before this. A small scar usually remains.

It will be noted that the primary lesion resembles that of syphilis, except that it does not usually occur on the genitals, is not transmitted by sexual contact, and is most commonly found in children.

Secondary lesions. After several months a rash appears on the body. This is macular. Some of these lesions disappear but others become papular. They increase in size, attaining a diameter of $\frac{1}{4}$ to $\frac{1}{2}$ inch. They are covered with a crust. If this is removed, the lesions are noted to be lobulated, reddish in color, and resembling a raspberry; hence the name frambesia. They occur on the skin all over the body as well as on mucous membranes. Where the skin is moist, lesions coalesce, forming condylomas as in syphilis. Where the skin is thick, as on the soles of the feet, the lesions form hard, calluslike plaques, known as crab yaws. Fissures and craterlike structures are seen in these plaques, and walking becomes difficult and painful. The second stage continues for weeks or months and may clear up even without treatment. This stage is very contagious, since organisms are present in the exudate beneath the crusts.

Tertiary lesions. If the disease is untreated it may go on to the tertiary stage. The lesions that result are gummas, as in syphilis. They are found chiefly in the bones and begin as a periostitis. The tibia is a common site, but other bones are also involved. The bone is destroyed, and deformities result. If the nasal bones are affected, a saddle nose or more marked deformity may result. Unlike syphilis, visceral and neural lesions are not common in the third stage.

Diagnosis

The diagnosis is made on the basis of the characteristic appearance of the lesions, on the finding of *Treponema pertenue* in the primary and secondary lesions, and on a positive serologic test.

Immunity

An attack confers immunity, so that reinfection does not occur while the disease is in progress. There is some evidence that immunity may last for many years even after recovery. There is also evidence that an attack of yaws confers a certain amount of immunity against syphilis, and that syphilis may confer a certain amount of immunity against yaws.

The Environment

Yaws is a widespread disease occurring on all the continents. In hot, humid climates it is readily communicable, affecting chiefly children. However, no age or race is immune, and males and females are both susceptible. Transmission is apparently by direct contact, though it appears that gnats or nonbiting flies may also play a part in spread. The disease is not venereal, and spread depends on close-ness of contact and lack of personal hygiene. It is not transmitted congenitally.

Although the origin of the disease is not definitely known, it is believed to have occurred first in the Mediterranean area and to have spread to the Americas with the slave trade. In the Western Hemisphere it is endemic in many parts of South and Central America and in the West Indian islands, but it does not occur in the United States or Canada.

Control

The control of the disease offers difficulties which are chiefly social and economic. In those areas where it is endemic and widely prevalent, the economic and sanitary conditions of the people are so low that any attempt at control by altering the environment and educating the people is so Herculean a task that it can be considered only in long-range plans. For the immediate control, an attempt at the elimination of the disease from the area by means of treat-ment must be considered. This is the plan adopted by the World Health Organization in its campaign to eliminate yaws in three demonstration areas—Haiti, Indonesia, and Thailand.

A survey group consisting of three nurses and a secretary goes to a village. By enlisting the aid of the headman, all the inhabitants are observed and diagnosed during a 2-day period, and the positive cases are registered. On the third day the rest of the team, consisting of a doctor and four nurses, arrives. The doctor confirms the diagnoses, and these are registered. The patients then proceed to the treatment room where injections of penicillin (procaine penicillin G in oil with 2 per cent aluminum monostearate) are given. Adults receive 4 cubic centimeters (1,200,000 units); children, 2 cubic centimeters (600,000 units), and infants, 1 cubic centimeter (300,000 units). A week after the first injection the team returns to give follow-up treatment and to administer penicillin to those patients who had been missed before.

In Indonesia it was possible to examine more than 80,000 persons, and to treat 15,000 per month by this method. By the two-dose method, about 97 per cent of those treated were cured or improved (two thirds cured, one third improved). By the use of a single-dose treatment schedule, about 95 per cent were cured or improved. For mass control this a highly satisfactory result.

Medical Care Plans

Treatment

The treatment of individual cases of yaws is similar to that of syphilis in the primary or secondary stages. An initial dose of 4 cubic centimeters (1,200,000 units) of penicillin G in oil with 2 per cent aluminum monostearate is given intramuscularly and is followed by daily treatments of 2 cubic centimeters (600,000 units) for 2 weeks. The use of the broad-spectrum antibiotics has not yet been sufficiently evaluated.

Diet

No dietary restrictions are necessary.

Supportive Nursing Care

In endemic areas, the nurse's responsibilities are similar to those in the care of syphilis in this country. In the individual case they are largely concerned with assistance in treatment and with education of the patient and his family. In mass control the public health nurse plays a very important part. Since large areas in primitive countries must be covered and since there is lack of medical personnel, the nurse must take on duties which are usually not assigned to her, such as screening for diagnosis and administering treatment. These are discussed under Control, page 458.

REFERENCES

1. Dwinelle, J. H.; Sheldon, A. J.; Rein, C. R.; and Sternberg, T. H.: "Evaluation of Penicillin in the Treatment of Yaws," *Am. J. Trop. Med.*, 27:633, 1947.
2. Kumm, H. W., and Turner, T. B.: "The Transmission of Yaws from Man to Rabbits by an Insect," *Am. J. Trop. Med.*, 16:245, 1936.
3. Simmons, J. T.; Whayne, T. F.; Anderson, G. W.; and Horack, H. M.: *Global Epidemiology*, J. B. Lippincott Company, Philadelphia, Vol. I, 1944, and Vol. II, 1951.
4. "Yaws Control in Indonesia," *Chronicle of the World Health Organization*, 5:249, 1951.

Chapter 54   DISEASES TRANSMITTED
BY ARTHROPODS

GENERAL CHARACTERISTICS

AN arthropod is an invertebrate animal with a segmented body in a firm integument, and with jointed limbs. The phylum Arthropoda is subdivided into classes, two of which are Insecta and Arachnida. Insects have their bodies divided into three regions—head, thorax and abdomen, while arachnids have their bodies divided into two regions—thorax and abdomen. Flies, mosquitoes, fleas, lice, and bugs are insects; ticks and mites are arachnids.

A vector is an organism (usually an arthropod) which carries and transmits microorganisms of disease. All arthropod vectors are blood-sucking. They are usually not made ill by the agent of disease which they harbor.

Manifestations of disease are usually systemic. The arthropod introduces the agent of the disease into the blood stream while biting, and a general infection results. Occasionally, the disease is localized at the point of inoculation, as in Oriental sore, or transmitted to a particular organ system, as in St. Louis encephalitis.

THE CAUSATIVE AGENT

Symptoms

The incubation period varies with the agent. Two incubation periods must be considered, one in the host (intrinsic) and one in the vector (extrinsic). The intrinsic incubation period varies with the causative agent and is given under the separate diseases. The extrinsic incubation period varies not only with the causative agents but also with the physical factors of temperature and humidity.

Viability

The organism does not go through a free-living phase, so that the viability depends on the viability of the host and vector.

Prevalence

This depends on the abundance of the agent and vector and on the number of susceptible hosts.

Reservoir

Since arthropod vectors live on animal blood, they infect the animal while taking a blood meal. The infected animal now acts as a reservoir of disease and, if bitten by a noninfected arthropod, will transmit the disease to it. The animal acting as the reservoir varies with the agent of disease. In some of the arthropod-borne diseases only one host exists, as in epidemic typhus; in others, a favored host is found, but if this host is unobtainable, the vectors adapt themselves to other hosts, as in malaria.

Life Cycle

In most of the arthropod-borne diseases the agent must go through a necessary stage of development in the arthropod. The occurrence of disease in the human depends on whether that cycle has occurred.

Pathogenicity

This differs with the agent of disease, although all are pathogenic. The agents of epidemic and of endemic typhus are closely related, yet the former causes a much severer disease than the latter. Even in the same disease different strains cause disease of different severity. In malaria, for instance, the disease caused by some strains of *Anopheles gambiense* is much worse than those caused by other strains.

THE HOST

Symptoms

These vary with the different agents and are described under the diseases.

Custom and Habits

Household sanitation plays a considerable part in transmission of arthropod-borne disease. Screening of windows keeps out many vectors. In the tropics it is a common practice to have a net around the bed so as to keep out any mosquitoes that may have got into the room. Mosquitoes breed in stagnant water, and it is important to keep the house and exterior free from puddles of water, uncovered rain barrels, pails, and cans into which rain water may settle. Rodents, which frequently act as reservoirs, are particularly difficult to keep out, and houses must be built properly to prevent their entry. Harborages must be eliminated.

Personal hygiene is also a factor. Flies and mosquitoes are attracted to clothes with recent stains of sirupy foods. Repellants, like citronella, keep mosquitoes away. Frequent bathing and change of clothes discourage lice. In epidemics of typhus, dusting the body with DDT will prevent lice from getting a foothold. In endemic tick areas, clothes that protect the legs and arms should be worn, particularly when working in brush. In the Orient soldiers were cautioned about sleeping on cots close to the ground, to avoid the bite of mites.

Recreational activities determine exposure to some extent. Mosquitoes are present only in places where there is opportunity for breeding, so that they are usually more abundant in the country than in urban communities. The number of trips taken to such places on picnics, vacations, etc., influences the opportunity for infection.

Defense Mechanisms

Individuals have varying sensitivity to the bite of an insect. The more sensitive the skin, the more apt the person is to kill the insect before it has bitten.

Constitutional factors play a small part in determining bites by insects. Age and sex may play a part merely because they may be factors in determining the role in certain occupations.

The carrier state exists in some arthropod-borne diseases and may be responsible for perpetuation of the disease in a certain locality. Persons infected with malaria may become chronic carriers of the disease. If a sufficient number moves into an area where the anopheles mosquito is prevalent, malaria may become an endemic disease although it had not existed there before.

Immunity

Immunity after recovery from disease caused by arthropod transmission varies. It is solid and permanent in some, as in yellow fever; less permanent in others, as in the typhus group of diseases; and only temporary in others, as in plague. In some of the diseases, as in typhus fever, a certain amount of cross immunity may result between different species, as between the epidemic and endemic types; in malaria, however, not only is there no cross immunity between different species, but two of them may infect an individual at the same time. Immunization procedures are available for some diseases, such as typhus and plague, but not for others, for example, malaria or dengue.

The Environment

Physical Environment

The geography of a country as well as its climate are very important determining factors in the survival and multiplication of arthropods. Mosquitoes require a certain amount of heat and moisture. They are most prevalent in hot, humid countries, as in the tropics, and hardly a problem in very cold countries. Even where they survive, indigenous strains may be kept from spreading by barriers like mountains or lakes. *Anopheles gambiense,* for instance, is common in Africa but not in Brazil. When it was introduced into that country it began to multiply and spread; and only by the use of heroic measures was it completely exterminated.

Social and Economic Environment

The economic status of the individual determines the type of housing he has and what protection it offers to arthropods. It also determines his occupation, which may expose him to certain types of arthropods. Woodcutters, for instance, may be exposed to infected wood ticks carrying Rocky Mountain spotted fever or to *Haemogogus* mosquitoes carrying yellow fever. The economic level of a community determines to a large extent the actions it will take in controlling animal reservoirs, like rats, and breeding places of arthropods. The procedures needed for such controls are usually expensive.

The density of the population determines the availability of susceptible hosts. However, the more people are crowded together in a community, the less opportunity for plant growth and moisture, which is needed by many arthropods. In the home, crowding frequently determines the opportunity for infestation with certain vectors, for instance, lice.

The social awareness of a community, the alertness of the governing group, and the level of education determine to a considerable extent the measures that will be taken to control the breeding of arthropods or the extermination of rodents. These measures require, however, the expenditure of money, often in large sums, and unless the community can afford it, projects cannot be undertaken unless outside assistance is obtained. An effective health department acts not only as a spearhead for such projects but as an important center for education and for initiation of treatment centers to cure those infected and provide prophylactic measures for those exposed.

Social upheavals are the great disrupters of health programs.

Wars come first in this category, followed closely by internal rebellions and natural catastrophes. Frequently, measures already taken are disrupted and destroyed, crowding is increased, sanitary standards are lowered, treatment is discontinued, and a program which offered possibilities of improvement is suspended. Add to this the migrations of people from and into the community, the loss of key personnel, and the importation of agents of disease and infected hosts and the picture is not a pretty one.

Biological Environment

The biological environment is more important in arthropod-borne diseases than in those transmitted in other ways. First, the vectors, themselves, must be present and be able to exist and multiply. The vectors concerned are as follows.

Mosquitoes. There are many genera and about 1,600 species. For transmission of diseases in humans, three genera are important: (1) *Anopheles,* (2) *Culex,* and (3) *Aedes.* All lay eggs but do not transmit the disease to them. The larvae and pupae are aquatic. Mosquitoes show discrimination in the selection of breeding sites, some requiring sun, others shade; some preferring clear water, others brackish water. They vary in flight range, most of them breeding near the sites where they feed, others flying considerable distances. Some survive ocean voyages or plane rides for several days. Those of medical importance have mouth parts adapted to piercing the skin and sucking blood. Some prefer to feed on humans, others on animals.

They respond to sound vibrations, and the use of this characteristic has been suggested by some observers for attracting mosquitoes to an electrically charged wire which would destroy them. They have a keen sense of smell and are repelled by odors like citronella.

Fertilization occurs after a blood meal, the male dying after copulation, the female surviving for 2 weeks to several months. Ovulation is dependent on a blood meal. Most eggs are laid in water, usually at night, although some are laid in mud. *Anopheles* and *Aedes* eggs are laid singly, *Culex* eggs are laid in rafts. Anopheline eggs have air sacs or floats, preventing them from sinking. *Aedes* eggs will sink if the surface of the water is disturbed, and *Culex* eggs will sink if separated from the float.

Hatching takes place in water, in from 24 to 96 hours, depending on the type of egg and the temperature. The larvae of anophelines lie parallel to the surface and just a little below and receive oxygen from the air through a pair of tracheal openings. The *Culex* and *Aedes* larvae are submerged at an angle to the surface and obtain air through a siphon tube. The larvae feed on plankton and organic debris. Usually, 10 days are needed for development into the pupal stage and another few days for the emergence of the adult mosquito. *Anopheles* adults rest at an oblique angle to the resting surface; *Culex* and *Aedes* adults rest with their bodies parallel to the resting surface and humped.

Lice. Lice are small, wingless insects, flattened from front to back. Those responsible for disease in man have mouths adapted to sucking blood, and legs provided with claws for clinging to hairs and fibers. They lay eggs which become cemented to hairs and body clothing. Normally, they spend their entire life on the host. When taking a blood meal, the louse inserts its teeth into the upper layers of the skin, inserts a stylet through the skin, deposits saliva in the wound, and draws blood into its pharynx. Eggs (nits) are laid within 1 or 2 days after fertilization and they are cemented to hairs or clothing. They hatch in 4 to 14 days. They feed, molt, and go through several stages and emerge as adults in 12 to 38 days after being laid as eggs. The adults live about 1 month, and the female lays from 150 to 300 eggs. They are easily transferred from one to another host of the same species. Human lice are of three types: (1) *Pediculus capitis,* or head louse, (2) *Pediculus corporis,* or body louse, and (3) *Phthirus pubis,* or crab louse. The body louse is the one chiefly concerned in the transmission of disease; the other two types cause irritations of the skin.

Fleas. Fleas are wingless, bloodsucking insects, with long hind legs adapted to jumping. After feeding on the host the fertilized female drops her eggs on the ground or floor, and they hatch, after a few days, into larvae. These feed on organic debris. The larva develops into a pupa in a period varying from 1 week to 3 months. From the pupal to the adult stage the period may be only 1 week or as long as 1 year. The adult usually survives 1 year or more. The flea most commonly involved in the transmission of human disease is *Xenopsylla cheopis* (the tropical rat flea). Fleas do not have transovarian passage of the agent.

Sand Flies. The bloodsucking sand flies belong in the genus *Phlebotomus.* They are small and humpbacked, with conspicuous black eyes and hairy bodies, wings, and legs. Only the females feed on blood, usually at night. By day the flies hide in dark places. In some species the female feeds once, lays eggs, and dies; in others she takes two or more blood meals, laying eggs after each. The eggs are laid in dark, moist places, and hatch after 9 to 12 days. The larvae look like worms. They feed on organic debris. They go through a pupal stage and emerge as adults after 30 to 40 days. Sand flies do not have a long flight range.

Ticks. Ticks are bloodsucking animals, covered with a hard shell. Oviposition occurs off the host, as many as several thousands eggs being laid at one time. The female usually dies after laying the eggs. The male dies after insemination. The larva, after hatching, obtains a blood meal from some host to which it has attached itself and then drops off. The larva molts to produce a nymph, which also feeds on a host and then drops off and becomes transformed into an adult. The complete development from egg to adult takes 1 to 2 years.

Mites. Mites are tiny acarids, often difficult to see with the naked eye. They have a soft shell. Some are colorless, while others, like chiggers, are colored red. Some, like the *Sarcoptes scabiei,* live in burrows in the skin of animals where the females lay eggs. The larvae develop in the skin and build other tunnels. They feed on the tissues of the host. Others, like *Liponyssus bacoti,* feed on blood and drop off their hosts after each meal. Still others, like *Trombidium akamushi,* feed on vegetables during the nymph and adult stage and on blood from a host during the larval stage. Transovarian transmission of disease usually occurs in ticks and mites.

Various considerations enter into the probability of transmission of disease by certain vectors. The environment must be suitable for the complete development of the vector. There must be proper breeding focuses and opportunities for the eggs to remain viable. The ability of the vector to fly or creep and the flight range are determining factors in the extent of the area that may be involved. The animal host needed by the vector for the blood meal must be available for the arthropod to survive. Finally, the transmission or failure to transmit of the causative agent transovarially is a factor to be considered in the opportunities for infection.

The fauna and flora must be favorable for the survival and multiplication of the vectors. Not only do these offer food, but they also offer shelter, needed by some arthropods, and moisture, which is needed by most.

Control

Methods of attack are directed against the adult arthropod as well as against the various stages of its development and the animal reservoir. Other tools used in control are education in personal hygiene, treatment of infected individuals, and prophylactic immunization. The method that is most effective in one disease need not necessarily be so in another; prophylactic immunization is quite effective in the control of yellow fever but not at all in malaria. Methods are frequently combined, as in epidemic typhus, where spraying with DDT, prophylactic immunization, and health education in personal hygiene are all carried on at the same time. Each problem has to be analyzed separately, and the methods best suited in the case must be applied. Most often a co-operative team, consisting of a doctor trained in epidemiology, a sanitary engineer, an entomologist, and a nurse, is needed. Plans can then be mapped out, and additional personnel can be added as needed.

Control of arthropods. Attacks on adult arthropods include the following procedures:

1. Destruction by hand, such as swatting mosquitoes or picking off ticks and destroying them
2. Screening of doors and windows; for small insects like sand flies, fine mesh must be used
3. Closing cracks and holes and openings around doors and windows
4. Using traps, such as impregnated or gummy paper to catch insects
5. Destroying them by poisons mixed with honey
6. Using repellants, like oil of citronella
7. Using DDT or other types of insecticide spray
8. Building the house beyond the flight range of the insect
9. Wearing clothes that are not penetrated by the arthropods

Attacks on breeding focuses are accomplished as follows:

1. Drainage and filling are used to do away with swamps where water is stagnant and where vegetation abounds
2. Impounded waters or reservoirs must be so constructed that they will not act as breeding places. Frequently an arrangement is made so that the water level can be alternately raised and lowered so as to discourage the growth of plants at the edges and kill ova that are caught above the water level. The addition of small fish life, such as minnows or guppies that feed on larvae, is frequently practiced
3. The removal of stagnant waters near the home such as in ruts, open cans, and rain barrels is a simple measure which offers high returns for the little work involved
4. Where other measures cannot be used to remove stagnant waters, or in addition to other measures, larvicides are frequently sprayed. The cheapest is petroleum oil which probably kills larvae by entering the trachea. Others are oil-pyrethrum mixtures, Paris green, and DDT powders. The latter two are frequently sprayed by low-flying airplanes. In the dilution used, neither is harmful to fish or man

Various naturalistic methods are used in control, such as altering flora to a kind that is objectionable to the insect, cutting down brush that harbor ticks or mites, agitating water in pools by introducing it from pipes above the surface, shading streams if the insect requires sunlight, introducing into water small fish that feed on larvae, and bringing into a community animals that are preferred to man by the insects.

Control of animal reservoir. In some diseases this is more effective than attempts to control the insects. It is particularly true in diseases like plague or endemic typhus, where the reservoir is a rodent. The various methods used against these animals, such as trapping, poisoning, protecting food sources adequately, and destroying rat harborages are frequently quite effective.

Treatment of patients. This is an important part of control, since patients and carriers act as effective reservoirs. The sooner they are treated and cured, the sooner will an active reservoir be eliminated.

Immunization. Prophylactic immunization is effective in only a few of the arthropod-borne diseases. These are chiefly viral and bacterial diseases. Effective methods have not yet been obtained for immunization against protozoan disease. An effective vaccine can be used in the prophylaxsis of yellow fever. Vaccines are available for horses in endemic areas of western equine encephalitis, and for man against epidemic typhus, Rocky Mountain spotted fever, and plague.

The diseases which are transmitted by arthropod vectors, their causative agents, and the arthropod involved are listed in the accompanying table.

Diseases Transmitted by Arthropods

A. *Transmitted by Mosquitoes*

DISEASE	CAUSATIVE AGENT	ARTHROPOD
1. Dengue	Virus	*Aedes aegypti*
2. Yellow fever	Virus	*Aedes aegypti*
		Haemagogus (jungle yellow fever)
3. Equine encephalitis	Virus	
a. Western		*Culex tarsalis*
b. Eastern		*Aedes*
4. St. Louis encephalitis	Virus	*Culex tarsalis*
5. Japanese B encephalitis	Virus	*Culex* (?)
6. Malaria	*Plasmodium vivax*	*Anopheles*
	Plasmodium malariae	
	Plasmodium falciparum	
	Plasmodium ovale	
7. Filariasis	*Wuchereria bancrofti*	*Culex, Aedes,* and *Anopheles*

B. *Transmitted by Flies*

DISEASE	CAUSATIVE AGENT	ARTHROPOD
1. Pappattaci fever (sand fly or phlebotomus fever)	Virus	*Phlebotomus papatasii*
2. Poliomyelitis	Virus	*Musca domestica* (?)
3. Typhoid fever	Salmonella typhi	*Musca domestica*
4. Bacillary dysentery	*Shigella*	*Musca domestica*
5. Bartonellosis (Oroya fever, verruga peruana, Carrión's disease)	*Bartonella bacilliformis*	*Phlebotomus* (sand fly)
6. Leishmaniasis (kala-azar) Leishmania tropica (Oriental sore)	*Leishmania donovani*	*Phlebotomus*
7. Trypanosomiasis (African sleeping sickness)	*Trypanosoma gambiense*	*Glossina palpalis* (tsetse fly)
8. Onchocerciasis	*Onchocerca volvulus*	*Simulium*

C. *Transmitted by Lice*

DISEASE	CAUSATIVE AGENT	ARTHROPOD
1. Epidemic typhus	*Rickettsia prowazeki*	*Pediculus corporis*
2. Pediculosis capitis	No agent of disease	*Pediculus capitis*
3. Pediculosis pubis	No agent of disease	*Phthirus pubis*
4. Trench fever	*Rickettsia* (?)	*Pediculus corporis*
5. Relapsing fever	*Borrelia recurrentis*	*Pediculus corporis*

D. *Transmitted by Fleas*

DISEASE	CAUSATIVE AGENT	ARTHROPOD
1. Murine typhus	*Rickettsia mooseri*	*Xenopsylla cheopis* (rat flea)
2. Plague	*Pasteurella pestis*	*Xenopsylla cheopis*

E. *Transmitted by Ticks*

DISEASE	CAUSATIVE AGENT	ARTHROPOD
1. Russian Far East Encephalitis (spring-summer encephalitis)	Virus	*Ixodes persulcatus*
2. Louping ill	Virus	*Ixodes ricinus*

DISEASE	CAUSATIVE AGENT	ARTHROPOD
3. Colorado tick fever	Virus	*Dermacentor andersoni*
4. Rocky Mountain spotted fever	*Rickettsia rickettsi*	*Dermacentor andersoni* *Dermacentor variabilis*
5. Boutonneuse fever	*Rickettsia conori*	*Rhipicephalus sanguineus*
6. Q fever	*Coxiella burnetii*	*Dermacentor andersoni* (?)
7. Tularemia	*Pasteurella tularensis*	*Dermacentor andersoni*
8. Relapsing fever	*Borrelia recurrentis* (spirochete)	*Ornithodorus*

F. *Transmitted by Mites*

DISEASE	CAUSATIVE AGENT	ARTHROPOD
1. Scrub typhus (tsutsugamushi fever)	*Rickettsia orientalis*	*Trombicula akamushi* *Trombicula deliensis*
2. Rickettsialpox	*Rickettsia akari*	*Allodermanyssus sanguineus*
3. Chiggers	No agent of disease	*Trombicula irritans*
4. Scabies	No agent of disease	*Sarcoptes scabei*

G. *Transmitted by Bugs*

DISEASE	CAUSATIVE AGENT	ARTHROPOD
1. Chagas' disease	*Trypanosoma cruzi*	*Triatoma* (kissing bug; assasin bug)
2. Bedbug bite	No agent of disease	*Cimex lectularius*

H. *Transmitted by Spiders*

DISEASE	CAUSATIVE AGENT	ARTHROPOD
1. Spider bite	Venom	*Latrodectus mactans* (black widow)

MEDICAL ASEPTIC TECHNIQUES

Gowns and Caps

Gowns and caps are essential in those diseases where close contact with the patient increases the danger of transmission of the vector to the nurse.

Concurrent Disinfection

Since the diseases under discussion are transmitted only through an intermediate arthropod, concurrent disinfection is concerned chiefly with care of the body of the patient and his linen to see that no disease-carrying vector remains alive. In those diseases where the vector remains on the body or linen of the patient, the patient should be disinfested as described on pages 493–494, and the linen should be adequately laundered before it is used by others. The windows of the room should be screened. In communities where there is difficulty in keeping out mosquitoes from the sickroom, the walls should be sprayed with an insecticide like DDT.

Terminal Disinfection

No special procedures are needed for terminal disinfection. The patient is bathed, his scalp and body are examined for parasites or ova, his linen is sent to the laundry, and his room is aired.

REFERENCES

1. Craig, C. K., and Faust, E. C.: *Clinical Parasitology*, 5th ed., Lea & Febiger, Philadelphia, 1951.
2. Harvey, W. C., and Hill, H.: *Insect Pests*, 2d ed., H. K. Lewis & Co., Ltd., London, 1947.
3. Herma, W. B., and Gray, H. F.: *Mosquito Control*, Commonwealth Fund, Harvard University Press, Cambridge, Mass., 1940.
4. Moulton, F. R.: *Human Malaria*, American Association for the Advancement of Science, Washington, D.C., 1941.
5. Ross, H. H.: *A Textbook of Entomology*, John Wiley & Sons, Inc., New York, 1948.
6. Simmons, J. S.; Whayne, T. F.; Anderson, G. W.; and Horaek, H. M.: *Global Epidemiology*, J. B. Lippincott Company, Philadelphia, 1944.
7. U.S. Department of Agriculture: "DDT and Other Insecticides and Repellants Developed for the Armed Forces," Miscellaneous Publication No. 606.

Chapter 55 DENGUE

GENERAL DESCRIPTION

DENGUE is an acute febrile disease, transmitted by infected mosquitoes and characterized by pain, fever, prostration, enlargement of the lymph glands, and a rash. The pain is sometimes quite severe, which explains the name of breakbone fever sometimes given to the disease.

THE CAUSATIVE AGENT

Dengue is caused by a small virus, approximately 12 to 25 millimicrons, and is transmited from man to man by a mosquito, *Aedes aegypti*. The virus can be recovered from the serum of patients by centrifugation and can be preserved by freezing at $-70°$ C. or by drying from the frozen state. Human blood remains infectious for several weeks if it is kept in an ordinary refrigerator. The virus is destroyed by ultraviolet light and by Formalin. In nature, only humans are infected, although certain species of monkeys may harbor inapparent infection. The virus can be grown in mice by intracerebral passage and has been grown in embryonated eggs after many passages in mice. It has also been grown in hamsters.

There appear to be more than one strain of dengue. At least two strains, the Hawaiian and the New Guinea C, are immunologically distinct, so that it is possible to be infected with dengue virus more than once. The probabilities are that infection with one strain confers partial immunity against other strains.

THE HOST

Symptoms

The incubation period may be from 3 to 15 days, although it is commonly 5 to 8 days. The onset is usually abrupt, with high fever, severe headache, pain in the eyeballs, and general pains in the muscles, joints, and back. Chilliness may also occur. The fever lasts 5 or 6 days and falls by crisis. Sometimes the temperature falls to normal during the middle of the febrile period; this causes the so-called "saddleback" type of fever curve. The pulse rises with

472

the fever, but toward the end of the acute period the pulse may be slow in comparison with the fever. A slow pulse may continue during convalescence. During the febrile period the patient has no appetite and may have abdominal discomfort. He has general malaise and may have sore throat or cough. Sweats are not uncommon. The lymph nodes are usually enlarged, but the spleen is not.

On the third to fifth day a rash appears, first on the chest, trunk, and abdomen, and then spreading to the extremities and the face. It is maculopapular or scarlatiniform in appearance and lasts a few days. It may be itchy. In some cases a petechial rash may also occur toward the end of the febrile period or early in convalescence. It is usually limited to the backs of the feet, legs, wrists, hands, and fingers and may also occur on the mucous surfaces of the cheeks and palate. Recovery is the rule in dengue.

There is a leukopenia with a relative lymphocytosis during the acute phase of the disease. The blood picture returns to normal within 1 week after the fall of temperature. There are no changes in the urine or in the cerebrospinal fluid.

In about half the cases there is a prodromal period from 6 to 12 hours before the onset of fever. The prodromal symptoms consist of general malaise, headache, backache, and loss of appetite.

Diagnosis

In the course of an epidemic, the diagnosis is readily made by the characteristic onset, fever, rash, muscle pains, and leukopenia. In sporadic cases, diagnosis by the clinical picture is more difficult, especially since not all cases fit into a textbook description. Laboratory confirmation is a protracted procedure and requires special skills. It consists of (1) transmitting the disease to volunteers by intradermal injection of the patient's serum; (2) adapting the virus to mice by repeated passages intracerebrally; (3) growing the virus on chick embryos, after passage in mice.

Laboratory confirmation can also be made serologically. A rising titer of neutralizing antibodies can be demonstrated in the serum of a patient with dengue if an early and a later specimen of his blood are obtained. The test is made in mice with mouse-adapted virus.

Immunity

Immunity results from an attack of dengue. It is not known how long the immunity lasts. Tests have indicated that it is at least as long as 18 months. While the immunity is solid against the strain that caused the illness, it is only partial to heterologous strains.

A vaccine has been prepared from infected mouse brain for active immunization. However, it has not yet been tried out sufficiently.

The Environment

The disease has been recognized since 1779, but the term "dengue" was first used by the British in 1869. The disease has been reported from every continent, and an epidemic in the southern part of the United States in 1922 affected between 1 and 2 million people, more than half a million of them in Texas. During World War II a considerable number of the troops stationed in the Pacific area contracted the disease.

Vector

Bancroft was the first, in 1906, to transmit the disease by the bite of the mosquito *Aedes aegypti*. Since then it has been shown that a few other species of *Aedes* mosquitoes may transmit the disease. The mosquito may become infected if it bites a patient as long as 18 hours before to 3 days after onset. The mosquito does not become infectious until after an incubation period of 8 to 14 days. It remains infectious for the rest of its life, which is about 1 to 3 months, but does not transmit the infection to the next generation. The virus multiplies in the body of the mosquito during the extrinsic incubation period and permeates the tissues, including the salivary glands. When it next bites an individual to obtain a blood meal, the virus is introduced with its saliva.

Like other mosquitoes, the *Aedes* requires warmth and moisture to multiply and survive. For this reason dengue is found chiefly in tropical and subtropical regions. The disease has not been seen in the United States for many years.

Aedes aegypti is a domestic mosquito and breeds close to human habitation. However, it has been shown that at least two other species, *Aedes albopictus* and *Aedes scutellaris* exist in the jungle and infect monkeys. The disease can thus be kept alive. Human beings going into the jungle can become infected. When they return home the infection can be maintained by the domestic *Aedes aegypti*. This sort of cycle is similar to that of yellow fever, where it has been established that, in addition to the urban type, there exists a jungle type, and that the latter may be the reservoir from which the domestic type draws its new cases.

Control

Isolation of a patient is not necessary, since the disease is transmitted by a mosquito. However, particularly in the summer, windows should be screened. Control depends on the elimination of the *Aedes* mosquitoes. This is not an impossible task, as was shown in Brazil in the elimination of yellow fever. It is accomplished by the suppression of breeding places and by spraying of houses in endemic areas with DDT or some other insecticide. In the face of an epidemic the use of a vaccine must be considered. Such a vaccine has been prepared and has been used safely in human volunteers.

MEDICAL CARE PLANS

Treatment

There is no specific treatment for dengue. Various sedative and antipyretic measures are used to control the fever and pains. Other symptoms are treated as they arise.

Diet

No special diet is required. The diet is the same as in other acute febrile illnesses. Liquids are given during the stage of fever, and solids are introduced as the patient is able to take them.

Supportive Nursing Care

The patient remains in bed during the acute stage and is made comfortable with frequent sponges to relieve the fever and an ice cap for the headache. If there is itching, calamine lotion may be applied to the rash. If insomnia is present the nurse should report it to the physician so that a sedative may be prescribed. Convalescence may be slow, and the patient may be depressed. The nurse should plan activities which will interest the patient and relieve his anxieties.

REFERENCES

1. Bancroft, T. L.: "On the Etiology of Dengue Fever," *Australasian M. Gaz.*, **25**:17, 1906.
2. Hotta, S.: "Experimental Studies in Dengue," *J. Infect. Dis.*, **90**:1, 1952.
3. Meiklejohn, G.; England, B.; and Lennette, E. H.: "Adaptation of Dengue Virus to the Hamster," *Am. J. Trop. Med. Hyg.*, **1**:59, 1952.
4. Sabin, A. B.: "Research on Dengue during World War II," *Am. J. Trop. Med. Hyg.*, **1**:30, 1952.
5. Sabin, A. B.: "Dengue" in Rivers, *Viral and Rickettsial Infections of Man*, J. B. Lippincott Company, Philadelphia, pp. 445–453, 1948.

Chapter 56 ENCEPHALITIS, VIRAL

General Description

THE term encephalitis does not refer to a specific disease but rather to a syndrome resulting from a common pathological condition, which is an inflammation of the brain. Various agents—physical, chemical, and biological—may cause inflammation of the brain or encephalitis. Electrical shock and alcohol are examples of physical and chemical agents. Encephalitis may occur in the course of such varied specific diseases as malaria, syphilis, typhoid fever, and typhus. The diseases that will be considered in this chapter are those in which encephalitis is the primary disease. In all of them a specific virus is the cause. The reason for grouping them together under one heading is that in most of them the symptoms are so alike as to make a definitive diagnosis possible only after laboratory examination of the blood or nervous tissue.

The diseases that will be discussed are (1) von Economo, or acute lethargic encephalitis; (2) St. Louis encephalitis; (3) equine encephalitis, Western, Eastern, and Venezuelan types; (4) Japanese B encephalitis; and (5) Russian Far East, or spring-summer, encephalitis. While the term "encephalitis" refers strictly to inflammation of the brain only, the spinal cord is also involved in most of these diseases so that the term "encephalomyelitis" is frequently used.

The Causative Agent

In all of the encephalitides listed except in von Economo encephalitis, a specific virus has been demonstrated to be the causative agent. The laboratory characteristics of the virus vary in the different diseases. In all of them the virus is found in nature in certain lower animals, while man is infected accidentally. Laboratory animals can, as a rule, be infected by the different agents and produce neutralizing and complement-fixing antiserums. All of the viruses can be kept for long periods of time at a temperature of $-70°$ C. and can be grown in tissue mediums and on chick embryos. They are all filterable.

The Host

Symptoms

The incubation period is 5 to 15 days. Onset is sometimes sudden but may be gradual, with fever, anorexia, irritability, drowsiness, and stiffness of the neck. Fever may mount to 103° or 104° F., and a variety of symptoms may occur. These include headache, lethargy, insomnia, confusion, disorientation, stupor, or coma. Paralyses of different parts of the body, alterations of reflexes, difficulties in speech, tremors, and convulsions are not uncommon. In Russian Far East encephalitis, flaccid paralysis of the shoulder girdle muscles is a characteristic feature. In von Economo encephalitis, ocular paralyses and psychotic disturbances are common, and later stiffness of the muscles, rigidity, and tremors frequently develop, and are followed by Parkinsonism.

The duration of illness may be very long in the von Economo type; it may progress from the acute to a subacute stage lasting for months, or to the chronic stage which merges with Parkinson's disease and continues for the rest of the patient's life. In St. Louis encephalitis the severity of the disease bears a relation to age, the mortality being highest in infants and adults, and lowest in children. Sequelae, in the form of mental retardation, hydrocephalus, and epilepsy may occur in a large percentage of infants. In a smaller percentage of older children and adults, there may remain tremors, weaknesses, and mental disturbance. Although Western equine encephalitis resembles the St. Louis type clinically, the prognosis is much better, most cases recovering completely. This is not so in Eastern equine encephalitis, where mortality may be very high in children (65 per cent in Massachusetts, 1938) and sequelae, consisting of paralyses, mental deterioration, or instability, are fairly common. The symptoms in Venezuelan equine encephalitis are rather mild, and recovery is the rule. Japanese B encephalitis, like St. Louis and Eastern equine encephalitis, is more severe in children than in adults. In all of these diseases, cases that recover are usually sick for 1 to 3 weeks.

All of these diseases occur in epidemic form, although sporadic cases may also be seen. The equine encephalitides are frequently preceded or accompanied by epizootics in horses. Epidemics of the diseases vary in severity, and the cases in each epidemic may also vary greatly. Mild cases occur, with fever, meningeal and slight cerebral symptoms, and recover in about 1 week. The more severe cases vary from the moderate to the fulminating type and may exhibit any of the symptoms mentioned. Mortality varies from 5 to 60 per cent.

As in poliomyelitis, a considerable number of persons in an epidemic area are found who have not had any symptoms referable to the nervous system but only such indefinite signs as fever of short duration. There are also individuals who have apparently had a subclinical infection. In both of these two groups a diagnosis is made by the demonstration of antibodies in the blood.

Diagnosis

A clinical diagnosis of encephalitis can be made without too great difficulty. It is not possible, however, to differentiate one type from another clinically, with the exception of the severer form of von Economo encephalitis which is characterized by rigidities and by the frequent occurrence of the parkinsonian syndrome. Nor can a differentiation be made pathologically, since in all types the same picture is seen: congestion and edema of the brain and cord, acute inflammation with predominance of lymphocytes, perivascular lymphocytic infiltration, small hemorrhages, and proliferation of glial tissue to replace necrotic neuroglia. The blood count usually shows a moderate leukocytosis with increase in the percentage of polynuclear cells. The spinal fluid is under pressure, clear, and usually shows from one hundred to several hundred cells. These may be polymorphonuclears at first but later are predominantly mononuclears. The protein is usually increased, but the sugar is normal.

The diagnosis of the specific type of encephalitis may be made in fatal cases by recovery of the virus from the brain or spinal cord by injecting a 10 or 20 per cent emulsion into the proper laboratory animal. If a filtrable agent is recovered, it is identified by serologic methods or by inoculation into immune mice. In the living individual the virus cannot be recovered, since it is not found in body discharges and only rarely in body fluids. Specimens of blood are obtained during the acute and the late convalescent stages. Both are tested at the same time for the presence of antibodies by the complement-fixation or neutralizing method. A fourfold increase in titer in the second specimen for a specific antigen is usually considered diagnostic of disease caused by that agent. If both specimens have the same titer, the individual probably had the disease caused by the specific agent at a previous time, the current illness being due to some other agent. If both specimens are negative, the individual probably did not have the disease tested for, although occasionally, experience with a disease is not manifested by the production of antibodies. Crossing with other types of encephalitis may occur, but as a rule the titer for the causative virus is higher than for a related virus.

Immunity

Immunity usually follows recovery from encephalitis, but only to the type caused by the specific virus. Such immunity results whether the individual has had an apparent or inapparent infection. The use of a vaccine made from the causative virus for active immunization is being experimented with in all the encephalitides discussed except the von Economo type, from which no virus has, as yet, been recovered. In the equine encephalitides a chick-embryo killed vaccine is at present being employed to immunize horses in epidemic areas. The use of specific antiserum for passive immunization is also in the experimental stage, although it has been used successfully in lower animals.

THE ENVIRONMENT

Von Economo encephalitis. This disease was first recognized in Vienna in 1917 and appeared in the United States in 1918, at the same time as the pandemic of influenza. Thereafter, epidemics were reported all over the world until 1926 when they suddenly ceased. Since no recent epidemics have occurred, there has been no opportunity to study the disease by modern laboratory methods, and no specific virus has been recovered. The disease occurred chiefly in winter and spring and the assumption has, therefore, been made that it was probably not spread by insects. Although it occurred in all age groups, children and young adults were most commonly affected, males somewhat more than females. About a fifth of infected individuals had residual symptoms, usually referable to the nervous system and frequently developing into frank cases of paralysis agitans, or Parkinson's disease. The mortality in epidemics was about 30 per cent.

St. Louis encephalitis. Epidemics of this disease were first recognized in the early 1930's, chiefly in and around St. Louis. The cases occurred for the most part in the summer and early fall. It has occurred in other parts of central and western United States. The incidence has varied for different age groups in different epidemics. In general, the attack rate appears to be highest in infants and adults and lowest in the 5–14 age group. Males are apparently more susceptible. Mortality varies in different epidemics from 5 to 30 per cent.

The vectors of the disease appear to be mosquitoes of the culicine family, chiefly *Culex tarsalis*, from which virus has been recovered in nature. The reservoir is believed to be the chicken, in which the infection is kept going by infected mosquitoes or chicken mites (*dermanyssus avium et gallinae*), from which the virus has been recovered. Infected chickens do not become ill and develop antibodies.

Western equine encephalitis. This disease was first recognized in horses in Western United States in the early 1930's, and soon thereafter in humans. Epidemics in humans and in horses have been occurring since then, chiefly in the West, the Middle West, and lower Canada. However, cases have also been recognized in the eastern part of the country and in Argentina. The epidemiologic pattern is similar to that of St. Louis encephalitis. It occurs mainly in the summer and early fall, it attacks chiefly infants and adults, and males more than females. The mortality is about 10 per cent.

The vectors appear to be similar to those of St. Louis encephalitis, chiefly *Culex tarsalis,* in which the virus has been recovered in nature, and the reservoir seems to be the chicken, in which the virus is kept going by infected mosquitoes or chicken mites.

Eastern equine encephalitis. In the early 1930's the virus of the Eastern equine encephalitis was recovered from horses in the eastern part of the United States, and a few years later it was recovered from humans. Massachusetts had an epidemic of the disease in horses and in humans in the summer and fall of 1938. Children were chiefly attacked, with a mortality of about 65 per cent. The sexes were about equally involved. The mortality in horses was about 90 per cent. The disease is caused by a virus different from the western type. It has been found in horses in Mexico, Cuba, Panama, and Brazil, in addition to the eastern part of the United States and adjacent Canada.

The method of transmission has not been definitely worked out, but *Aedes* mosquitoes appear to be the vectors, of which *Aedes sollicitans* seems to be the most important. It is believed that birds are the reservoir; virus was recovered from pheasants and pigeons.

Venezuelan equine encephalitis. In the late 1930's the virus of this disease was recovered from horses that died in an epizootic in Venezuela. Since then, the disease has been reported in Ecuador, Trinidad, Panama, and Argentina. Few cases have been reported in humans, and little is known of the epidemiology of the disease, including its method of transmission.

Japanese B encephalitis. This disease has been known in Japan in epidemic form for a great many years, but the specific virus was not recovered until 1934. Like St. Louis and Western equine encephalitis, it occurs chiefly in the summer. In some epidemics the older population has been chiefly attacked, but in other areas the cases are mainly in children. It is believed that the older people have had inapparent infection, since a large percentage of them have antibodies in the circulating blood. Males have a higher attack rate than females. The disease is found in Japan, China, Korea, Indo-China, Philippines, and eastern Siberia.

Epidemiologically, the disease behaves very much like St. Louis encephalitis, so that mosquitoes have been suspected to be the vectors. No definite reservoir has been implicated, but chickens are suspected.

Russian Far East (spring-summer) encephalitis. This disease was also first observed in the early 1930's, but the virus was not recovered from human cases until about 5 years later. As its name indicates, it is seen chiefly in the spring and summer. Epidemics have occurred in lumber camps and among forest workers. Male adults are most commonly attacked, and the mortality is about 30 per cent.

The epidemiology differs considerably from the other encephalitides in the age groups attacked, in its limitation to certain occupational groups, and in its seasonal occurrence. The vector is believed to be a tick, *Ixodes persulcatus,* from which virus has been recovered in nature and by the bite of which the disease has been transmitted to mice. Transovarian transmission from adult ticks to larvae has been demonstrated. The reservoir is believed to be small woodland mammals and birds.

Control

No method of control is known for von Economo encephalitis. In the others, control depends on the use of a vaccine in horses in epidemic areas for the equine encephalitides. Measures commonly used for mosquito and tick control are applicable here, too. These have been discussed on pages 466–468. The development of a vaccine for active immunization of susceptible persons in endemic areas is still in the experimental stage.

Since the diseases are not transferred from person to person, patients need not be isolated, nor do contacts have to be quarantined.

MEDICAL CARE PLANS

Treatment

There is no specific treatment for encephalitis. The antibiotics are of no value. All therapy is symptomatic. Since the symptoms are largely neurologic, the drugs used are mainly sedatives, to alleviate excitability or restlessness and to prevent, if possible, the occurrence of convulsions. Spinal taps are performed for diagnosis only.

Diet

No special diet is necessary. As long as there is fever, the patient is fed a liquid or soft diet. If the patient is stuporous it may be necessary to keep up the fluid requirements with 5 per cent glucose solution given intravenously.

During convalescence, carefully selected foods high in nutritive values are given.

Supportive Nursing Care

In the early stage of the disease, general comfort of the patient is directed toward the alleviation of headache, generalized muscular aches, and catarrhal or gastro-intestinal symptoms. As there are wide variations in symptomatology, the nurse's skill in observation and accurate recording of changes in the condition of the patient are indispensable.

The plan for nursing care should be well organized and uninterrupted wherever possible. Consideration should be given to a separate room and factors in the environment which lessen tension and excitability. The lighting may need adjustment, as some patients complain of photophobia. Complete bed rest and maintenance of good body mechanics are essential.

Muscular twitching, choreiform movements, and tremors occur in severe infections. Sideboards for adults and padding of the sides of the crib for young children may be necessary to prevent injury. Restraints should not be used. Sedation may be prescribed for restlessness and for control of excitability.

Routine oral hygiene prophylaxis should be used. Cleansing the mouth with a mouthwash is indicated. Sordes can be prevented by swabbing the tongue with equal parts of glycerin and lemon juice. Cold cream, liquid petrolatum, or camphor ice may be applied to the lips to prevent fissures and dryness.

Because of the accompanying stupor, the patient prefers to remain undisturbed. His position should be changed frequently to prevent decubitus and pulmonary complications. Bony prominences should be inspected daily and should receive special care.

Retention and suppression of urine occur frequently, and it may be necessary to catheterize the patient. If the patient is constipated, enemas may be necessary.

In severe forms of the disease the patient may be irritable and suspicious, and may exhibit hostility to a marked degree. His complaints are numerous, and these may be highly exaggerated. Behavior changes which may occur include unusual drowsiness, mental disorientation, irritability, difficulties in speech, blurring of vision, and changes in facial expression and personality. These changes in behavior during illness may become permanent and affect the patient's ability to adjust to his family and the ordinary everyday activities.

Rehabilitation of the patient following recovery is dependent upon the extent of organic injury to the brain. The nurse's knowledge and understanding of organic changes contribute to effective handling of these patients. In some instances, physiotherapy may be helpful.

Mild and abortive cases of encephalitis are discovered periodically during outbreaks. Home visits by the public health nurse may be requested by the family or physician to give nursing care to the patient and to assist the family with other pressing problems. Upon discharge from the hospital, the nurse may make periodic visits to assist the family with nursing care and rehabilitation of the patient.

REFERENCES

1. Ayres, J. C., and Feemster, R. F.: "The Sequelae of Eastern Equine Encephalitis," *New England J. Med.*, **240**:960, 1949.
2. Blattner, R. J., and Heyes, F. M.: "St. Louis Encephalitis," *J.A.M.A.*, **129**:854, 1945.
3. Bredeck, J. F.: "The Story of Epidemic Encephalitis in St. Louis," *Am. J. Pub. Health*, **23**:1135, 1933.
4. Casals, J. M.: "Diagnosis of Epidemic Encephalitis by Complement Fixation Tests," *Am. J. Pub. Health*, **31**:1281, 1941.
5. Hammon, W. McD.: "Encephalitis," *J.A.M.A.*, **121**:560, 1943.
6. Muckenfuss, R.: *Epidemic Encephalitis*, reprint. Samuel D. Gross Lecture delivered before Philadelphia Pathological Society, Nov. 11, 1937.
7. Rollings, H. E.: "Encephalitis," in Pullen's *Communicable Diseases*, Lea & Febiger, Philadelphia, 1950.
8. von Economo, C.: *Encephalitis Lethargica*, Oxford University Press, New York, 1931.
9. Wesselhoeft, C.; Smith, E. C.; and Branch, C. F.: "Human Encephalitis," *J.A.M.A.*, **111**:1735, 1938.
10. Zentay, P., and Basman, J.: "Epidemic Encephalitis Type B in Children," *J. Pediat.*, **14**:323, 1939.

Chapter 57 MALARIA

MALARIA is a disease of world-wide distribution, caused by a protozoan, transmitted by the anopheline mosquito, and characterized by attacks of chills, fever, and sweats and other constitutional symptoms.

THE CAUSATIVE AGENT

The cause of malaria is the *Plasmodium,* a protozoan organism of the class of Sporozoa. It lives in the blood and tissues of man, having sexual and asexual forms, the former of which have their cycles in the mosquito and the latter in man. During the asexual cycle, pigment is produced in the red blood cells of man. When the sexual forms are ingested by an anopheline mosquito, they complete their cycle in the insect and produce sporozoites which are infective for man. In addition to man, other animals, such as monkeys, birds, and bats, may be infected with various species of plasmodia.

Life Cycle in Man

This is known as *schizogony* and takes place in the red blood cells. After an infected mosquito has bitten a man, and the *Plasmodium* has been inoculated by the bite, a period of 4 to 5 days elapses before it is seen in the circulating blood. It probably goes through a stage of development in the liver during this time. It is first seen in the red blood cell as a small, ringlike form known as *trophozoite.* It enlarges, develops pigment, and becomes a *schizont.* This enlarges until it fills the blood corpuscle and divides into a number of smaller bodies known as *merozoites.* The blood cell bursts, and the merozoites escape into the plasma. They enter other red corpuscles, where some become *trophozoites* and go through the same cycle again. Others develop into male or female sexual forms or *gametocytes.* These increase in size in the corpuscle but do not divide. When the cell ruptures, they remain free in the blood and disintegrate in a few days unless taken up by a mosquito. The cycle takes approximately 48 to 72 hours, depending on the species of *Plasmodium.*

Life Cycle in the Mosquito

This is known as *sporogony*. The gametocyte is ingested by the female anopheline mosquito when it takes its blood meal. It goes through a process of maturation in the mosquito's stomach, becoming a *gamete*. Fertilization occurs by fusion of the male and female gametes, resulting in a *zygote*. This goes through a process of development, penetrates the lining of the mosquito's stomach, and comes to rest between the layers, forming a cyst, known as *oocyst*. In the oocyst many tiny, spindle-shaped, slender bodies develop, known as *sporozoites*. The oocyst ruptures, and the sporozoites are released and travel to all the tissues of the mosquito, including the salivary glands and ducts. When the infected mosquito bites man, the saliva is injected into the wound and the sporozoites with it. After the exo-erythrocytic phase in the liver, they invade the blood stream and become trophozoites and start the human cycle. The sexual cycle in the mosquito takes about 2 weeks.

Four species of *Plasmodium* may cause malaria in man. These are: (1) *Plasmodium vivax,* the cause of tertian malaria; (2) *Plasmodium malariae,* which causes quartan malaria; (3) *Plasmodium falciparum,* the cause of estivo-autumnal or malignant malaria; and (4) *Plasmodium ovale.*

Plasmodium Vivax

The human or schizogonic cycle is completed in 48 hours. The trophozoite begins as a ring form and becomes actively ameboid in its early stages. The schizont divides into twelve to twenty-four merozoites. The red blood cell enlarges as the organism enlarges. In a stained smear the cytoplasm is blue, while the nuclear chromatin is red. Small pink dots may be seen in the red-cell cytoplasm. These are known as "Schüffner's dots." Multiple infections of the same cell are not common.

Plasmodium Malariae

This species completes its cycle in man in 72 hours. Gametocytes are not produced until schizogony has gone on for several generations. The trophozoite is smaller than *Plasmodium vivax* and less actively motile. The red blood cell does not enlarge as in *Plasmodium vivax infection.* The schizont divides into six to twelve meozoites. The staining is similar to that of *Plasmodium vivax.* Some of the older trophozoites are shaped like a ribbon or band and are known as "band forms." Schüffner's dots are not found in the red blood cells. Multiple infections of the same cell are rare.

Plasmodium Falciparum

The cycle in man is completed in 36 to 48 hours. Only tropho-zoites and gametocytes appear in the peripheral blood. The develop-ment of the gametocytes into schizonts occurs in the capillaries of the internal organs. The gametocytes are readily recognized because they have a crescentic shape which stains blue with red chromatin in the center. In the trophozoite or ring forms, there are sometimes two chromatin dots, close together or separated. The schizont divides into eight to thirty-six merozoites, the average being eighteen to twenty-four. Appliqué forms are much more frequently seen than in *Plasmodium vivax* or *malariae*. They are ring forms which are applied to the periphery of the red cell. Multiple infections of the same cell are very common.

Plasmodium Ovale

Infections with this species are less frequent than with the other plasmodia. The cycle in man is completed in 48 hours. The infected red corpuscle is often ovoid in shape and ragged at the edges, and contains many Schüffner granules. The trophozoites are slightly motile. The red cells increase in size but not to the same extent as in *Plasmodium vivax* infections. The segmenting schizonts do not fill more than about three quarters of the red cell and divide into six to twelve merozoites.

THE HOST

Symptoms

There are two incubation periods in malaria, the *intrinsic* in man and the *extrinsic* in the mosquito. The intrinsic incubation period varies with the type of infection. It is about 14 days in *vivax* malaria, which is the most common. The extrinsic incubation period varies with the temperature, being longer in cold and shorter in warm climates. At 18° C. a mosquito has an extrinsic incubation period of 20 days, while at 25° to 30° C., the incubation period is 8 days.

The symptoms are characterized by the occurrence of attacks of chills, fever, and sweating at regular intervals, depending on the time needed for segmentation of the *Plasmodium* to occur. In *vivax* and *ovale* malaria, where schizogony is completed in 48 hours, attacks occur every other day, but in quartan malaria where seg-mentation of schizonts occurs every 72 hours, the attacks occur every 3 days. In *falciparum* malaria, attacks tend to occur every 36 to 48 hours.

The onset is sudden, with a severe, shaking chill, followed by a fever of 104° to 105° F. The patient complains of headache, pain in the muscles, and general malaise. After a few hours there is a sudden drop in fever, accompanied by profuse sweating. The spleen becomes enlarged in cases of malaria, and the liver is also enlarged. Anemia results from destruction of red cells.

In *falciparum* malaria pernicious symptoms may arise as a result of blocking of the capillaries in the brain or other organs with segmenting schizonts. As a result, the typical chills and fever may be masked by sudden delirium or convulsions or coma or symptoms referable to some other organ of the body. *Blackwater fever* occasionally occurs in malaria. It is characterized by the passage of dark-red urine, usually preceded by chills and fever.

Untreated cases of malaria usually relapse. Relapses, occasionally after many years, may occur also in cases apparently treated adequately.

Diagnosis

An accurate diagnosis is made only by the demonstration of the *Plasmodium* in the blood. A thin film is made similarly to one for the differentiation of white blood cells. Thick films are preferable since there may be few plasmodia present in the blood. A large drop of blood is placed on a clean slide and is smeared with a needle over an area about 1 centimeter in diameter. The stain commonly used for thin and thick smears is Giemsa. Serologic tests are not available for diagnosis.

Immunity

No race or color appears to be immune to malaria. Immunity to a particular strain may result after infection with it, but the individual can still be infected with other strains. Infection with more than one strain at the same time is not unusual. In some endemic areas, certain adults appear to be immune. This is probably due to the fact that they have exhausted infections with all strains in that area. There is no method for active or passive immunization to malaria.

THE ENVIRONMENT

Malaria has been recognized as a disease since ancient times. The *Plasmodium* was first seen in human blood by Laveran, in 1880. Sir Ronald Ross proved its transmission from bird to bird by mosquitoes in 1897 and he, Grassi, and Manson proved the transmission by mosquito from man to man in 1898 and 1899. The sexual forms were first recognized by MacCallum in 1897. Cinchona or Peruvian bark was used in treatment as far back as the seventeenth century;

quinine was prepared from it in 1823. Atabrine was synthesized in 1933.

Malaria is world wide in distribution and may occur in any region where the mean summer temperature does not fall below 24° C. (72° F.). *Vivax* malaria is found chiefly in Central and West Africa, around the Mediterranean, in the Near East, in China, and in Central and South America. *Falciparum* malaria is found chiefly in the tropics and in some subtropical areas. *Plasmodium ovale* has a limited distribution in the Near East, India, Philippines, East Africa, and South America.

In addition to an isotherm of 60° to 70° F., the anopheles mosquito requires moisture for its survival and development. About 30 inches of precipitation are needed. In desert areas the anopheles cannot breed. The seasonal prevalence of malaria is dependent on temperature and moisture.

The anopheles is the only mosquito transmitting malaria in man. Transmission may occur by direct infection from man to man as in transfusion, and infections have occurred in drug addicts as a result of the use of a common infected needle.

No race is immune to infection. Apparent immunity in certain races is due to the fact that they have been indigenous to the area and have had infections with all available strains. Similarly, children appear to be more readily infected than adults because they have not had sufficient opportunity to exhaust all strains. More men than women are infected because they spend more time outdoors. An occupation that brings man closer to the breeding places of the mosquito is more apt to allow infection to occur.

Not all anopheles mosquitoes can transmit malaria. There are about 200 species, and only about 60 have been proved to harbor *Plasmodium*. In the United States *Anopheles quadrimaculatus* is the most common transmitter of malaria.

Mosquitoes may show a preference for human (anthropophilism) or for animal blood (zoophilism). Some zoophilic mosquitoes will feed on humans if animals are not available. This fact is used in control measures by importing animals into the area.

Malaria surveys are made by the use of two indexes: (1) the *splenic index* and (2) the *parasite index*. In the former, the spleens of a sample of the population are palpated and the rate is determined for the sample. In some endemic areas the rate is 90 to 100 per cent in school children. The first attack of malaria causes an enlarged spleen. After repeated infections the spleen reduces in size. A high splenic index in children and a low one in adults indicates an area of high endemicity. A high index in both adults and children indicates an epidemic of malaria. A *parasite index* is obtained by taking

thin and thick blood smears and examining them for malaria in a
sample of the population and then arriving at a rate. It is a more
exact index but more time-consuming and difficult to carry out.

Surveys are also made by trapping mosquitoes and examining the
stomach walls of females for oocysts and the salivary glands for
sporozoites. This is specialized and slow work and gives an index
of infection in the mosquito rather than in man.

Control

Methods of control of malaria are similar to those discussed for
arthropods in general. Since malaria is probably the most important
disease on earth in terms of numbers infected and number of deaths
every year, control has become a specialized training. The science
of malariology has become a specialty in public health work.

MEDICAL CARE PLANS

Treatment

Treatment may be curative or suppressive. A number of drugs
are available for both. As a rule the same drug is used for both but
in different doses and at different intervals. The drug first used in
malaria was *quinine*. It is still a good drug but has been largely
replaced by others. It is used in a dose of 0.65 gram (10 grains) of
the sulfate three times a day, by mouth, for a week. In pernicious
malaria quinine dihydrochloride is given by vein, about 0.65 gram
(10 grains) diluted in 250 to 500 cubic centimeters of saline. This
may be repeated, if necessary.

Atabrine or Quinacrine hydrochloride. This drug is now used very
widely. It is a rapidly curative drug and less likely to be followed
by a relapse than is quinine. It is administered by mouth in a dose of
two tablets of 0.1 gram (1½ grains) five times the first day, and then
one tablet three times a day for 6 days. It destroys the asexual forms
of all species of malaria and the gametocytes of *Plasmodium vivax*
and *malariae* but not those of *Plasmodium falciparum*. Following
the use of Atabrine, the skin is often colored yellow. This disappears
within a few weeks.

Aralen (chloroquine disphosphate). This drug has been introduced more recently and rivals Atabrine in its effectiveness. It is
administered in a dose of two tablets of 0.25 gram each, three times
a day for the first 24 hours and then two tablets a day for two days
more.

For suppressive treatment Aralen is given in a weekly dose of
0.5 gram. Quinine and Atabrine can both be used, but the latter is
the more effective of the two. It is administered in a dose of 0.1 gram

per day. Suppressive treatment does not prevent infection. It merely suppresses the symptoms and is thus of value in keeping individuals in hyperendemic areas at their jobs until they can get out of the region. It is of special value in military operations in such areas. Individuals leaving such areas should discontinue the drug and, if symptoms develop and they have a positive smear, should be treated with adequate, curative doses.

Diet

No special diet is required. While the fever is elevated, liquids in large amounts are given. As soon as the temperature declines, a balanced diet fortified with essential nutrients, iron, and vitamins is given.

Supportive Nursing Care

Complete bed rest is essential during malarial paroxysms. Because chills and fever are characteristic of the infection, the room should be warm and sudden temperature changes should be avoided. The bed should be adequately protected with a full-length rubber sheet. When chilly sensations arise, they begin in the extremities, progress upward, and are accompanied by general shivering and shaking. The patient should be provided with extra blankets, and hot-water bottles should be applied to the extremities and to the sides of the body. A rise in temperature may occur prior to or during the chill.

With the onset of the hot stage, the face is flushed, and there is a generalized sensation of heat throughout the entire body. The patient complains of feeling very hot. An ice bag is applied to the head to relieve headache, and tepid sponge baths may be given to lessen discomfort from high temperature. Vomiting, abdominal pain, severe backache, and mild delirium may be present during this stage. Small pillows propped against the back often relieve backache. Careful recording of temperature, pulse, respiration, and the character of the chill are important as they are significant aids in diagnosis. All temperatures should be taken by rectum and recorded at the bedside.

With the decline in temperature and cessation of chills, the attack terminates spontaneously. The patient perspires profusely. The gown and bed linen should be changed when necessary, and alcohol rubs should be given to stimulate skin circulation. The avoidance of sudden removal of bed covering and exposure to draughts is important. In relative proportion to the amount of sweating, the patient feels better, becomes relaxed, and falls into a deep sleep. The temperature drops to the normal or subnormal range, the pulse becomes slower, and recovery is imminent.

In *falciparum* malaria, the onset is characterized by symptoms simulating influenza, and the paroxysms are more severe. The temperature cycle may be irregular and the fever continuous rather than intermittent. Psychic disturbances and delirium may be more pronounced than in tertian and quartan malaria.

During the paroxysm, the mucous membranes of the mouth are dry, and fissures may develop. Mouthwashes should be used.

In general, all patients experience a transient mental depression during paroxysmal attacks. The degree of anxiety depends upon the personality makeup of the individual. The behavior and personality of the patient are not altered to any great extent unless relapses occur at frequent intervals. Latent infections and recurring attacks may influence attitudes toward acceptance of illness and predispose one to melancholia.

Although recovery from malarial attacks is rapid, work activities should be modified for some time. Continuous medical care is vital for the maintenance of optimal health and for supervision of suppressive therapy.

REFERENCES

1. Allyn, L. G., and Steiner, J.: "Nursing Care in Malaria," *Am. J. Nursing*, 46:675, 1946.
2. Andrews, J. M., *et al.:* "Malaria Eradication in the U.S.," *Am. J. Pub. Health*, 40:1405, 1950.
3. Arbuse, D. I.: "Neuropsychiatric Manifestations in Malaria," *U.S. Nav. M. Bull.*, 45:304, 1945.
4. Boyd, M. F.: *Malariology*, Vols. I and II, W. B. Saunders Company, Philadelphia, 1949.
5. Coggeshall, L. T.: "Malaria," *Am. J. Nursing*, 45:673, 1946.
6. Einhorn, Colonel N. H.: "Tertian, Quartan and Mixed Malarial Infections," *Am. J. Dis. Child.*, 73:55, 1947.
7. Faust, E. C.: "Malaria in the United States Today," *Modern Med.*, 16:35, 1948.
8. Funkenstein, D. H.: "Tertian Malaria and Anxiety," *Psychosom. Med.*, 11:158, 1949.
9. McCracken, L.: "New Victory over a Mass Killer," *Hygeia*, 28:44, 1950.
10. Moulton, F. R.: Symposium on Human Malaria, American Association of Advancement and Science, Washington, D.C., 1941.
11. Russel, P. F.; West, L. S.; and Manwell, R. D.: *Practical Malariology*, W. B. Saunders Company, Philadelphia, 1946.
12. "The Therapeutics of Malaria, Third General Report of the Malaria Commission," *Quarterly Bull., Health Organ., League of Nations*, 2:181, 1933.
13. Walker, A. J.: "Malaria Therapy, 1950," *Bull. Tulane M. Fac.*, 9:48, 1950.
14. World Health Organization: "The Fight against Malaria," *W.H.O. Newsletter*, 10:2, 1950.

Chapter 58 PEDICULOSIS (LOUSINESS)

GENERAL DESCRIPTION

PEDICULOSIS means the infestation of the scalp or other parts of the body with lice.

THE CAUSATIVE AGENT

Three trypes of lice infest human beings: (1) the head louse, *Pediculus capitis,* (2) the body louse, *Pediculus corporis,* and (3) the crab louse, *Phthirus pubis.* They are all wingless insects, flattened from front to back, which cling to hairs or fibers, bite their hosts, and suck blood for their meals. They normally spend their entire lives on their hosts. Eggs are laid within 1 or 2 days after the adult female has been fertilized. Head lice deposit their eggs on the hairs of the head or neck, pubic or crab lice on the pubic hairs and occasionally on eyebrows and the hairs of the chest or axillae. Body lice usually attach their eggs to the fibers of underclothing. The eggs are ovoid and are cemented to the hairs or fibers so that they are not easily removed by brushing or combing. The eggs hatch in about 1 week after they are laid. Adults live about 1 month. Body lice may transmit disease to man. Examples are typhus fever and relapsing fever. Head and pubic lice do not commonly transmit disease, but may do so on occasion. All lice cause an irritation of the skin which is intensified by scratching.

THE HOST

Symptoms

The saliva which is introduced by the louse when it bites an individual causes a reddish papule which is itchy. Scratching results, and is often severe enough to cause bleeding. Infection may follow, so that it is not uncommon to see on the skin of infested individuals scratch marks, impetiginous lesions, and infected sores. The skin may become indurated as a result of repeated scratching, and the regional lymph glands may become enlarged.

Diagnosis

This is readily made by identifying the insect or its ova. In the scalp, the latter can be differentiated from dander by the fact that the egg is not easily brushed off, whereas dander is.

Immunity

No immunity results from infection. Repeated attacks of lousiness may occur if the opportunities for infestation exist.

THE ENVIRONMENT

Infestation with pediculi has been recognized for many centuries. At the present time it is known to accompany crowding and filth and is usually found chiefly among the very poor and in insanitary places where people are herded together, such as jails and some institutions. In the Middle Ages, when bathing was a luxury and personal hygiene was at a low level, lousiness was common in all classes of society. It is found in all parts of the world, in cold as well as hot climates, and is most commonly widespread when wars and other calamities disorganize life and cause the dislocation of people and their crowding in makeshift quarters without proper sanitary arrangements. Although lousiness is in itself not a serious or dangerous disease and is commonly considered merely as an index of cleanliness, widespread infestation with pediculi, particularly in times of war, always carries the danger of typhus fever. Disinfestation of troops, or delousing, used to be a complicated task. At present delousing is done by means of a hand spray with a 5 to 10 per cent DDT powder. This is dusted into the scalp, up the sleeves, and under the clothing in the belt region. The experience in Naples, in World War II, indicated that it is a cheap, quick, and effective method of preventing an epidemic of typhus.

Control

The patient with pediculosis should be kept out of school until treated and should sleep alone. It is rare to find only one person in a family infested, so that when a child is found to have pediculosis, all members of the family should be examined and all those infested should be treated.

MEDICAL CARE PLANS

Treatment

Head lice. The hair should be cut short, if possible. Formerly, treatment consisted in killing adult lice with kerosene and olive oil applied to the scalp and then combing out the nits or eggs with a fine-tooth comb. The modern treatment is with DDT powder. A 10 per cent DDT powder is rubbed into all parts of the scalp; usually 1 or 2 teaspoonfuls suffice for a boy, and 2 to 4 teaspoonfuls for a girl.

DDT is best applied to the hair by means of a powder puffer or container with a perforated cover. When applying the insecticide, the mouth and eyes should be closed and the head tilted forward. A paper or cloth towel may be used to cover the eyes as an additional protective measure against irritation. The powder is spread evenly through the hair, the hair is combed thoroughly, and the head is covered with a towel or snug-fitting white cap. The hair should be combed every day to prevent matting. After 7 days, the hair is shampooed and rinsed with a warm diluted solution of vinegar or lemon juice to loosen nits. The hair is then combed with a fine-tooth comb. A second application is usually necessary. The insecticide kills the adults, but not the nits. However, as these hatch, they are destroyed by the residual DDT. The scalp should be examined to make sure that all ova are gone. Otherwise the treatment should be repeated.

Pubic lice. The same treatment may be applied.

Body lice. With an atomizer, 10 per cent DDT powder should be applied to the patient's body. Although such treatment will usually kill the lice in the underclothing which come in contact with the body, it is a wise precaution to sterilize the underwear before using it again. A 25 per cent emulsion of benzyl benzoate may be used instead of DDT for pediculosis of the body. This is applied as in scabies. There are several other drugs on the market which are useful in treatment, such as Cuprex and Kwell.

Supportive Nursing Care

The problem of pediculosis is of concern to school authorities, public health school nurses, and agencies giving care to children. Although essentially a hygienic problem, it has public health implications, particularly in wartime and in areas where typhus is endemic. Poor practices in personal hygiene as well as inadequate facilities and overcrowding within the home are contributory factors to susceptibility and spread. In recent years there has been a tendency to shift responsibility for instruction in hygiene of the hair and scalp to the classroom teacher on the assumption that it is strictly a hygienic problem and can be handled adequately in this way. While the use and distribution of nursing time has been a factor in this philosophy, control of and responsibility for health counseling remains a nursing function. Printed instructions given by teachers are often not read or understood by parents, particularly if there are language barriers. Home visits by the nurse may be necessary to demonstrate care of the hair, and to teach the family the need for personal hygiene and treatment of all infested members.

A practical way of meeting the problem in the school may be by group instruction. Children inspected routinely by the teacher and discovered to have pediculosis may be isolated until the nurse is free to discuss the problem with all the children together. In the higher grades, disinfestation may be carried out in the school under the direction of the nurse or the hygiene teacher. When the nurse is not available in the school, the responsibility should be shifted to a teacher or health counselor.

REFERENCES

1. Davis, W. A., and Juvera, P. M.: "Studies on Lice Control in Civilian Populations," *Am. J. Hyg.,* **29**:177, 1944.
2. Kaiser, A. D.: "Treatment of *Pediculosis Capitis* in School Children with DDT Powder," *Am. J. Pub. Health,* **36**:1133, 1946.
3. Peck, S. M.; Wright, W. H.; and Grant, J. Q., Jr.: "Cutaneous Reactions Due to the Body Louse," *J.A.M.A.,* **123**:832, 1943.
4. Weiss, M.: "Who Said Lice," *Am. J. Nursing,* **46**:225, 1946.

Chapter 59 PLAGUE

GENERAL DESCRIPTION

PLAGUE is an acute infectious disease caused by the plague bacillus, which is transmitted by fleas. Plague is evidenced as an inflammation of the lymph glands, or the lungs, or as a general sepsis.

THE CAUSATIVE AGENT

The causative agent is *Pasteurella pestis,* a gram-negative bacillus with rounded ends, which grows readily in cultures containing bile salts. In smears from fresh specimens it shows bipolar staining. The organism is not motile. It is destroyed by sunlight in 3 to 4 hours and by heat and the usual antiseptics. In dried sputum it may remain alive for 3 months, and in dry flea feces, for several weeks. *Pasteurella pestis* elaborates a toxin which is lethal for mice and rats. The organism can usually be recovered from the buboes of patients of bubonic plague, from the sputum in pneumonic plague, and from the blood stream in both types. The disease can be transmitted without difficulty to guinea pigs.

THE HOST

Symptoms

The incubation period is 3 to 6 days. Three types of the disease are commonly recognized: (1) bubonic, (2) pneumonic, and (3) septicemic. In bubonic plague, cases may be mild so that they are overlooked, and the diagnosis will be made only by bacteriological examination of the swollen glands or buboes. In the more severe cases of bubonic plague the onset is often acute, with fever, rapid pulse, restlessness, and prostration. Pain develops in the affected glands and calls the patient's attention to them. On examination they are found to be enlarged and firm and surrounded by edematous tissues. Blood-stream invasion may supervene, or the disease may start as a septicemia. There are then increased restlessness and nervous symptoms, and there may be hemorrhagic signs such as epistaxis and hematuria. The course is usually short, from a few days to 1 week. In pneumonic plague the onset is also acute, with fever, chills, headache, nausea, and prostration. Respirations are rapid and shallow, and there is cough with expectoration. The sputum is watery and becomes blood-tinged. The mortality is not known accurately, since mild cases escape detection. For moderate to severe cases of bubonic plague the case fatality rate runs to about 50 per cent. Pneumonic and septicemic types have a much higher fatality.

Diagnosis

Diagnosis based on the clinical picture alone is not easy. When the epidemiological data are included, the probabilities of a correct diagnosis are increased. Laboratory confirmation is important. This can be obtained by culture of a bubo or of sputum, and by blood cultures.

Immunity

The immunity conferred by the disease is only relative, since second attacks are not rare. A vaccine has been prepared from killed plague bacilli and is commercially available. It is administered subcutaneously in two doses of 0.5 and 1.0 cubic centimeter at a weekly interval. The immunity conferred by the vaccine is of short duration. Booster doses should be given at 6-month to yearly intervals to exposed individuals.

THE ENVIRONMENT

The plague has an old history, going back to the period before Christ. It was in the fourteenth century, however, that bubonic plague spread over Europe, striking down all in its path and earning for itself the unenviable reputation of being a greater killer than any other disease. As the Black Death it spread all over Europe, returning periodically later. At the present time the disease is confined largely to the continents of Asia and Africa, being endemic in some countries and occurring sporadically in others. In Europe it is present in rats and occasionally in humans. In the United States it has occurred since the beginning of the century in ground squirrels and other field rodents in California and has been gradually spreading eastward as far as Kansas. Occasional human cases have been reported.

From an epidemiological point of view, plague should be divided into the urban and sylvatic types. The urban type is spread by the rats. It occurs in heavily populated communities, particularly if insanitary conditions prevail. It spreads overland, and also across water by means of ships. Sylvatic plague is spread by ground squir-

rels, chipmunks, and other field rodents and is transmitted to man
if he comes into intimate contact with infected animals, usually as
a result of his occupation. The division is similar to that of urban
and jungle yellow fever. Urban plague attacks both sexes and all
ages and races. The rapidity of spread is dependent on the presence
of rats, and this, in turn, depends on crowding and insanitary conditions. Actual transfer of the disease to man occurs through the
intervention of the rat flea which becomes infected when it bites a
sick rat and transmits the disease to humans when it bites them. The
most common vector is *Xenopsylla cheopis.* The type of disease transmitted by fleabites is probably always bubonic plague. Primary cases
of pneumonic plague occur most probably in patients with bubonic
or septicemic plague by spread to the lungs. Once infected, an individual with pneumonic plague can transmit the disease to susceptible individuals directly by coughing, kissing, etc.

Control

The patient should be isolated until recovery and should be
promptly treated. His room should be screened and sprayed with
DDT solution. Great care should be taken to dispose of purulent discharges, if possible by burning. In the pneumonic form, spread may
occur by droplet infection. The nurse caring for the patient should
wear a mask, in addition to a gown, to protect herself against this
possibility. Rubber gloves should be worn when dressing purulent
buboes to obviate the possibility of contact infection. Since plague
bacilli may live for some time in dried discharges, all linen should
be sterilized by boiling after use. Contacts to cases of plague should
be disinfected with DDT or other insecticide and kept under surveillance for 6 days. The use of antibiotics as a prophylactic should
be considered.

General control in communities where urban plague occurs consists of measures to help break the cycle of spread, which is rat to
flea to rat, and, accidentally, to man. Efforts should be directed
toward the destruction of fleas by dusting with DDT or other insecticide, toward the eliminiation of rats by poisoning and by ratproofing
of houses, and toward the strengthening of the resistance of the
human host by immunization. There should be a continued program for the bacteriological examination of rodents and fleas. In
areas where sylvatic plague is prevalent, individuals who, as a result
of their occupation, may come in contact with wild rodents should
be immunized, and measures should be adopted for the routine
bacteriologic sampling of wild rodents and the insects that prey on
them. In ports where boats arrive from all parts of the world,
special precautions should be taken to destroy all rats on ships

before docking, and bacteriologic sampling of rats should be a routine measure. The ratproofing of ships should be insisted upon. Spraying of airplanes before arrival at the terminal should also be a routine practice.

MEDICAL CARE PLANS

Treatment

Treatment for the general symptoms is symptomatic, emphasis being laid on fluid-loss replacement, sedatives for the restlessness, and proper nutrition. Specific treatment has become available with the introduction of antibiotic drugs. Those found most effective so far are sulfadiazine and streptomycin, used alone or, preferably, in combination. Both drugs are given in large doses and kept up for about 2 weeks after the drop in fever. No reports are yet available on the use of the newer antibiotics.

Diet

Fluids are given during the acute stage, and light nourishment is added as soon as the patient is sufficiently well to take solid food.

Supportive Nursing Care

Skilled nursing care and comfort of the patient are essential. The patient is isolated in a verminproof room, and rigid aseptic nursing techniques are observed. Tepid sponge baths may be given for high elevations in temperature. The application of an ice cap to the head may relieve headache.

Nursing care of pneumonic plague is the same as for other pneumonias. The nurse giving care to plague patients should be immunized.

In areas where plague is present, the public health nurse assists in an educational program. The principles of personal and environmental hygiene must be stressed, and the nurse should demonstrate the use of insecticides. She may also assist with immunization of the population.

REFERENCES

1. Huang, C. H., and Chu, L. W.: "Treatment of Bubonic Plague with Sulfadiazine," *Am. J. Trop. Med.*, 26:831, 1946.
2. Smith, G.: *Plague on Us*, Commonwealth Fund, Harvard University Press, Cambridge, Mass., 1941.
3. Zinsser, H.: *Plague, Rats and History*, Little, Brown & Company, Boston, 1935.

Chapter 60 THE RICKETTSIAL DISEASES

THESE diseases are caused by microorganisms known as "rickett-siae." They are intermediate in size and have characteristics similar to both the bacteria and the viruses. They are large enough to be seen under the microscope, where they appear as coccobacillary organisms which stain unevenly and are gram-negative. They do not take the color well with the usual stains but can be seen clearly with special stains, of which the commonest used are the Giemsa and the Macchiavello.

Like viruses, they multiply only within cells of susceptible species in the cytoplasm or in both cytoplasm and nucleus. Generally, the typhus group of rickettsiae grows in cytoplasm only, and the spotted fever group grows in both. Rickettsiae may be cultured in chick embryos and in tissue cultures. Some are filterable and others are not. In the natural state the rickettsiae are found in man, in a number of animals, and in arthropods; the latter are the vectors in most of the rickettsial diseases.

Rickettsiae are readily destroyed by heat and the usual antiseptics. They die at room temperature in a few hours but remain viable in the refrigerator for 1 or 2 days and, when rapidly frozen to −70° C., will remain alive for several years. Rapid freezing is done by placing sealed-glass ampules of the rickettsiae in an alcohol–dry-ice mixture. The ampules are kept in the frozen state in a dry-ice cabinet or a deep-freeze unit. The rickettsiae may also be preserved by desiccation from the frozen state. The rickettsia of Q fever is more resistant to destruction by heat, desiccation, and chemicals than are the other rickettsiae.

The pathology of rickettsial infections is quite characteristic. The rickettsiae multiply in the endothelial cells lining the small blood vessels. As a result, the cells swell. There is an accumulation of leukocytes and other blood cells around the lesions in the capillaries. These lesions occur chiefly in the skin and also in the central nervous system, but they may occur in other organs. The capillaries become thrombosed, and the thrombosis may extend to the small arteries and veins. It is as a result of such lesions that petechiae and hemor-rhages occur in the skin.

Animals and humans infected with rickettsiae develop a number of specific antibodies, the most important of which are the complement-fixing, agglutinating, neutralizing, and precipitin antibodies. They also develop agglutinating antibodies against certain strains of *Bacillus proteus*. The test for the latter is the Weil-Felix test. It consists in mixing serum from a patient suffering from a rickettsial disease with a strain of *Bacillus proteus*. Agglutination of the organism results in all rickettsial diseases except Q fever and rickettsialpox. The reason for the reaction is not known, since *Bacillus proteus* has no etiological relationship to rickettsial diseases. It is believed that there is a common antigenic substance in *Bacillus proteus* and in certain rickettsiae. Different strains are aggultinated in the different rickettsial diseases. They are discussed under the separate diseases. The Weil-Felix and the complement-fixation reactions are the commonest serologic tests used.

Rickettsiae can be recovered from the blood of patients early in the disease without too much difficulty by injecting the blood into mice or guinea pigs or embryonated hen's eggs. The organisms are identified by characteristic lesions in experimental animals and by serological reactions.

The most important rickettsial diseases are listed below and are discussed individually:

1. The Typhus group
   a. Epidemic (louse-borne)
   b. Brill's disease
   c. Murine (endemic, flea-borne)
2. Scrub typhus (tsutsugamushi fever)
3. The spotted fever group
   a. Rocky Mountain spotted fever
   b. Rickettsialpox
   c. Boutonneuse fever
4. Q fever

The Typhus Group

Epidemic Typhus Fever (Louse-borne)

GENERAL DESCRIPTION

Epidemic typhus fever, also known as "jail fever," "camp fever," or "war fever," is an acute infectious disease caused by a rickettsia and characterized by fever, headache, and a generalized rash.

The Causative Agent

The causative agent is *Rickettsia prowazeki*. It has the general characteristics discussed on page 500. It grows only in the cytoplasm of infected cells.

The Host

Symptoms

The incubation period is 12 days. There is usually an abrupt onset, with headache, chilly sensations, pains in the muscles, and fever. This rises during the next 2 or 3 days to a level of 103° to 104° F. and the remains elevated for about 2 weeks, when it drops by crisis. During the early febrile period there may be a slight cough. The severe frontal headache and the prostration are, however, the marked symptoms. The face is flushed, the pulse rapid, and the tongue thick and coated. There may be excitement or delirium. About 4 to 5 days after onset a rash appears, which is generalized, occurring first on the trunk and spreading to the extremities, sparing the hands, feet, and face. The rash is at first macular and fades on pressure. Later it becomes petechial or hemorrhagic. In severe cases the hemorrhagic areas may be extensive and there may be hematuria or melena. During the second week the patient may be quite ill, dull, delirious, stuporous, or even comatose. The blood pressure is low, and the cough may persist, with signs of bronchitis. There are muscular twitchings and incontinence. The rash may be quite extensive and hemorrhagic. Death occurs in about 20 per cent of the cases.

Diagnosis

The diagnosis is made by the clinical picture and positive Weil-Felix reaction with Proteus OX 19 at the end of the first week of illness, in a titer of 1:160 or over. The complement-fixation reaction differentiates epidemic typhus from murine typhus and from Rocky Mountain spotted fever, which it resembles. It begins to be positive at the end of the first week of illness and reaches a peak titer during early convalescence. Another test that may be used is the specific agglutination of washed rickettsiae by the patient's serum. The white blood count is usually reduced in the first week but normal in the second week.

Immunity

An attack of epidemic typhus usually confers a permanent immunity against epidemic and murine typhus. However, the rickettsiae may remain dormant in the patient's cells and, many years later, cause a recrudescence of the disease which is milder in type. This is known as Brill's disease and is discussed below. Active immunization can be performed with a vaccine of rickettsiae grown in the yolk sac of embryonated eggs and activated with Formalin. It is administered in two doses of 1 cubic centimeter each, a week apart. Reimmunization with a dose of 1 cubic centimeter should be given every 6 to 12 months if there is danger of typhus.

THE ENVIRONMENT

Although typhus has probably existed since ancient times, it was confused with other fevers and was not recognized as a specific disease until the sixteenth century. Even after that it was confused with typhoid, which, in European countries, is called *typhus abdominalis* to distinguish it from typhus, which is called *typhus exanthematicus.* The disease has always been a companion in wars, jails, asylums, camps, and in other situations where humans are closely congregated and where sanitation is poor. It has been said that typhus has killed more soldiers than bullets. In World War I more than 1 million people died from typhus in Rumania, and several millions died from the disease in Russia. Even in World War II extensive epidemics occurred in the Balkans, on the eastern front, and in Japan.

In 1909, Nicolle, Compte, and Conseil established the fact that typhus was transmitted by lice. The following year Ricketts and Wilder discovered the agent of the disease in a smear of the intestinal contents of lice. In honor of this work the organisms were given the generic name of *Rickettsia.*

Typhus fever occurs in all countries and in all climates, but it is more common in cold countries and during the winter, when people live indoors more, crowd closer together, and bathe and change their garments less often. Focuses exist in central and eastern Europe, the Middle East, central Asia, China, and South America. Although it attacks all ages, the case fatality rises with age. Both sexes and all colors are equally susceptible. The extent of infection is directly proportional to the amount of lousiness. Epidemic typhus fever is one of the few diseases which can be eliminated by strict personal hygiene. Unfortunately, there are situations in which this is not possible.

Vector

The vector of epidemic typhus is the body louse, *Pediculus corporis.* The head louse, *Pediculus capitis,* may also serve as a vector. The body louse lives only in the clothes of man. It lays its eggs in the seams of underclothes. The eggs hatch in about 1 week and become adults in about 2 weeks. They take five to six blood meals a day from their host, and become infected from the blood of patients which contains rickettsiae early in the disease. The rickettsiae multiply so rapidly in the louse's intestines that the intestinal cells may swell and burst. The infected lice usually die in about 1 week to 10 days. If the lice are transferred to another human and get a blood meal from him, they infect him with the disease. The rickettsiae are excreted in the louse's feces and may cause infection by being rubbed into the abraded skin in scratching. Rickettsiae may survive in dried feces for as long as 2 months. The possibility exists that they may be scattered in dust and inhaled. The infection is not transmitted by lice to their offspring.

Control

The patient should be isolated until deloused. The nurse or attendant performing this process should be suitably gowned, preferably in a one-piece overall with close-fitting neck and wristbands. Caps should be worn, and gloves should fit closely at the wrist. The patient should be undressed and his clothing sprayed with DDT or fumigated. The hair of his body and head should be clipped, and he should be bathed with soap and water. Scalp and skin should be examined for the presence of lice or nits. If these are present they should be removed with forceps and placed in a jar of kerosene or DDT solution. The outerclothing of the nurse or attendant should be removed after the patient has been cleaned up; it should be fumigated or impregnated with DDT. Nurses and attendants should be immunized with typhus vaccine. All contacts in the family should be likewise deloused.

When typhus fever breaks out in a community, all cases should be sought out and hospitalized, and mass prophylaxsis should be instituted in the population. Its effectiveness was demonstrated in Naples during World War II. It consists of hand dusting the population with a dust gun, using a 10 per cent DDT powder. The powder is introduced beneath the clothing at several strategic points and into the hair. If the community is large, delousing stations are established, and the DDT dusting is done by motor-driven dust guns.

Public health nurses should participate in such a program as members of a team with other workers. They should take part in the educational program. They may also be called upon to care for patients remaining at home and to teach the family nursing procedures.

Medical Care Plans

Treatment

The first specific drug for the treatment of rickettsial diseases which offered considerable promise was para-aminobenzoic acid (PABA), which was introduced in the early 1940's. It is given orally in fairly large doses. While its value was being tested, the antibiotics were introduced and these were soon tried out. Penicillin and streptomycin have not been found to be of great value, but Aureomycin, chloramphenicol, and Terramycin are of distinct value and have brought about a marked change in the prognosis of the rickettsial diseases, similar to that brought about by penicillin in pneumococcus pneumonia. Aureomycin, Terramycin, and Chloromycetin are given in a daily dose of 20 to 30 milligrams per kilogram of body weight, or about 2 grams a day for an adult and half the amount for a child, in four or six divided doses. A priming dose of 2 grams in an adult and 1 gram in a child should be given initially. Frequent blood counts should be made if Chloromycetin is employed, since aplastic anemia has been reported after its use.

Diet

The diet should be chiefly liquid during the acute stage and should be liberalized as soon as the patient improves. The daily fluid requirement should be given by mouth, in small quantities frequently repeated. If the required amount cannot be taken, fluid in the form of 5 per cent glucose solution should be given intravenously.

Supportive Nursing Care

Complete bed rest and skilled nursing care are essential. Tepid sponge baths may be given to lessen discomfort from high elevations in temperature. The mouth should be kept clean with simple mouthwashes.

As hemorrhages in the subcutaneous tissues may be present, a daily cleansing bath is necessary for maintenance of circulation. Frequent change of bed linen may be necessary, as sweating may be profuse. Catheterization may be necessary when there is urinary retention. In the terminal phase of the disease, muscular twitching and urinary and fecal incontinence may be present.

For the relief of headache, the application of an ice cap may be effective. Sedative drugs may be prescribed for restlessness and insomnia, and codeine for cough.

The patient is usually in a stuporous condition, and delirium is a common occurrence. To safeguard the patient against injury, sideboards may be necessary.

The public health nurse may be called upon to give nursing care to patients at home during an epidemic, and to give instructions to families regarding preventive measures.

Brill's Disease

GENERAL DESCRIPTION

In 1898, Brill reported 17 cases in New York City of a disease resembling typhoid fever which differed from the latter disease because the Widal test appeared to be negative. In 1910 he reported a total of 255 cases. They were mainly in immigrants from Russia or Poland. The chief symptoms were fever, headache, and malaise. A rash occurred on the fourth or fifth days, and the blood cultures and the Widal test were negative. In 1912, Anderson and Goldberger showed the immunological relationship of this disease to Mexican typhus fever. However, lice were never implicated in its transmission. When murine typhus was shown to be a different variety of typhus from epidemic typhus, the idea occurred to some that Brill's disease was a form of murine typhus. However, the latter disease is transmitted by the rat flea, and in the cases in New York no vector seemed to play a part.

Zinsser suggested, in 1934, that Brill's disease was a recrudescent form of epidemic typhus. All cases had occurred in individuals who were born in a foreign country where typhus was endemic, there was no connection between the cases and no vector could be implicated. Three strains of rickettsia were isolated by him from patients, and these strains resembled epidemic rather than murine typhus. In 1943, when specific antigens for epidemic and murine typhus became available, Plotz performed complement-fixation tests with serums from patients with Brill's disease, and these gave higher titers against epidemic than endemic typhus.

In 1950, a study was made of a group of fourteen patients with Brill's disease in New York, Boston, Philadelphia, and Montreal. All were foreign-born persons who had lived years ago in an epidemic area, and all had fever, severe headache, and a rash on the fourth to the sixth day of illness. Rickettsiae were recovered from the blood of several patients early in the disease, and from body lice allowed to feed on them. The Weil-Felix reaction was frequently negative, but the complement-fixation reaction and the rickettsial agglutination test were positive in higher dilutions for epidemic than for endemic typhus. It appears very likely that Brill's disease is a recrudescent form of epidemic typhus. This offers an explanation for the occurrence of epidemics of typhus fever, although no animal reservoir for the disease is known. Man, himself, is the reservoir; the rickettsiae remain alive but inactive in his body. They may, however, become reactivated later. It also indicates that a host and an agent of disease may live in equilibrium for a great many years and still have equilibrium destroyed and serious disease set in.

The Causative Agent

As indicated above, the agent is probably *Rickettsia prowazeki,* similar to the agent of epidemic or classical typhus, which has remained dormant in the host's cells.

The Host

Symptoms

The symptoms of Brill's disease are similar to those of epidemic typhus, but milder. There is usually a sudden onset, with fever, chills, and malaise, and severe headache. The latter is the most constant symptom, as in epidemic typhus. A rash occurs on the fourth to the sixth day after onset. It is macular or maculopapular and does not usually become petechial as in epidemic typhus. It begins on the chest, spreads rapidly to the rest of the trunk, and then to the extremities, the height being reached on the seventh or eighth day. It disappears with convalescence. Bronchitis may occur. Neurologic symptoms are not common; when they occur they are usually those of apathy or confusion. Stupor and coma are extremely rare. The blood pressure is usually low.

Diagnosis

The occurrence of a typhuslike disease in a community where no focus of classical or murine typhus exists should make the clinician suspect Brill's disease. If the disease occurs in an individual who has lived in a region where classical typhus is endemic, if the Weil-Felix test is negative or positive in low titer, and if the complement-fixation test with convalescent serum is positive in a higher titer with epidemic than with endemic typhus antigen, a definite diagnosis of Brill's disease may be made.

Medical Care Plans

These are similar to those described under Epidemic Typhus, page 505.

Murine Typhus

GENERAL DESCRIPTION

Murine typhus, also known as "endemic typhus," is an acute rickettsial disease of rats and mice, transmitted to man by the rat flea and causing a disease resembling louse-borne typhus, but milder.

THE CAUSATIVE AGENT

The causative agent is *Rickettsia mooseri* and resembles *Rickettsia prowazeki,* from which it can be distinguished by its reaction in animals and by serological reactions.

THE HOST

Symptoms

The incubation period is 12 days. The symptoms of murine typhus are similar to but milder than those of epidemic typhus. The onset is usually not as abrupt as in classical typhus, and the symptoms are less severe. As in the latter disease a rash appears on the fourth or fifth day after onset. It is usually macular or maculopapular and there are not, as a rule, petechial or hemorrhagic lesions. Involvement of the central nervous system is uncommon and, when present, is milder in type. Complications are infrequent. The temperature comes down by lysis after 10 days to 2 weeks, and complications are rare. The mortality is about 2 per cent, chiefly in older people.

Diagnosis

Murine typhus cannot be distinguished from epidemic typhus clinically, except that the course is usually milder. The Weil-Felix reaction with Proteus OX 19 is also positive. Differentiation is made on the basis of serological reactions. The serums of patients recovering from murine typhus show a higher titer in the complement-fixation reaction with homologous than with heterologous antigens.

Immunity

An attack of murine typhus confers immunity for long periods of time against both murine and epidemic typhus. There are no vaccines available for immunization.

THE ENVIRONMENT

The occurrence of sporadic cases of typhus fever has been noted since the early twentieth century. Cases of the disease were considered to be epidemic typhus. In 1925 and 1926, Maxcy made an intensive investigation of such cases in southern United States and for epidemiological reasons postulated the theory that the disease found there was transmitted by fleas or ticks and that the reservoir was probably the rat or mouse. This was later proved to be the case. At first it was thought that murine typhus was the same as Brill's disease. This was disproved later.

Endemic or murine typhus is a disease of rats and mice and is transmitted from rat to rat by the rat louse, *Polyplax spinulosa* and by the rat flea, *Xenopsylla cheopis*. Man is accidentally infected by the rat flea. Infected rats usually recover. The flea becomes infected when feeding on an infected rat in the acute stage. The rickettsiae multiply in the flea without damaging it, and the flea continues to excrete the organisms in its feces until it dies. If it bites a human and the feces are rubbed into the broken skin, infection occurs.

Murine typhus is world wide in distribution and attacks people of all colors, both sexes, and all ages. Infection depends on the accessibility of infected rats. The greatest incidence is in the summer and fall when fleas are most abundant. In the United States most of the cases are reported from nine southern states. Up to 1947 a total of 44,819 cases was reported. The disease is commonest in adult males living in urban areas and working in establishments where rats are common.

Control

The disease is not transmitted from person to person, so that isolation of the patient and quarantine of contacts is unnecessary. The control of the disease in man depends on its control in rats. The measures that have been taken are (1) the elimination of harborages and food supply for rats by adequate waste disposal and food storage; (2) the ratproofing of buildings to prevent rats from entering; (3) the trapping and poisoning of rats to reduce the rat population; and (4) the dusting of rat runs and ratholes to kill the rat fleas which act as vectors. Such a program has been in effect in the states where murine typhus is endemic and has yielded good results.

MEDICAL CARE PLANS

Treatment

This is the same as in Epidemic Typhus, page 505.

Diet

As in epidemic typhus and Brill's disease, fluids only are given in the acute febrile stage. As the patient improves, soft foods are added, and with onset of recovery a general diet is given.

Supportive Nursing Care

This is similar to the nursing care for patients with epidemic typhus fever or Brill's disease. (See page 505.)

Scrub Typhus (Tsutsugamushi Fever)

GENERAL DESCRIPTION

Scrub typhus is an acute rickettsial disease occurring in the Far East. It is transmitted by a mite.

THE CAUSATIVE AGENT

The etiologic agent of scrub typhus is *Rickettsia orientalis (Rickettsia tsutsugamushi)*. It has properties similar to those of other rickettsiae.

THE HOST

Symptoms

The incubation period is 7 to 10 days. The onset is sudden, with fever, chilliness, and headache. A small necrotic lesion or eschar is seen at the site of attachment of an infected mite. From the fifth to the eighth day a maculopapular eruption, dull red in color, appears on the trunk and spreads to the arms and legs; it persists for several days. Fever is present throughout this time, and general lymphadenopathy, more pronounced in the glands draining the eschar. As in epidemic typhus, cough may be present. During the second week fever continues high, there may be signs of pneumonia, and the patient may be dull, apathetic, or delirious. By the third week there is a gradual fall in fever, the eschar heals, symptoms abate, and the patient becomes convalescent. In others, symptoms continue and death supervenes. The mortality varies in different places from a low of 1 or 2 per cent to a high of 60 per cent.

Diagnosis

Except for the eschar the clinical picture is similar to that of epidemic typhus. The eschar should be searched for, since it may be located on any part of the body. The white blood count is usually normal. The Weil-Felix test is important in diagnosis since it is positive with the OXK strain and not with the OX 19 strain. It becomes positive by the end of the second week. The rickettsiae may be recovered from the blood early in the disease. Specific complement-fixation tests may be performed but are technically difficult.

Immunity

An attack of scrub typhus gives prolonged immunity, as with other rickettsial diseases. The development of a vaccine for prophylactic immunization is still in the experimental stage.

The Environment

The disease was described in Japan early in the nineteenth century, and later in Malaya, the Dutch East Indies, India, Indo-China, New Guinea, and Australia. In World War II many cases occurred in American soldiers stationed in the Pacific area.

The disease is transmitted to man by the bite of mites, *Trombicula akamushi* or *Trombicula deliensis*. They are tiny, red in color, and feed on lymph or tissue juice of animals to which they attach themselves when in the larval stage. The infection in mites is transmitted from female to offspring. Only the larvae are parasitic on animals; the other stages of the mite develop in scrub growth. The reservoir is a small rodent such as the field mouse, rat, shrew, or vole.

The disease is found in the South Pacific area. Infection is not confined to either sex or to any particular age group, race, or color. It depends rather on the presence of susceptible hosts, animal reservoirs, the presence of low brush in which the mites can develop, and the presence of the organism.

Control

Since the disease is transmitted only by the bite of a larval mite, isolation of the patient and quarantine of contacts is not necessary. Control is directed toward killing the mite and making the environment unacceptable to mites and rodents. The former is done by impregnating clothes with anti-mite chemicals such as benzyl benzoate. The latter is achieved by burning or cutting vegetation very low or by spreading oil on the ground. Sleeping cots in the field should be kept at some distance from the ground. The use of prophylactic vaccines is still in the experimental stage.

Medical Care Plans

Treatment

Treatment is the same as in other rickettsial diseases. It is discussed under Epidemic Typhus, page 505.

Diet

No special diet is used. As in other febrile diseases, a fluid diet is used in the acute stage and is gradually liberalized by the addition of solids. If fluids cannot be taken orally, the requirement must be made up with parenteral injections.

Supportive Nursing Care

This is similar to the care given to patients with epidemic typhus.

The Spotted Fever Group

This is a group of tick- and mite-borne diseases of rickettsial origin of which Rocky Mountain spotted fever is the most important. Among other diseases in the group are boutonneuse fever and rickettsialpox.

Rocky Mountain Spotted Fever

GENERAL DESCRIPTION

Rocky Mountain spotted fever is an acute disease of rickettsial origin which is transmitted by a tick and which occurs chiefly in the western part of the United States but also in the rest of the continent and in South America.

THE CAUSATIVE AGENT

The causative agent is *Rickettsia rickettsi* which grows in the nucleus as well as the cytoplasm of infected cells. Its characteristics are similar to those described for rickettsiae in general. The organism is not filterable.

THE HOST

Symptoms

The incubation period is from 3 to 10 days. The onset is usually abrupt, with chills, sweating, fever, headache, and prostration. Pains in the muscles and joints are complained of. There often are photophobia and pain on pressure over the eyeballs. On the third or fourth day a red, maculopapular rash appears, first on the ankles and wrists and then spreading to the arms and legs and trunk. The rash frequently becomes petechial. Fever continues for 2 to 3 weeks, with morning remissions. The tongue is dry and coated, and the breath is often foul. The rash is fainter during the periods of remission, but generally becomes more intense, and petechial or hemorrhagic in character. Neurologic symptoms, such as headache, restlessness, and insomnia, usually occur. There may be lethargy or delirium, stupor, and even coma. Convalescence begins about the third week and continues to recovery. Death occurs in about 20 per cent of cases. It is much higher in adults (25 per cent) than in children (7 per cent).

Diagnosis

Clinically, it is difficult to differentiate spotted fever from typhus. The rash in spotted fever usually starts in the extremities and involves the trunk later, while the reverse is true of typhus. The white blood count shows a leukocytosis, while in typhus there is usually a leukopenia at first and a normal count later. In spotted fever there is often a history of exposure to ticks or a tick bite. In typhus there is no such history, but in endemic typhus there is a history of exposure to rats, and in epidemic typhus there is evidence of lousiness.

Early in the disease rickettsiae can be recovered from a patient's blood by injecting the blood into a guinea pig. The Weil-Felix reaction becomes positive at the end of the second week with the Proteus OX 19 antigen but is often also positive with OX 2 antigen. The complement-fixation reaction differentiates spotted fever from typhus. The virus neutralization test may also be used for this purpose.

Immunity

An attack of the disease confers a fairly solid immunity. A vaccine made either from infected ticks or from rickettsiae grown in the yolk sac of embryonated eggs confers protection. It is given in three weekly doses of 1 cubic centimeter or two weekly doses of 2 cubic centimeters. The immunity is not absolute and is stronger in children than in adults; in the latter it is more effective against mild than against severe infections. Booster doses are advisable yearly if the individual remains exposed to the disease.

The Environment

The disease was first described by Maxcy in 1899 in the Rocky Mountain area of the United States, hence its name. Howard Ricketts first transmitted the disease from humans to guinea pigs in 1906 and indicated the part played by the wood tick. At first it was thought that the disease was limited to the northwestern part of the United States. However, the disease has been reported from nearly all the states as well as from Canada, Mexico, and South America. In America about 400 to 500 cases are reported yearly.

In the western United States the vector is the wood tick, *Dermacentor andersoni,* which is active in the spring and early summer. In the eastern United States the vector is the brown dog tick, *Dermacentor variabilis,* which is most active in the summer. Cases in the West occur largely in the spring, while in the East they occur in the summer. In the West the disease is largely an occupational one among adult males who work as woodsmen, foresters, miners, trappers, huntsmen, and sheep handlers. In the East the disease is commonest in children who are in closest contact with dogs.

The death rate is highest among adults and is consequently higher in the West than in the East. Women are more frequently infected in the East than in the West for the same reason that children are.

A variety of other ticks, in addition to those mentioned, have been found infected in nature. Infected ticks transmit the rickettsiae to their offspring. The larvae and nymphs feed on rodents and small carnivores, and the adults feed chiefly on larger animals, such as sheep, dogs, deer, and cattle. Their life cycle takes about 2 years. Man is infected accidentally as the ticks are brushed off from plants or animals. When infected ticks attach themselves to man or an animal, they do not transmit the infection until they have fed for several hours.

Control

Most important in control is personal hygiene. Individuals should avoid tick-infested areas, if possible, particularly during the tick season. If this is not possible, suitable clothing should be worn. This includes high boots and leggings worn outside the trouser legs. Head and neck should be as well covered as the rest of the body. Body and clothing should be examined twice daily, and attached ticks should be removed with forceps. If removed with bare fingers they may be crushed, and infection may result. The tick bite should be touched with an antiseptic.

Individuals who, by occupation or residence, are exposed to ticks in infected areas should be immunized with vaccine preceding the tick season and receive booster doses annually. If infection occurs, treatment with chloramphenicol should be undertaken. Since the disease is not transmitted from man to man, isolation of the patient and quarantine of contacts are not necessary.

MEDICAL CARE PLANS

Treatment

The broad-spectrum antibiotics have been used in spotted fever as in the typhus group, with similar good results. Aureomycin, Terramycin, and Chloromycetin are all effective. For the average adult an initial dose of 2 to 3 grams is given. This is followed by a dose of 2 grams a day in four or six divided doses until the temperature remains normal for 12 hours. For children, approximately half the dose is used. If Chloromycetin is employed, the patient should be followed with frequent blood counts, since aplastic anemia has been reported after its use.

Diet

As in the typhus group, no special diet is indicated. The food given depends on the patient's general condition. When fever is high, liquids are given. These are supplemented with solid foods as the condition improves. If the patient is very ill and is unable to take his fluid requirements by mouth, they should be given intravenously in the form of 5 per cent glucose solution.

Supportive Nursing Care

The patient should be kept in bed during the febrile stage and made comfortable. The usual routine of mouth care and bathing should be carried out. The light in the room may need to be subdued, if photophobia is present. If the lips are dry or cracked, cold cream or liquid petrolatum should be applied. Headache is often relieved by an ice cap. If there is restlessness or insomnia, a sedative drug may have to be prescribed.

Rickettsialpox

GENERAL DESCRIPTION

Rickettsialpox is an acute disease of rickettsial origin transmitted by the bite of a mite.

THE CAUSATIVE AGENT

The causative agent is *Rickettsia akari,* which grows in the cytoplasm and nucleus of infected cells and has the characteristics of other rickettsiae.

The Host

Symptoms

The incubation period is 7 to 14 days. An initial lesion appears at the site of the bite. It is firm, red, and papular, but becomes vesicular. The vesicle dries, and an eschar is formed, which falls off after about 3 weeks from the beginning, leaving a small scar. Regional lymphadenopathy is usually present. About 1 week after the initial lesion there is an abrupt onset, with fever, headache, chilliness, backache, and sweating. The fever has a remittent course and continues high for about 1 week when it gradually subsides. About 2 to 4 days after the acute onset, a red rash appears on the body, which persists for about 1 week. It is first maculopapular, but in a few days it becomes papulovesicular. The vesicles later dry, the scabs fall off, and the rash disappears in about 1 week from onset, without leaving scars. There have been no deaths or complications from the disease.

Diagnosis

Rickettsialpox is a much milder disease than Rocky Mountain spotted fever and is of shorter duration. Clinically, it can be distinguished from that disease and from typhus by the occurrence of a primary lesion and by the character of the rash, which is papulovesicular. This fact and also the fact that the rash rarely occurs on the palms and soles distinguish it from boutonneuse fever. During the acute stage of rickettsialpox there is a leukopenia of 2,000 to 5,000 white blood count. The rickettsiae can be recovered from blood of patients early in the disease by injection into mice. The Weil-Felix reaction is not positive in significant titers in rickettsialpox as it is in typhus, Rocky Mountain spotted fever, and during convalescence in boutonneuse fever. The complement-fixation reaction with specific antigen becomes positive in the second week and continues positive for a long time. It distinguishes the disease from typhus and most other rickettsioses, but there is crossing with Rocky Mountain spotted fever.

Immunity

Since the discovery of the disease in 1946 there has been no instance of a second attack in the same person. No prophylactic vaccines are available.

The Environment

The disease was first discovered in New York City in 1946. About 170 cases occurred in a housing development in one of the boroughs, and the physicians attending the cases suspected that they were dealing with a rickettsial disease, possibly a mild form of Rocky Mountain spotted fever. An investigation was undertaken by the New York City Department of Health in conjunction with the U. S. Public Health Service, and the clinical and epidemiological aspects were completely worked out. The name Rickettsialpox was given to the disease. Since 1946, from 75 to 100 cases have been reported yearly in all boroughs of the city except Richmond. In 1951, the first cases found outside of New York City were reported from Boston. The disease attacks all ages and both sexes and has been seen in Negroes as well as whites.

The vector of the disease is a tiny, colorless mite, *Allodermanyssus sanguineus,* and the reservoir is the field or house mouse, *Mus musculus.* Man is infected accidentally. In the original outbreak, the reservoir was maintained by food allowed to accumulate in incinerators. These were not fired frequently enough and, in effect, became mouse harborages. In all houses in other parts of the city where cases were found later, mice were seen in considerable numbers.

Control

Rickettsialpox is not transmitted from person to person. Patients need not be isolated, nor do contacts have to be quarantined. Control of the disease depends, as in murine typhus, on eliminating the animal reservoir. This consists of proper refuse disposal, care in food storage, elimination of rodent harborages, and trapping of rodents. Dusting of ratholes and rat runs with DDT in order to destroy the mites clinging to mice and dusting with DDT of locations where mites are found in a building are necessary measures of value.

MEDICAL CARE PLANS

Treatment

The disease is self-limited. The symptoms are rarely severe enough to require heroic treatment. However, symptomatic and specific treatment is similar to that of other rickettsial disease and is detailed under Rocky Mountain spotted fever. (See page 515.)

Diet

Dietary restrictions are not necessary. During the period of fever the diet should be accommodated to the patient's desires.

Supportive Nursing Care

With an illness as short as that of rickettsialpox, no uncommon nursing procedures are needed. The important steps are to keep the patient in bed during the pyrexia, to sponge him in order to reduce the discomforts of the sweating, to apply cold applications to his head for the relief of headache, and to keep the room darkened if there is photophobia or pain in the eyeballs. General malaise is usually relieved with aspirin.

Boutonneuse Fever

GENERAL DESCRIPTION

Boutonneuse fever is an acute disease of rickettsial origin occurring in the Mediterranean area and transmitted by a tick.

THE CAUSATIVE AGENT

The causative agent is *Rickettsia conori* which grows in the nucleus as well as the cytoplasm of infected cells. It passes a Chamberland filter. Its characteristics are similar to other rickettsiae.

THE HOST

Symptoms

The incubation period is 5 to 6 days. Onset is sudden, with fever, chilliness, headache, and pains in the bones and joints. A small ulcer with a black, necrotic center (tache noir), the size of the tick bite, usually precedes the onset of symptoms and persists until defervescence of fever. Regional adenopathy is present. Three to four days after onset of fever a rash appears on the body. It is red and maculopapular, and spreads to the entire body, including palms, soles, and face. The fever and other symptoms continue for about 1 or 2 weeks after onset. The rash persists until after the fever is gone and disappears without leaving scars. The disease has a mortality of about 2 per cent.

Diagnosis

The disease is much milder than spotted fever and resembles rickettsialpox. Clinically, it is distinguished from the latter by the character of the rash, which is not vesicular, and by its frequent occurrence on the palms and soles. Serologically, it can be distinguished from other rickettsial disease by the complement-fixation reaction with specific washed rickettsiae. The Weil-Felix reaction with OX 19 and OX 2 becomes positive late in convalescence, distinguishing this disease from rickettsialpox in which the Weil-Felix reaction remains negative.

Immunity

An attack of the disease confers immunity. There are no available prophylactic vaccines.

THE ENVIRONMENT

The disease was first described in Tunis in 1910 by Conor and Bruch. Since then it has been described in other Mediterranean countries. It is transmitted by the brown dog tick, *Rhipicephalus sanguineus,* the dog serving only as the transmitter of the tick, but not being infected by it. No reservoir other than man has been found.

Control

The avoidance of tick-infested areas and the disinfestation of dogs are the most important control measures. The disease is not transferred from man to man so that isolation of patients and quarantine of contacts are not necessary.

MEDICAL CARE PLANS

These are the same as for rickettsialpox. (See pages 517–518.)

Q Fever

GENERAL DESCRIPTION

Q fever is an acute disease of rickettsial origin characterized by fever and pulmonary signs.

THE CAUSATIVE AGENT

The causative agent is a rickettsia, *Coxiella burneti,* which is filterable and more resistant than, but otherwise similar to, other rickettsiae. Like rickettsialpox and unlike the other rickettsioses, the agent of Q fever does not stimulate the production of agglutinins to any of the antigens of *Bacillus proteus.* The Weil-Felix test is, therefore, negative.

THE HOST

Symptoms

The incubation period is 2 to 3 weeks. Onset is sudden, with headache, chilliness, fever, sweats, and general aches and pains. Insomnia is a common complaint. About the fifth or sixth day a dry cough develops and, with it, some chest pain. An X ray taken at this time shows patchy areas of consolidation. Physical signs are often absent or minimal, consisting of localized rales. The fever lasts about 1 week, but roentgenographic clearing of the lungs is not seen until a few days to 1 week later. The white blood count is usually normal. Recovery is uneventful. Deaths are rare.

Diagnosis

The differential diagnosis from other rickettsial disease is not difficult, since no rash occurs in Q fever, and pneumonic lesions do not, as a rule, occur in other rickettsial diseases. Differentiation from bacterial and atypical pneumonias, from influenza, psittacosis, and several other diseases can be made by the laboratory.

The organism can be recovered from the blood as well as the sputum of patients early in the disease by injection into guinea pigs, mice, or embryonated eggs. Serum from patients gives a positive complement-fixation reaction with specific rickettsiae by the second week. For diagnosis, an early and later specimen should be obtained, so that a rise in antibody titer may be demonstrated.

Immunity

An attack of Q fever confers immunity against the disease. There are at present no vaccines for active immunization against the disease.

The Environment

The disease was first described in Australia in 1935. Since then single cases and epidemics of the disease have been described in various parts of the world. In the United States several epidemics have been described, and a large endemic area has been studied in California. A number of laboratory epidemics have also been described.

The disease is not limited to any climate or season nor to any race or color. Although it is more common in men than in women, this appears to be due to occupation. The same holds true for age, the disease being more common in adults than in children.

Occupational exposure appears to play a large part in the transmission of the disease. Most of the cases have occurred in workers in stockyards, meat-packing plants, and dairies and in individuals living within a short distance of such places. Epidemics have also been described among workers in wool-sorting plants as well as among sheep tenders. The occurrence of epidemics in laboratories where the virus of Q fever is studied has already been mentioned. There appears to be evidence in California that a relationship exists between occurrence of illness and the consumption of milk from

Rickettsial Diseases

Disease	Causative Agent	Vector	Animal Reservoir	Weil-Felix Test	Specific Complement-Fixation Test
Epidemic typhus	*Rickettsia prowazeki*	Louse (*Pediculus corporis*)	Man only	OX 19 +++ OX 2 − 0 OX K − 0	Positive
Brill's disease	*Rickettsia prowazeki*	None (recrudescent)	Man	Usually negative	Positive with antigens of epidemic and endemic. In higher dilutions with former
Murine (endemic) typhus	*Rickettsia mooseri*	Flea (*Xenopsylla cheopis*)	Rat	OX 19 +++ OX 2 − 0 OX K − 0	Positive
Scrub typhus	*Rickettsia tsutsugamushi* (*orientalis*)	Mite (*Trombicula akamushi Trombicula deliensis*)	Wild rodents	OX 19 − 0 OX 2 − 0 OX K −+++	Positive
Rocky Mountain spotted fever	*Rickettsia rickettsi*	Tick (*Dermacentor andersoni Dermacentor variabilis*)	Rodents and small carnivores	OX 19 ++ OX 2 + OX K − 0	Positive
Rickettsialpox	*Rickettsia akari*	Mite (*Allodermanyssus sanguineus*)	Mouse	OX 19 − 0 OX 2 − 0 OX K − 0	Positive (crosses with R.M.S.F.)
Boutonneuse fever	*Rickettsia conori*	Tick (*Rhipicephalus sanguineus*)	Dog	OX 19 −++ (delayed) OX 2 + OX K − 0	Positive (crosses with R.M.S.F.)
Q fever	*Coxiella burneti* (*Rickettsia burneti*)	Tick?	Rodents? Cattle?	OX 19 − 0 OX 2 − 0 OX K − 0	Positive

522 MODERN CONCEPTS OF COMMUNICABLE DISEASE

infected cows. The virus appears in the milk of such cows but is destroyed by boiling or pasteurizing the milk. The latter process, as commercially performed, may allow some organisms to survive.

In nature the virus has been found in cows, sheep, goats, bandicoots, and ticks. The method of transmission to humans has not been worked out. Transmission by insects or other arthropods appears improbable. The weight of evidence is in favor of transmission by infected dust. Infected milk may play a part in certain regions. Direct transmission from person to person has not been demonstrated.

Control

Isolation of the patient is not necessary since the disease is not transmitted directly from person to person. All milk should be pasteurized. Since the virus is readily shed by animals, it does not appear that proper environmental protective measures can be found. It appears probable that control of the disease among individuals working with or living near infected animals will depend either on eliminating all infected animals or on proper immunization of cattle and, perhaps, of humans exposed as a result of occupation or contiguity. At present there is no effective vaccine for active immunization.

Medical Care Plans

The disease is comparatively mild and self-limited. There is evidence that the antibiotics effective for the other rickettsial diseases are effective in this disease also. Symptomatic treatment, diet, and general nursing measures are similar to those of other respiratory diseases.

REFERENCES

Rickettsial Diseases

1. Andrews, J. M., and Link, V. B.: "The Murine Typhus Problem in the United States," *Pests*, 15:12, 1947.
2. Bell, J. A.; Beck, M. D.; and Huebner, R. J.: "Epidemiologic Studies of Q Fever in Southern California," *J.A.M.A.*, 142:868, 1950.
3. Bishopp, F. C.: "Medical and Public Health Importance of Insecticide DDT," *Bull. New York Acad. Med.*, 21:561, 1945.
4. Blake, F. G.; Maxcy, K. F.; Sandush, J. F., Jr.; Kohls, G. M.; and Bell, E. J.: "Studies on Tsutsugamushi Disease (Scrub Typhus, Mite-borne Typhus) in New Guinea and Adjacent Island," *Am. J. Hyg.*, 41:243, 1945.
5. Blanc, G., and Caminopetros, J.: "Etudes Epidemiologiques et Experimentales sur la Fievere Boutonneuse, Faites a l'Institut Pasteur d'Athens," *Arch. Inst. Pasteur de Tunis*, 20:343, 1932.
6. Brill, N. E.: "Acute Infectious Disease of Unknown Origin," *Am. J. M. Sc.*, 139:484, 1910.

7. Cox, H. R.: "Rocky Mountain Spotted Fever," *Pub. Health Rep.*, **54**:1070, 1939.

8. Derrick, E. H.: " 'Q' Fever, a New Fever Entity," *Med. J. Australia*, **2**:281, 1937.

9. Dyer, R. E.: "Typhus Fever," *M. Clin. North America*, **27**:775, 1943.

10. Dyer, R. E.: "The Rickettsial Diseases," *J.A.M.A.*, **124**:1165, 1944.

11. Greenberg, M.; Pellitteri, O. J.; and Jellison, W. L.: "Rickettsialpox III. Epidemiology," *Am. J. Pub. Health*, **37**:860, 1947.

12. Greenberg, M.; Pellitteri, O. J.; Klein, I. F.; and Huebner, R. J.: "Rickettsialpox II. Clinical Observation," *J.A.M.A.*, **133**:901, 1947.

13. Heubner, R. J.; Stamps, P.; and Armstrong, C.: "Rickettsialpox I. Isolation of the Etiologic Agent," *Pub. Health Rep.*, **61**:1605, 1946.

14. Maxcy, K. F.: "An Epidemiological Study of Endemic Typhus (Brill's Disease) in the Southeastern United States," *Pub. Health Rep.*, **41**:2967, 1926.

15. Murray, E. S., and Snyder, J. C.: "Brill's Disease. Etiology," *Am. J. Hyg.*, **53**:23, 1951.

16. Murray, E. S.; Baehr, G.; Schwartzman, G.; Mandelbaum, R. A.; Rosenthal, N.; Doane, J. C.; Weiss, L. B.; Cohen, S.; and Snyder, J. C.: "Brill's Disease," *J.A.M.A.*, **142**:1059, 1950.

17. Parker, R. R.: "Rocky Mountain Spotted Fever," *J.A.M.A.*, **110**:1185, 1938.

18. Payne, E. H.; Knaudt, J. A.; and Palacios, S.: "Treatment of Epidemic Typhus with Chloromycetin," *J. Trop. Med.*, **51**:68, 1948.

19. Philip, C. B.; Woodward, T. E.; and Sullivan, R. R.: "Tsutsugamushi Disease (Scrub or Mite-borne Typhus) in the Philippine Islands during American Reoccupation in 1944–1945," *Am. J. Trop. Med.*, **26**:229, 1946.

20. Pike, G.; Cohen, S.; and Murray, E. S.: "Rickettsialpox," *New England J. Med.*, **243**:913, 1950.

21. Pincoffs, M. D., *et al.*: "The Treatment of Rocky Mountain Spotted Fever with Chloromycetin," *Ann. Int. Med.*, **29**:656, 1948.

22. Pinkerton, H.: "Diseases Caused by Rickettsiae," in Bercovitz's *Clinical Tropical Medicine*, Paul B. Hoeber, Inc., New York, 1944.

23. Plotz, H.: "Complement Fixation in Rickettsial Diseases," *Science*, **97**:20, 1943.

24. Plotz, H.; Reagan, R. L.; and Wertman, K.: "Differentiation between Fievre Boutonneuse and Rocky Mountain Spotted Fever by Means of the Complement Fixation Reaction," *Proc. Soc. Exper. Biol. & Med.*, **55**:173, 1944.

25. Pullen, R. L.: *Communicable Diseases*, Lea & Febiger, Philadelphia, 1950.

26. Rivers, T. M.: *Virus and Rickettsial Diseases of Man*, J. B. Lippincott Company, Philadelphia, 1948.

27. Rose, H. M.; Kneeland, Y., Jr.; and Gibson, G. D.: "Treatment of Rickettsialpox with Aureomycin," *Am. J. Med.*, **9**:300, 1950.

28. Ross, S., *et al.*: "Aureomycin Therapy of Rocky Mountain Spotted Fever," *J.A.M.A.*, **138**:1213, 1948.

29. Smadel, J. E.; Leon, A. P.; Ley, H. L.; and Varela, G.: "Chloromycetin in Treatment of Typhus Fever," *Proc. Soc. Exper. Biol. & Med.*, **68**:12, 1948.

30. Smadel, J. E.; Woodward, T. E.; Ley, H. L., Jr.; and Lewthwaite, R.: "Chloramphenicol (Chloromycetin) in the Treatment of Tsutsugamushi Disease (Scrub Typhus)," *J. Clin. Invest.*, **28**:1196, 1949.

31. Strong, R. P.: *Stitt's Diagnosis, Prevention and Treatment of Tropical Diseases*, 6th ed., The Blakiston Company, Philadelphia, 1943.

32. Stuart, B. M., and Pullen, R. L.: "Endemic (Murine) Typhus Fever," *Ann. Int. Med.*, **23**:520, 1945.

33. Topping, N. H.: "Rocky Mountain Spotted Fever," *Pub. Health Rep.*, **58**:757, 1943.

34. Wheeler, C. M.: "Control of Typhus in Italy, 1943–1944, by the Use of DDT," *Am. J. Pub. Health,* **36**:119, 1946.
35. Wolbach, S. B.: "The Rickettsial Diseases," in *Cecil's Textbook of Medicine,* 7th ed., W. B. Saunders Company, Philadelphia, 1947.
36. Zinsser, H.: "Varieties of Typhus Virus and the Epidemiology of the American Form of European Typhus Fever (Brill's Disease)," *Am. J. Hyg.,* **20**:513, 1934.

Chapter 61 SCABIES (ITCH)

GENERAL DESCRIPTION

SCABIES is a skin disease caused by the itch mite and characterized by burrows, made by the mite, and by vesicles and pustules, which are produced as a result of scratching.

THE CAUSATIVE AGENT

The *Sarcoptes scabei* is the mite responsible for the lesions. It is tiny, measuring from about $\frac{1}{60}$ to $\frac{1}{80}$ inch in length. The mites live on the skin, in burrows, which they dig and which are from about $\frac{1}{16}$ to $\frac{1}{2}$ inch in length. Fertilization takes place in the burrow and eggs are laid for several weeks, a total of about forty to fifty. The eggs hatch in 3 to 5 days, and the larvae emerge and produce lateral tunnels or new ones. They mature in about 2 weeks, the females are fertilized, and new deposition of eggs occurs. Adult males die soon after fertilizing the females, and the latter die after deposition of ova. The mites feed on the tissues of the host and deposit small fecal pellets.

The burrow is a superficial tunnel which is dug by the female itch mite on any part of the body but which is most commonly seen in the webs between the fingers, on the backs of the hands, in the axillae, groin, genitalia, and under the breasts in women. It appears like a thin, black, slightly raised line.

THE HOST

Symptoms

The incubation period varies. The main symptom is itching, and the chief physical sign is the burrow. Scratching causes a variety of lesions from bleeding and oozing to vesicle and pustule formation. The itching is very intense and is commonest at night when the patient is under warm covers. There are no constitutional symptoms.

Diagnosis

The diagnosis is made by inspection. Usually one burrow or more can be identified, and if the roof is removed with a pin the parasite can be obtained and identified.

Immunity

No immunity is conferred by an attack of scabies. Reinfection is common.

THE ENVIRONMENT

The disease has been recognized since Biblical times, but the itch mite was first described as the etiologic agent in 1687 by Bonomo and Cestoni. The infection is found all over the world and is not limited to any particular climate, to any race or age, or to either sex. It is most common where there is crowding and where there is lack of cleanliness.

Control

The infected individual should be kept away from contact with others until he is cured. It is especially important that he sleep alone. Quarantine of contacts is not necessary. Infected children should be excluded from school. As soon as a case is discovered, treatment should be instituted. Since infestation in a family group is not limited to a single individual, it is wise to examine all members of the group and to treat them if they are found to be infested.

MEDICAL CARE PLANS

Treatment

The time-honored treatment is the use of sulfur. After a hot cleansing bath, a 5 per cent sulfur ointment is rubbed into the skin of the entire body, with the exception of the face and scalp, and is repeated for 2 succeeding nights. On the fourth night a bath is again taken, and the body is cleansed with soap and warm water. A complete change of underclothing, pajamas or gown, and bed linen is made. The treatment may have to be repeated in 1 week.

While the treatment is effective, the sulfur may cause a dermatitis in some individuals, and in young children a half-strength ointment may have to be used. Furthermore, the treatment is messy and soils underclothing and bedclothes. In recent years a number of other drugs have been recommended. One that has met with considerable success is a 25 per cent emulsion of benzyl benzoate. After a bath, the emulsion is painted on the skin with a 2-inch brush and allowed to dry. A second coat is applied after 24 hours, and after 48 hours a bath is taken and the body is cleansed with soap and warm water. Underclothing, sheets, and pillowcases should be changed and should be sterilized by boiling.

REFERENCES

1. Cannon, A. B., and McCrae, M. E.: "Treatment of Scabies," *J.A.M.A.*, 138:557, 1948.
2. Friedman, R.: *Scabies, Civil and Military*, Froben Press, Inc., New York, 1941.
3. McElbenny, T. J.: "The Treatment of Scabies in Children with a New Sarcopticide," *J. Pediat.*, 29:189, 1946.
4. Mackenzie, I. F.: "Scabies Treated by Benzyl Benzoate Emulsion," *Brit. M. J.*, 2:401, 1941.
5. Mellanby, K.: *Scabies*, Oxford University Press, New York, 1943.

Chapter 62 TULAREMIA

TULAREMIA is a disease of wild animals, particularly rabbits and hares, which is caused by *Pasteurella tularensis,* and which may be transmitted to man directly or through an arthropod vector. In man the illness is acute, with fever, chills, and swollen glands.

THE CAUSATIVE AGENT

Pasteurella tularensis is a nonmotile, gram-negative bacterium which may appear in coccoid form. It grows readily on culture mediums. It shows a certain amount of cross agglutination with *Brucella.* It is fairly resistant, surviving in water and in carcasses for months. It is, however, destroyed by heat and the usual disinfectants.

THE HOST

Symptoms

Tularemia in man is caused by handling infected animals, particularly wild hares or rabbits, by eating their uncooked meat, by being bitten by infected animals, flies, or ticks, or by drinking infected water. The first is the most common method.

The incubation period is about 3 days. Onset is sudden, with chills, fever, and prostration. In most human infections there are ulceration at the site of infection and a spread by the lymphatics to the regional lymph glands which swell, are tender, and may break down and form an abscess. Bacteremia may occur early but is usually transitory. The symptoms may last for several weeks, and recovery is gradual and often drawn out. This type of the disease is referred to as the *ulceroglandular* type. In the *pneumonic* type there is a consolidation of the lungs resembling that of tuberculosis. In the *oculoglandular* type there are ulceration of the lower lid, conjunctivitis, and enlargement of the glands. The *septic* or *typhoidal* type is caused by the development of bacteremia and a general septic state.

About 5 per cent of the cases die.

Diagnosis

Specific antibodies appear in the blood during the second week and can be demonstrated by the agglutination test. A skin test may be used early in the disease. A specially prepared vaccine of *Pasteurella tularensis* is injected intradermally in 0.05-cubic-centimer amounts, and a positive reaction is indicated by redness and induration in 48 hours. Positive blood cultures may occasionally be obtained, and cultures should also be made from abscesses and from sputum or pleural effusion in cases of pneumonia. The organisms may also be recovered by injecting guinea pigs or mice.

Immunity

An attack confers immunity. Second attacks are rare, and when they do occur, are mild. There are no available vaccines or serums for immunization.

THE ENVIRONMENT

Many animals are naturally infected. The most common are wild hares and rabbits. However, other animals which may be infected are the muskrat, squirrel, skunk, cat, deer, dog, fox, hog, and hen. The disease may also be transmitted by infected ticks or deer flies. It is not transmitted from man to man.

Tularemia occurs in all parts of the United States. Infection is more common in the summer in Western states where it is usually transmitted by ticks and deer flies. In the East it is more common in the hunting season in the fall and winter. Ticks apparently keep the infection alive in animals since, once infected, they remain so for life and even transmit the infection to their offspring.

Control

To prevent tularemia, hunters should be careful in handling hares and rabbits that appear ill, butchers should use gloves in dressing their meat, and housewives should cook them thoroughly. Care should be taken to avoid bites by ticks and deer flies. Raw water should not be drunk in areas where tularemia is prevalent.

MEDICAL CARE PLANS

Treatment

Penicillin is of no value. Streptomycin is highly effective for treatment. It is given in a dose of 1 gram a day intramuscularly for about 1 week. Aureomycin, chloramphenicol, and Terramycin also appear to be effective.

Diet

A soft diet should be given and increased to a full diet as the patient improves.

Supportive Nursing Care

During the febrile period the patient is on bed rest, and nursing care is similar to that of other acute infections. Tepid sponge baths and antipyretics may be given for elevated temperatures and to relieve general discomfort. To control pain, codeine may be prescribed.

The patient may be placed in an upright position, supported by backrest and pillows, if he is more comfortable. Wet dressings or compresses may be applied to swollen lymph nodes. Soiled dressings should be removed and handled with forceps or gloves, placed in a paper bag, and burned.

The debilitating effects of the disease and the slow recovery often restrict participation in work and social activities. Orientation of the patient to his illness, constant reassurance, and an understanding attitude of the family will aid in lessening fears and worries. The nurse should provide suitable diversion for the patient and encourage occupational therapy. Frequent rest periods should be planned to offset fatigue and depression.

In rural areas a physician or the family may request the services of a public health nurse to give or supervise nursing care of the patient. She should help the family with plans for the convalescent period and stress the preventive aspects of the disease.

REFERENCES

1. Ayres, J. C., and Feemster, R. F.: "Epidemiology of Tularemia in Massachusetts with a Review of the Literature," *New England J. Med.*, **238**:187, 1948.
2. Cry, E. M.: "Tularemia," *Am. J. Nursing*, **48**:387, 1948.
3. Foshay, L., and Pasternack, A. B.: "Streptomycin for Tularemia," *J.A.M.A.*, **130**:393, 1946.
4. Lindeke, H. I., and Maiden, S. D.: "Tularemia Treated with Aureomycin," *J.A.M.A.*, **142**:99, 1950.
5. Pullen, R. L., and Stuart, B. M.: "Tularemia, Analysis of 225 Cases," *J.A.M.A.*, **129**:495, 1945.
6. Rausmeier, J. C.: "The Effect of Aureomycin against Bacterium Tularense," *J. Clin. Investigation*, **28**:977, 1949.
7. Tillman, S. G.: "Nursing Care of the Patient with Tularemia," *Am. J. Nursing*, **48**:389, 1948.

Chapter 63 YELLOW FEVER

GENERAL DESCRIPTION

YELLOW FEVER is an acute infectious disease of viral origin, transmitted by mosquitoes and characterized by fever, bleeding, and jaundice, and by liver damage.

THE CAUSATIVE AGENT

The cause of yellow fever is a small virus which grows in tissue culture and in developing chick embryos. It is readily destroyed by heat and the usual antiseptics. The virus is both neurotropic and viscerotropic, different strains having different affinities. Monkeys are more commonly affected by the viscerotropic strains and albino mice by the neurotropic ones. By continued growth in tissue culture, some strains lose their infectivity. This has happened to the so-called "17D strain," which is widely used for immunization.

THE HOST

Symptoms

The incubation period of yellow fever is 3 to 6 days. Onset is acute, with fever, chills, headache, and backache. The fever continues high for 3 or 4 days. The patient feels ill, is nauseous, and may vomit. The eyes are injected, and the face is congested. The pulse is slow in relation to the fever (Faget's sign), and the blood pressure is low. After the fourth day the temperature may drop, but the patient remains ill. The temperature then rises again, and there are marked nausea and vomiting, bleeding from the mouth and rectum, albuminuria, and prostration. Occasionally, the fever continues through this stage. Jaundice may appear, and oliguria or anuria may develop. Death may occur, usually about 1 week from onset, or the patient may improve and make a complete recovery. Many cases are mild, with few or no symptoms. These are diagnosed by serological methods. Considering all types, the mortality is about 5 per cent.

Leukopenia is the rule in yellow fever. The main pathological changes are in the liver and kidney. In the liver there occurs a midzone necrosis of the lobules, which is quite characteristic and is used

diagnostically in surveys. In the kidney the picture is that of degeneration of the tubules, and in the spleen the malpighian corpuscles
are destroyed.

Diagnosis

The laboratory procedures which assist in diagnosis are isolation
of the virus and demonstration of specific antibodies in the blood.
In fatal cases the liver can be examined for the presence of mid-zone
necrosis. Virus can be isolated from a patient in the acute phase,
up to the fifth day of illness, by injecting his serum intracerebrally
into mice. For serological diagnosis two specimens of serum from the
patient are needed, one early in the disease and the other about
2 or 3 weeks later. Neutralization antibodies are tested for by mixing
the serum with virus and injecting the mixture into the brains of
mice. If the disease is yellow fever, the first specimen will not protect
the mouse but the second specimen will, or both specimens will
protect, but the second in a much higher titer than the first. The
examination of liver sections from the cadavers of persons dying of
acute diseases of short duration is widely practiced in countries
where yellow fever is endemic. Sections of the liver are obtained
readily by means of a small cutting instrument, the viscerotome.

Immunity

An attack of yellow fever usually confers immunity for life. Vaccination with living virus made from an attenuated strain, such as
the 17D, grown in chick embryo, is widely practiced among people
living in or going to an endemic region. Immunity lasts for about
4 years. In this country the vaccine is not produced commercially but
will be administered by the Public Health Service to anyone who
requires it. The dose is one injection of 0.5 cubic centimeter.

Another method of vaccination, used largely by the French in
Africa, is to employ a mouse-adapted strain of virus which has lost
its power to cause disease in monkeys. The dried mouse brain is suspended in gum arabic before use and is applied to the skin by the
multiple-puncture or scarification methods. Often, vaccinia virus
is mixed with the gum, so that the individual is vaccinated against
yellow fever and smallpox at the same time.

The Environment

Yellow fever is found in America and in Africa. It is not known in
which of these it first occurred, but a definitely identified epidemic
took place in Mexico in the seventeenth century. The disease was
widely distributed in the Americas in the seventeenth, eighteenth,
and nineteenth centuries and caused many deaths. In the Spanish-

American War 1,575 cases and 231 deaths occurred in American troops stationed in Cuba. It was as a result of this that Walter Reed was put in charge of a yellow fever commission to discover the cause and method of spread of the disease. The dramatic findings of the commission have become part of the popular lore. The commission proved that the agent was filterable, that it was present in the blood of patients early in the disease (in the first 3 days), and that it was transmitted by the bite of the mosquito, *Aedes aegypti,* after an incubation period of 12 days in the mosquito.

Yellow fever was a widely prevalent disease in the Americas. In the nineteenth century about half a million cases occurred in the United States. By the use of anti-aegypti measures, Gorgas eradicated yellow fever in Cuba, and others, largely through the aid of the International Health Division of the Rockefeller Foundation, eliminated it in North America, the Caribbean Islands, and Central America above Panama. An unexpected hitch occurred in South America when it was found that, in addition to the cycle of man—mosquito—man, there existed another cycle, chiefly in jungles. This was the cycle from monkey to mosquito to monkey. The mosquitoes involved in this cycle are different from the *Aedes aegypti* and spread the disease from monkey to monkey in the absence of man, who becomes infected only if he strays into the jungle. In South America, the *Haemagogus* genus is chiefly involved. However, once infected, man can transmit the disease to other men through the *Aedes aegypti* mosquito. This form of the disease is known as "jungle yellow fever" and offers a new problem in control.

The *Aedes aegypti* is a domestic mosquito, which breeds chiefly in or near houses. Once infected, it remains infected for life but shows no evidence of illness. It does not transmit the infection to its off-spring. Mosquitoes become infected by biting a patient during the first 3 days of the disease, and are able to transmit the disease after an incubation period of 12 days. Urban yellow fever, which is transmitted by the *Aedes aegypti,* is a household disease and affects both sexes and all ages. Jungle yellow fever, on the other hand, affects adult males chiefly, since, as a rule, they are the only ones who enter the jungle to hunt or clear the forest. In the absence of the *Aedes aegypti,* which has been largely wiped out in many areas, the disease is not transmitted to the women and children. Urban yellow fever, although largely eliminated in South America, is still quite prevalent in Africa.

Control

The patient should be isolated for the first 3 or 4 days, when he is infective for the mosquito. Quarantine of contacts is unnecessary.

The main control measures are those directed at the elimination of the *Aedes aegypti* mosquito and the immunization of the exposed, susceptible population. The first consists of the suppression of breeding places and the spraying of houses in endemic areas with DDT or other insecticides. Immunization of the population is carried out with yellow fever vaccine in a single dose of 0.5 cubic centimeter. As a method of survey to determine the extent of the disease in an area, liver sections are collected, by means of the viscerotome, from fatal cases of illness of short duration, and are examined for the typical pathology. In countries like the United States, where yellow fever has been eliminated, control is largely a matter of keeping out infected persons. This can be done by quarantining individuals who arrive from an epidemic region for 5 days from the time of departure, unless they have been immunized within the past 4 years. As an added means of control all ships and airplanes arriving from yellow fever areas should be sprayed with insecticide prior to arrival.

Medical Care Plans

Treatment

No specific treatment is available. Drugs are used symptomatically.

Diet

Maintenance of good nutrition is essential. Fluids in liberal quantities should be given if they can be retained. If they cannot be taken by mouth, these requirements should be made up by parenteral injections.

Supportive Nursing Care

Skilled and constant nursing care is required for all patients ill with yellow fever. As prostration and restlessness are very severe, comfort of the patient is of primary importance, and every effort should be made to disturb the patient as little as possible.

Complete bed rest in quiet surroundings is highly desirable. However, if the patient is severely ill and transportation to a hospital is difficult, a decision to keep the patient in his present environment should be made. Nausea and vomiting are more or less persistent. The patient becomes very apprehensive and anxious when the vomitus becomes "coffee ground," and he believes impending death is near.

Constant mouth care is essential. The gums bleed easily, and cleansing with a mouthwash such as sodium perborate will ease soreness. The tongue should be swabbed to prevent accumulation of sordes. Cold cream or mineral oil should be applied to the lips.

Suppression and retention of urine is a common symptom, so that catheterization may be necessary. A purgative may be prescribed at the onset of the disease to offset constipation.

Analgesics may be prescribed for headache, and an ice cap may be applied to the head. Once established, convalescence is rapid with supportive nutrition.

In endemic areas the public health nurse may assist in an immunization program for the prevention of the disease and may participate with a corps of other professional workers in education of the community.

REFERENCES

1. Fox, S. P., and Cabral, A. S.: "The Duration of Immunity Following Vaccination with 17D Strain of Yellow Fever Virus," *Am. J. Hyg.*, **37**:93, 1943.
2. Richard, E. R.: "The Organization of the Viscerotome Service of the Brazilian Cooperative Yellow Fever Service," *Am. J. Trop. Med.*, **17**:163, 1937.
3. Shannon, R. C.; Whitman, L.; and Franca, M.: "Yellow Fever Virus in Jungle Mosquitoes," *Science*, **88**:110, 1938.
4. Soper, F. L.: "Recent Extensions of Knowledge of Yellow Fever," *Quarterly Bull. Health Organ., League of Nations*, **5**:1, 1935.
5. Theiler, M.: "Yellow Fever," in Rivers, *Viral and Rickettsial Infections of Man*, J. B. Lippincott Company, Philadelphia, pp. 420–440, 1948.
6. Whitman, L.: "The Multiplication of the Virus of Yellow Fever in *Aedes Aegypti*," *J. Exper. Med.*, **66**:133, 1937.

Index

537